Pediatric Musculoskeletal Imaging

Guest Editor

SANDRA L. WOOTTON-GORGES, MD

MAGNETIC RESONANCE IMAGING CLINICS OF NORTH AMERICA

www.mri.theclinics.com

August 2009 • Volume 17 • Number 3

SAUNDERS an imprint of ELSEVIER, Inc.

W.B. SAUNDERS COMPANY
A Division of Elsevier Inc.

1600 John F. Kennedy Boulevard • Suite 1800 • Philadelphia, Pennsylvania 19103-2899

http://www.theclinics.com

MRI CLINICS OF NORTH AMERICA Volume 17, Number 3
August 2009 ISSN 1064-9689, ISBN 13: 978-1-4377-1238-4, ISBN 10: 1-4377-1238-X

Editor: Joanne Husovski
Developmental Editor: Theresa Collier

Magnetic Resonance Imaging Clinics of North America (ISSN 1064-9689) is published quarterly by Elsevier Inc., 360 Park Avenue South, New York, NY 10010-1710. Months of issue are February, May, August, and November. Business and Editorial Offices: 1600 John F. Kennedy Blvd., Suite 1800, Philadelphia, PA 19103-2899. Customer Service Office: 11830 Westline Industrial Drive, St. Louis, MO 63146. Periodicals postage paid at New York, NY and additional mailing offices. Subscription prices are $276.00 per year (domestic individuals), $414.00 per year (domestic institutions), $134.00 per year (domestic students/residents), $308.00 per year (Canadian individuals), $520.00 per year (Canadian institutions), $400.00 per year (international individuals), $520.00 per year (international institutions), and $194.00 per year (international and Canadian students/residents). International air speed delivery is included in all *Clinics* subscription prices. All prices are subject to change without notice. **POSTMASTER:** Send address changes to *Magnetic Resonance Imaging Clinics*, 11830 Westline Industrial Drive, St. Louis, MO 63146. Customer Service (orders, claims, online, change of address): Elsevier Periodicals Customer Service, 11830 Westline Industrial Drive, St. Louis, MO 63146. Tel: 1-800-654-2452 (U.S. and Canada). Fax: 314-523-5170. E-mail: journalscustomerservice-usa@elsevier.com (for print support); journalsonlinesupport-usa@elsevier.com (for online support).

Reprints. For copies of 100 or more of articles in this publication, please contact the Commercial Reprints Department, Elsevier Inc., 360 Park Avenue South, New York, NY 10010-1710. Tel.: 212-633-3812; Fax: 212-462-1935; E-mail: reprints@elsevier.com.

Magnetic Resonance Imaging Clinics of North America is covered in the *RSNA Index of Imaging Literature, MEDLINE/PubMed (Index Medicus),* and *EMBASE/Excerpta Medica.*

Printed in the United States of America.

Contributors

GUEST EDITOR

SANDRA L. WOOTTON-GORGES, MD
Associate Professor of Radiology and Director of Pediatric Imaging, Department of Radiology, University of California, Davis Medical Center, UC Davis Children's Hospital; Medical Director of Imaging, Department of Radiology, Shriner's Hospital of Northern California, Sacramento, California

AUTHORS

ALVARO BURDILES, MD
Associate Instructor of Radiology, Hospital Clínico, Pontificia Universidad Católica de Chile, Santiago, Chile

PAUL S. BABYN, MD
Associate Professor of Radiology, Radiologist-in-Chief, Department of Medical Imaging, University of Toronto, Hospital for Sick Children, Toronto, Ontario, Canada

HEIKE E. DALDRUP-LINK, MD
Department of Radiology and Biomedical Imaging, University of California, San Francisco, San Francisco, California

JERRY R. DWEK, MD
Department of Radiology, Rady Children's Hospital and Health Center-San Diego, San Diego, California

KATHLEEN H. EMERY, MD
Clinical Professor of Radiology, Department of Radiology, Cincinnati Children's Hospital Medical Center, Cincinnati, Ohio; Clinical Professor of Pediatrics, Department of Pediatrics, Cincinnati Children's Hospital Medical Center, Cincinnati, Ohio

SIDDHARTH P. JADHAV, MD
Assistant Professor, Department of Radiology, University of Texas Medical Branch, Galveston, Texas

PARITOSH C. KHANNA, MD, DMRE
Assistant Professor, Department of Radiology, Seattle Children's Hospital, University of Washington School of Medicine, Seattle, Washington

CHIRAG V. PATEL, MD
Assistant Professor of Radiology, Division of Pediatric Imaging, Department of Radiology, University of California, Davis, Medical Center and UC Davis Children's Hospital, Sacramento, California

SUMIT PRUTHI, MD
Department of Radiology, Seattle Children's Hospital, University of Washington School of Medicine, Seattle, Washington

RAMON SANCHEZ, MD
Section of Pediatric Radiology, C.S. Mott Children's Hospital, University of Michigan Health System, Ann Arbor, Michigan

THOMAS RAY S. SANCHEZ, MD
Assistant Professor, Division of Pediatric
Radiology, Department of Radiology,
University of California, Davis Medical Center
and UC Davis Children's Hospital,
Sacramento, California

LYNNE STEINBACH, MD
Department of Radiology and Biomedical
Imaging, University of California, San
Francisco, San Francisco, California

REBECCA STEIN-WEXLER, MD
Associate Professor of Radiology, Department
of Radiology, University of California, Davis,
Sacramento, California

PETER J. STROUSE, MD
Section of Pediatric Radiology, C.S. Mott
Children's Hospital, University of Michigan
Health System, Ann Arbor, Michigan

LEONARD E. SWISCHUK, MD
Professor of Radiology & Pediatrics; Director,
Pediatric Radiology and Residency Program;
Director, Department of Radiology, University
of Texas Medical Branch, Galveston, Texas

MAHESH M. THAPA, MD
Assistant Professor, Department of Radiology,
Seattle Children's Hospital, University of
Washington School of Medicine, Seattle,
Washington

SANDRA L. WOOTTON-GORGES, MD
Associate Professor of Radiology and Director
of Pediatric Imaging, Department of Radiology,
University of California, Davis Medical Center,
UC Davis Children's Hospital; Medical Director
of Imaging, Department of Radiology, Shriner's
Hospital of Northern California, Sacramento,
California

Contents

The knee is one of the joints most commonly injured during sport-related activities in the pediatric population. Although physical examination and conventional radiography remain the most important tools for determining the extent of the injury, clinical assessment of the knee may be limited in patients with pain, swelling, and effusion, and conventional radiology may overlook serious injuries. MR imaging is an excellent modality for pediatric knee disorders given its lack of ionizing radiation, multiplanar capabilities, and high resolution, which provides accurate assessment of bone, cartilage, menisci, ligaments, and adjacent soft tissues. This article describes MR imaging findings of unique disorders of the pediatric knee, common traumatic injuries, frequent developmental abnormalities, and benign incidental findings.

MR imaging of the foot and ankle in children poses unique challenges, not only because of technical issues, but also because of the variations produced by age related changes. However, because of its excellent soft tissue contrast (especially helpful in delineating cartilage related abnormalities), MR imaging offers a distinct advantage over other imaging modalities. This article discusses MR imaging techniques for examining the pediatric foot and ankle, and reviews some common conditions encountered in a child's foot and ankle. This includes lesions such as osteochondritis dissecans; tarsal coalition; soft tissue and bony tumors of the foot and ankle; infection; and clubfoot.

Various congenital and acquired disorders can affect the upper extremity in pediatric and adolescent patients. MR imaging can provide unique anatomic and diagnostic information in the evaluation of many of these disorders, including inflammatory, infectious, neoplastic, and arthritic conditions. This article rounds out the issue on pediatric musculoskeletal MR imaging. It focuses on the evaluation of more common congenital disorders, and mainly sports-related injuries of the shoulder, elbow, and wrist in children. MR imaging can be more challenging in diagnosis of some of these disorders. Features of overuse injuries in skeletally immature athletes are a unifying theme throughout the article.

Magnetic Resonance Imaging Clinics of North America

FORTHCOMING ISSUES

MR Imaging of the Athlete
George Koulouris, MD,
Guest Editor

Select Topics in MR Imaging

Breast MR Imaging

Neonatal Brain Imaging

RECENT ISSUES

May 2009

Clinical Applications of MR Diffusion and Perfusion Imaging
Scott B. Reeder, MD, PhD and
Pratik Mukherjee, MD, PhD, *Guest Editors*

February 2009

Emerging Concepts in MR Angiography
William Weadock, MD and
Thomas L. Chenevert, PhD, *Guest Editors*

RELATED INTEREST

Neuroimaging Clinics of North America May 2007 (Vol. 17, No. 2)
Pediatric Neurovascular Disease: Diagnosis and Intervention
Pierre Lasjunias, MD, *Guest Editor*

THE CLINICS ARE NOW AVAILABLE ONLINE!

Access your subscription at:
www.theclinics.com

GOAL STATEMENT

The goal of *Magnetic Resonance Imaging Clinics of North America* is to keep practicing physicians up to date with current clinical practice by providing timely articles reviewing the state of the art in patient care.

ACCREDITATION

The *Magnetic Resonance Imaging Clinics of North America* is planned and implemented in accordance with the Essential Areas and Policies of the Accreditation Council for Continuing Medical Education (ACCME) through the joint sponsorship of the University of Virginia School of Medicine and Elsevier. The University of Virginia School of Medicine is accredited by the ACCME to provide continuing medical education for physicians.

The University of Virginia School of Medicine designates this educational activity for a maximum of 15 *AMA PRA Category 1 Credits*™ for each issue, 60 credits per year. Physicians should only claim credit commensurate with the extent of their participation in the activity.

The American Medical Association has determined that physicians not licensed in the US who participate in this CME activity are eligible for a maximum of 15 *AMA PRA Category 1 Credits*™ for each issue, 60 credits per year.

Credit can be earned by reading the text material, taking the CME examination online at: http://www.theclinics.com/home/cme, and completing the evaluation. After taking the test, you will be required to review any and all incorrect answers. Following completion of the test and evaluation, your credit will be awarded and you may print your certificate.

FACULTY DISCLOSURE/CONFLICT OF INTEREST

The University of Virginia School of Medicine, as an ACCME accredited provider, endorses and strives to comply with the Accreditation Council for Continuing Medical Education (ACCME) Standards of Commercial Support, Commonwealth of Virginia statutes, University of Virginia policies and procedures, and associated federal and private regulations and guidelines on the need for disclosure and monitoring of proprietary and financial interests that may affect the scientific integrity and balance of content delivered in continuing medical education activities under our auspices.

The University of Virginia School of Medicine requires that all CME activities accredited through this institution be developed independently and be scientifically rigorous, balanced and objective in the presentation/discussion of its content, theories and practices.

All authors/editors participating in an accredited CME activity are expected to disclose to the readers relevant financial relationships with commercial entities occurring within the past 12 months (such as grants or research support, employee, consultant, stock holder, member of speakers bureau, etc.). The University of Virginia School of Medicine will employ appropriate mechanisms to resolve potential conflicts of interest to maintain the standards of fair and balanced education to the reader. Questions about specific strategies can be directed to the Office of Continuing Medical Education, University of Virginia School of Medicine, Charlottesville, Virginia.

The faculty and staff of the University of Virginia Office of Continuing Medical Education have no financial affiliations to disclose.

The authors/editors listed below have identified no professional or financial affiliations for themselves or their spouse/partner:

Paul S. Babyn, MD; Alvaro Burdiles, MD; Heike E. Daldrup-Link, MD; Eduard de Lange, MD (Test Author); Jerry R. Dwek, MD; Kathleen H. Emery, MD; Joanne Husovski (Acquisitions Editor); Siddharth P. Jadhav, MD; Paritosh C. Khanna, MD, DMRE; Chirag Vishrambhai Patel, MD; Sumit Pruthi, MD; Ramon Sanchez, MD; Thomas Ray S. Sanchez, MD; Lynne Steinbach, MD; Rebecca Stein-Wexler, MD; Peter J. Strouse, MD; Leonard E. Swischuk, MD; Mahesh M. Thapa, MD; and Sandra L. Wootton-Gorges, MD (Guest Editor).

Disclosure of Discussion of non-FDA approved uses for pharmaceutical products and/or medical devices:
The University of Virginia School of Medicine, as an ACCME provider, requires that all faculty presenters identify and disclose any "off label" uses for pharmaceutical and medical device products. The University of Virginia School of Medicine recommends that each physician fully review all the available data on new products or procedures prior to instituting them with patients.

TO ENROLL

To enroll in the Magnetic Resonance Imaging Clinics of North America Continuing Medical Education program, call customer service at 1-800-654-2452 or visit us online at: www.theclinics.com/home/cme. The CME program is available to subscribers for an additional fee of $99.95.

Preface

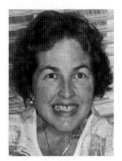

Sandra L. Wootton-Gorges, MD
Guest Editor

MR imaging has become a mainstay in the evaluation of pediatric musculoskeletal disorders. In addition to all the well-known advantages MR imaging offers to musculoskeletal imaging in the adult, MR imaging offers special advantages to children. First, MR imaging is superior in visualizing the cartilaginous aspects of the growing skeleton and in imaging the bone marrow. Second, and very importantly, it provides detailed imaging without radiation exposure. Relatively minor disadvantages to pediatric MR imaging include the need for sedation in younger, uncooperative patients and some technical limitations related to the small size of the patient.

It is important to remember that children are not small adults. Before one can successfully image children, one must understand the anatomy, physiology, and pathophysiology of the immature and growing skeleton. Unique musculoskeletal problems encountered within the pediatric population include imaging of congenital anomalies, tumors, and tumor-like conditions different than those encountered in the adult population; infections and inflammatory processes unique to the pediatric population; and traumatic lesions unlike those seen in the adult.

In this issue, the authors provide excellent reviews of important topics in musculoskeletal imaging in children and offer technical suggestions to optimize imaging in the pediatric patient. The issue begins with MR imaging of normal and abnormal marrow in children and normal and abnormal appearances of cartilage in the growing skeleton. Reviews of pediatric arthritis, infection and inflammatory disorders, tumors and tumor-like conditions of the bone and soft tissues, and trauma are provided. Then, uniquely pediatric issues of the hip, knee, ankle, foot, and upper extremities are discussed.

Sandra L. Wootton-Gorges, MD
Department of Radiology
University of California, Davis Medical Center
UC Davis Children's Hospital
4860 Y Street, Suite 3100
Sacramento, CA 95817, USA

E-mail address:
sandra.gorges@ucdmc.ucdavis.edu
(S.L. Wootton-Gorges)

Magn Reson Imaging Clin N Am 17 (2009) xi
doi:10.1016/j.mric.2009.04.001
1064-9689/09/$ – see front matter © 2009 Elsevier Inc. All rights reserved.

mri.theclinics.com

Pediatric Bone Marrow MR Imaging

Alvaro Burdiles, MD[a], Paul S. Babyn, MD[b],*

KEYWORDS

- Bone marrow • MR imaging • Children bone marrow
- Pediatric imaging • Neoplasia

One of the largest organs in the body, bone marrow is highly cellular and the main site of hematopoiesis, producing and regulating the supply of erythrocytes, platelets, and leukocytes.[1] At least some bone marrow is visible in every MR image, underscoring the importance of a good understanding of the MR imaging appearance of normal and abnormal bone marrow. MR imaging is superior to other imaging modalities in the assessment of bone marrow because of its high tissue contrast, especially its sensitivity in detection of fat and water. This unique soft tissue contrast of MR imaging can enable earlier assessment of bone marrow infiltration by tumor or other marrow disorders before osseous destruction becomes apparent on radiograph or CT or metabolic changes occur on bone scintigraphy or positron emission tomography scan.[2]

This article provides an overview of the MR imaging findings in normal marrow and in the most common focal and diffuse marrow lesions encountered in childhood.

NORMAL BONE MARROW

To interpret the MR imaging appearance of marrow accurately it is important first to review the normal constituents of bone marrow and the expected normal developmental and physiologic changes that occur with age.

The development of marrow tissue is dependent on the formation of the marrow cavity and surrounding bone. From the fetal period throughout early childhood, significant osteogenesis is occurring, accompanied by ongoing enlargement of the marrow space.[3] Hematopoiesis starts initially in the fetus in the yolk sac and then extends to the liver and, to a lesser degree, to the spleen by the second trimester.[1,4] In the fourth fetal month hematopoiesis begins within the bone marrow space as bone cavities develop.[1,4] Bone marrow soon becomes the exclusive site of granulocytic and megakaryocytic proliferation; however, it is not until the end of the third trimester that the marrow environment supports erythroblasts. At birth, the bone marrow is the major site of red cell production.[1,4]

On gross examination, bone marrow appears red (hematopoietic marrow) or yellow (fatty marrow) depending on its predominant components. Hematopoietic marrow is red because of the presence of hemoglobin within the erythrocytes and their precursor cells, and is actively involved in hematopoiesis. Fatty marrow is yellow because of its marked lipid content. Fat is a major component of both yellow marrow and (to a lesser extent) red marrow. The amount of fatty marrow is responsive to the need for hematopoietic marrow and can increase or decrease accordingly. When the need for hematopoietic marrow volume increases, as in response to severe blood loss, fatty adventitial cells lose fat and increase the space available for hematopoiesis.[5] During periods of decreased hematopoiesis, fat cells increase in size and number. Fat cells may be actively involved in hematopoiesis, supplying metabolic or nutritional support, possibly along with growth factors.[5] The cellular composition of red marrow consists of 60% hematopoietic cells and 40% adipocytes; its chemical composition is 40% to 60% lipid, 30% to 40% water, and 10% to 20% proteins.[6] In contrast, yellow marrow is almost entirely composed of adipocytes (95%),

[a] Hospital Clínico, Pontificia Universidad Católica de Chile, 367 Marcoleta Street, Santiago, Chile
[b] Department of Medical Imaging, University of Toronto, Hospital for Sick Children, 555 University Avenue, Toronto, Ontario M5G 1X8, Canada
* Corresponding author.
E-mail address: paul.babyn@sickkids.ca (P.S. Babyn).

Magn Reson Imaging Clin N Am 17 (2009) 391–409
doi:10.1016/j.mric.2009.03.001

with its chemical composition being 80% lipid, 15% water, and 5% protein.[6,7] Cancellous bone, composed of primary and secondary bridging trabecular bone, provides the underlying structural framework for the cellular elements of marrow and also serves as a mineral depot.[8]

Bone Marrow Conversion

The composition of the cellular marrow changes significantly with age and anatomic location. The rate and patterns of marrow conversion on MR imaging are now well understood and have allowed for the mapping of the expected age-related marrow distribution throughout the skeleton.[9] At birth, hematopoietic marrow is present throughout the entire skeleton. Various regions of hematopoietic marrow then rapidly undergo conversion to fatty marrow with the transition beginning in the periphery of the skeleton in the distal phalanges of the fingers and toes and extending in a symmetric, centripetal manner into the central skeleton (**Fig. 1**).[6,10] The cartilaginous epiphyses and apophyses lack marrow until they ossify. These centers, once ossified, initially contain hematopoietic marrow, followed by rapid conversion to fatty marrow within months of ossification. In the first decade of life, a superimposed additional sequence of marrow conversion begins in the long bones, starting in the diaphyses and progressing toward the metaphyses, particularly the distal metaphyses.[6,10] Persistence of significant hematopoietic marrow in the diaphyses after the first decade of life is abnormal. Prominent hematopoietic marrow in the metaphyses is normal, however, until the end of the second decade of life. Heterogeneous sharply demarcated linear areas or focal islands of red marrow can be encountered as normal variants (**Fig. 2**). Lack of red marrow in the proximal femoral metaphyses in the young child is abnormal and raises concern for myeloid depletion (**Fig. 3**). In the late third decade of life the bone marrow distribution achieves its mature state.[10]

Bone Marrow Reconversion

In the event of increased functional demand for hematopoiesis, yellow marrow may reconvert to red marrow. Conditions triggering reconversion include chronic anemias, such as sickle cell disease and thalassemia; stress; endurance running; obesity; extensive marrow replacement from marrow proliferative or replacement disorders; and chemotherapy with marrow stimulating agents, such as granulocyte colony–stimulating factor (**Figs. 4** and **5**).[9,10] The extent of reconversion depends on the severity and duration of the stimulus. The reconversion process proceeds in the reverse order from initial conversion (ie, from central to peripheral skeleton), and in the long bones from the metaphyses to the diaphyses.[6]

In clinical practice, prominent red marrow can be observed in some areas including in the epiphyses, most commonly in the distal femur, proximal

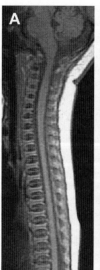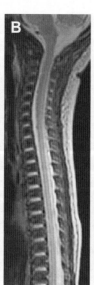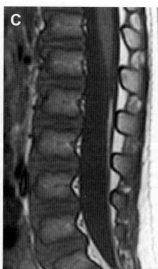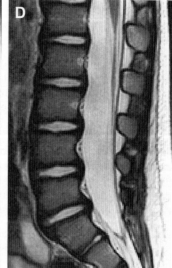

Fig. 1. Normal marrow conversion in the spine. Normal appearance of the upper spine in a 1-day-old baby. Note the appearance on T1-weighted (*A*) and T2-weighted sequence (*B*). Contrast this with the appearance in the lower spine in a 17 month old where there is increased fat present in the vertebrae especially adjacent to the basivertebral vessels on T1-weighted (*C*) and T2-weighted sequences (*D*).

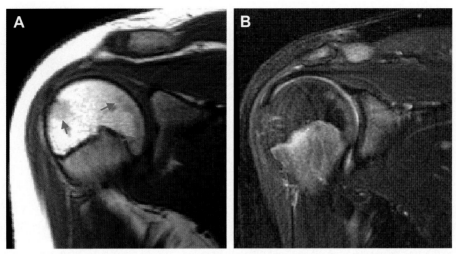

Fig. 2. Foci of normal hematopoietic marrow are present within the proximal humeral epiphysis especially in the subchondral region as shown on T1-weighted (*A, arrowheads*) and T2-weighted fast spin echo sequence (*B*).

tibia, and proximal humerus. This is often interpreted as evidence of marrow reconversion, but the lack of sequential studies does not allow documentation of reconversion. A better term for this finding may be an "extended hematopoietic marrow pattern."[11]

APPEARANCE OF BONE MARROW ON MR IMAGING

The MR imaging characteristics of bone marrow are influenced by a number of factors including choice of imaging sequence, and the cellularity, lipid content, surrounding trabecular bone, and iron content of the marrow and especially its hematopoietic tissues.[3]

Conventional T1- and T2-weighted spin-echo (SE) sequences remain the mainstay of clinical marrow MR imaging because differences in T1 and T2 relaxation times generally allow the differentiation of normal red and yellow marrow from pathologic marrow. Trabecular bone itself has little direct signal, but contributes to T2 shortening, producing local magnetic field gradients.[7,12] Because fatty marrow is composed primarily of lipids, with low cellularity, its signal characteristics are similar to those of subcutaneous fat on both T1- and T2-weighted SE sequences. Red marrow shows higher cellularity but still contains significant lipid. The signal characteristics of fat are averaged with the longer T1 and T2 relaxation times of water and protein.[7,9] On T1-weighted images, the

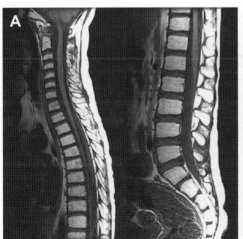
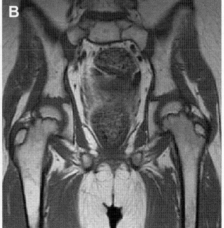

Fig. 3. Abnormal fatty marrow. (*A, B*) There is loss of the expected appearance of hematopoietic marrow within the spine and pelvis on the T1-weighted images. This child had received therapy for T-cell lymphoma.

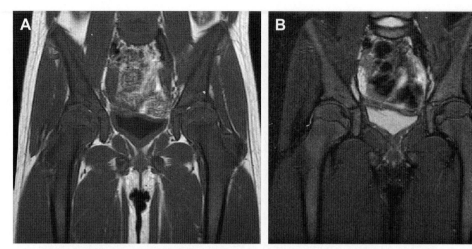

Fig. 4. Bone marrow reconversion. A 10-year-old girl with known sickle cell disease showing extensive low signal intensity on T1-weighted imaging with hematopoietic marrow within the pelvis and proximal femora (*A*) and slight increased signal on fast inversion recovery sequences (*B*). Note the complete replacement of expected fatty marrow within the proximal femoral epiphysis.

signal intensity of red marrow is considerably less than that of fatty marrow, but typically higher than muscles and intervertebral disks except for the very young child, where the fat content can be quite low. The exact signal intensity depends on the specific amount of marrow water and lipid content.[7,9] On T2-weighted images the signal intensity of red marrow is slightly brighter than adjacent muscle and approximates the signal intensity of fatty marrow. The contrast between red and fatty marrow is more evident on T1-weighted sequences. SE imaging leads to under-estimation of the proportion of hematopoietic marrow because the short T1 relaxation time of fat overwhelms the longer T1 relaxation time of

the red marrow, and alternative sequences must be used to identify subtle changes in bone marrow signal.

Fast spin echo (FSE) T2-weighted sequences have largely replaced conventional T2-weighted SE imaging because of the marked reduction in acquisition times and improved signal-to-noise ratio for similar acquisition times.[3] On T2-weighted FSE images, fat is markedly brighter compared with conventional T2-weighted images; selective fat suppression is generally applied to T2-weighted FSE images.[9] With fat-saturation, T2-weighted FSE images have been shown to be highly effective in the evaluation of marrow abnormalities improving the conspicuity of

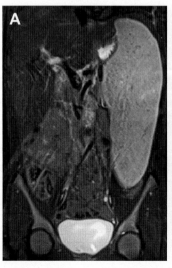
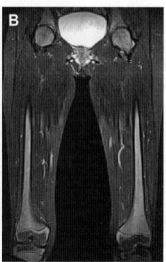

Fig. 5. Child with hypercellular marrow and abnormal marrow appearance. This is caused by peripheral destruction and consumption of red blood cells. Note the marked splenomegaly (*A*) and diffuse increased signal greater than adjacent muscles within the pelvis and femoral shafts and distal epiphysis from hypercellular marrow on coronal short-tau inversion recovery (STIR) images (*A, B*).

marrow lesions.[13] Because most marrow lesions are rich in free water, they are brighter than both red and yellow marrow on T2-weighted images and are easily detected;[9] most marrow lesions have a large quantity of slowly relaxing free water protons, resulting in a longer T2 relaxation value, so they are identified as areas of high signal intensity. Lesion visibility is poorer, however, in T2-weighted FSE images than that of short-tau inversion recovery (STIR) or FSE inversion recovery.

STIR is widely used for bone marrow imaging because it offers excellent detection of marrow abnormalities and improved lesion conspicuity compared with T2-weighted SE. STIR images have additive T1 and T2 characteristics, so lesions with long T1 and T2 relaxation times are bright on STIR. Normal fatty marrow is low in signal intensity, whereas red marrow demonstrates intermediate signal intensity similar to muscle.[3] The chemical shift-selective fat-suppression techniques used in fat-suppressed T2-weighted FSE images may cause field heterogeneity, particularly with large fields of view. With large field of view STIR images, the status of a large volume of the bone marrow can be assessed.[9] Fast STIR sequences can show marrow lesions with considerable savings in imaging time.

Intermediate proton-weighted images lack sufficient contrast resolution between normal marrow and pathologic processes to be useful for marrow evaluation.

Chemical shift imaging has become an important supplement to standard MR imaging techniques applied to the assessment of bone marrow, because most marrow lesions lack fat and show no chemical shift effect, as opposed to normal bone marrow.

Gradient echo sequences are often used in musculoskeletal imaging. Many factors influence the appearance of normal marrow on gradient echo, including tissue characteristics and acquisition technique. Unlike SE techniques, local magnetic field inhomogeneities are not rephased on gradient echo, making it more sensitive to susceptibility differences and signal loss, such as the effects induced by trabecular bone and marrow heterogeneity.[3] On gradient echo imaging this leads to a loss of marrow signal intensity that is greatest in the regions with the highest content of trabecular bone (eg, epiphyses, metaphyses, vertebrae) and is even greater when iron is adjacent, as in hematopoietic marrow.[14] Epiphyseal marrow signal intensity shows greater loss than metaphyseal marrow, which shows a greater degree of loss than diaphyseal marrow, because of the greater trabecular pattern.[14] In gradient

echo sequences, if fat and water protons are in phase, their signals are added; if they are opposed phase, they are subtracted. If normal marrow is replaced by a marrow lesion, fat can be obliterated, and no subtraction occurs on opposed-phase imaging.[15]

Marrow enhancement after intravenous administration of gadolinium contrast agents can be seen especially in infants and young children with highly vascular normal hematopoietic marrow. The degree of enhancement depends on the type of marrow present. Greater enhancement is visible with hematopoietic marrow than fatty marrow where enhancement is not visually evident. Normal marrow enhancement decreases with advancing age, paralleling an increasing proportion of marrow fat, and its decreasing vascularity.[3] A delay in scanning after gadolinium injection reduces the degree of enhancement obtained.[16] Enhanced MR images are particularly useful for the detection of diffuse marrow abnormality that may not be recognized on unenhanced MR imaging.[17] It should be noted that in the developing spine, enhancement of the bone marrow may be marked because of prominent blood supply, increased marrow cellularity, and an extensive extravascular space that allows contrast to pool. In young children care should be taken to avoid a diagnosis of a pathologic marrow based solely on enhancement of the spinal marrow on MR imaging.

Neoplastic involvement of bone marrow typically demonstrates increased marrow enhancement. Application of advanced MR imaging techniques, such as dynamic gadolinium-enhanced MR imaging, can be useful in this population. Peak marrow enhancement is most evident within the first minute after injection (between 45 and 60 seconds). Dynamic contrast-enhanced MR imaging reflects capillary blood flow, permeability, and the relative volume of the extravascular extracellular space. Such techniques are positive because of the presence of angiogenesis, a common finding in neoplastic involvement of the marrow.[11] Quantitative estimates of tumor necrosis obtained using dynamic contrast-enhanced MR imaging have shown strong correlation with the percentage of necrosis determined by pathologic evaluation, particularly in making the clinically relevant distinction between those tumors that are less or more than 90% necrotic.[18] This suggests that dynamic MR imaging could be of value for noninvasively assessing treatment response during neoadjuvant therapy, potentially allowing a change to be made in that therapy for those patients whose response is poor.[18]

Diffusion-weighted MR imaging reflects free mobility of water molecules in interstitial tissue. When measured, the apparent diffusion coefficient reflects the local water mobility in vivo. Preliminary studies in adults have indicated that diffusion-weighted MR images allow excellent distinction between neoplastic and benign causes of collapsed vertebral bodies.[11]

ABNORMAL BONE MARROW

MR imaging has proved to be a sensitive method for detecting focal, multifocal, or diffuse bone marrow lesions, including those of neoplastic, infectious, or ischemic origin. In diffuse marrow abnormalities there is extensive or complete replacement of normal bone marrow. The differential diagnosis of diffuse marrow disorders is broad and includes neoplastic disorders, such as the leukemias; lymphomas; and metastatic disease, especially neuroblastoma; and rhabdomyosarcoma. Other nonneoplastic conditions include aplastic anemia, myelodysplastic syndromes, myelofibrosis, hemosiderosis, Gaucher disease, and osteopetrosis.

Many pulse sequences are currently available for marrow MR imaging, and the appropriate choice depends not only on the suspected underlying condition, but also on the signal characteristics of the surrounding normal marrow so that lesion conspicuity may be enhanced.

On T2-weighted sequences most marrow lesions are brighter than either hematopoietic or fatty marrow because they contain increased amounts of free water.[7] Most marrow lesions (benign or malignant) have a T1-weighted SE signal intensity similar to or lower than that of muscle, and are conspicuous against the background of high signal intensity yellow marrow, as in adults, adolescents, and older children.[10] Marrow lesions may appear similar to red marrow on T1-weighted images, however, especially in younger children.[6,7,19] Because marrow lesions replace marrow fat, they show a longer T1 relaxation time decreasing the overall T1 signal intensity, similar to or lower than that of adjacent muscle. Normal red marrow in children older than 2 or 3 years shows signal intensity higher than that of muscle or nondegenerated intervertebral disks.[20]

Diffuse hematopoietic marrow may be difficult to distinguish from diffuse marrow disease in young children,[21] particularly in acute leukemias.

Quantitative serial assessment of the fat fraction of bone marrow may provide improved diagnostic discrimination in distinguishing normal from abnormal marrow. It may be useful for monitoring patients' response to therapy for leukemia, aplastic anemia, and Gaucher disease.[22]

NEOPLASIA

The inherent differences in the resonance frequencies of water and lipid protons can be used to evaluate the marrow for the presence of a tumor, using gradient echo chemical-shift imaging. When the appropriate echo time is used, the visualized signal intensity on the resultant opposed-phase image represents the difference between the signals from lipid and water: the result is a reduction of the overall signal from those voxels that contain both lipid and water.[10] The signal intensity from red or fatty marrow is decreased on opposed-phase imaging because both contain fat and water, but tumor deposits in marrow do not show signal loss on opposed-phase images because most tumor deposits do not contain fat.[10,23,24] This is also useful in evaluation of nonneoplastic processes, such as ischemia and injury, which do not obliterate marrow fat.[11]

Fat-suppression facilitates detection of marrow lesions by suppressing signals from surrounding fat marrow. This is essential when using FSE or turbo SE T2-wieghted images to evaluate the bone marrow. The STIR pulse sequence is less affected by inhomogeneous magnetic fields, compared with fat-suppressed T2, and is a highly sensitive technique in marrow lesion detection, considered superior to T1-weighted SE in some studies.[25]

Tumors affecting the bone marrow can be classified according to origin: from myeloid elements of marrow (leukemia, lymphoma); from mesenchymal elements of marrow (primary sarcomas of bone); or from hematogenous metastases to marrow. On T1-weighted sequences, tumor spread is identified by replacement of fat-containing marrow, resulting in a hypointense signal (**Fig. 6**). Fat-suppressed sequences, such as STIR, depict neoplastic lesions by virtue of the hyperintense signal because of increased content of water within the tumor cells. Osteoblastic metastases may be depicted in STIR sequences with variable signal intensities, however, from hypointense in dense sclerotic lesions to hyperintense when more cellular components are present.[2]

In adults, MR imaging has been reported to provide higher sensitivity to that of skeletal scintigraphy for detecting bone metastases.[26–28] Special diagnostic problems occur in children because of their highly cellular hematopoietic marrow, however, which may impair the detection of bone marrow lesions based on T1-weighted MR

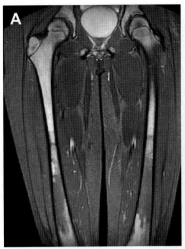
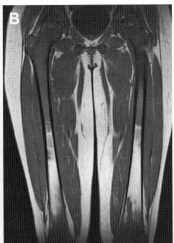
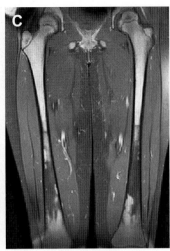

Fig. 6. Child with acute lymphoblastic leukemia showing diffuse patchy abnormal marrow signal intensity. There is high signal intensity on coronal STIR (*A*), low signal on coronal T1-weighted image (*B*), and increased enhancement following contrast administration (*C*) within the proximal and distal femora with relative sparing portions of the diaphyses bilaterally.

imaging sequences alone.[9,29] Multiple foci of red marrow must not be confused with multiple metastatic lesions. Foci of red marrow show feathery margins that interdigitate with fatty marrow, and typically show symmetric distribution; in contradistinction marrow metastases, aside from their focal abnormal signal intensity, tend to be more rounded and sharply defined.[10]

The differentiation of highly cellular hematopoietic marrow from neoplasia can be problematic in children, requiring knowledge of expected age-dependent conversion patterns of the bone marrow (**Fig. 7**).[29] The differentiation between highly cellular hematopoietic and neoplastic marrow may be facilitated by use of in- and out-of-phase pulse sequences, which display both entities with different signals. Reticuloendothelial system-specific contrast agents may also be helpful because they reduce the signal intensity of hematopoietic macrophage-containing marrow but not of neoplastic marrow.[30,31]

The skeletal system is a frequent target of metastatic spread from various primary tumors. Compared with other imaging modalities like radiography, CT, or bone scintigraphy, MR imaging is the most sensitive technique for the detection of bone metastases in children and young adults, even if the trabecular bone is not destroyed.[29,32]

In hematologic malignancies MR imaging provides information that aids in diagnosis, staging, and follow-up.[32] In leukemia the normal bone marrow is replaced by leukemia cells.[33] MR imaging has proved to be very sensitive for depicting changes in the bone marrow of patients with

acute leukemia. Three patterns of marrow infiltration depicted with MR imaging have been described in patients with leukemia: (1) diffuse uniform, (2) diffuse patchy, and (3) focal.[11] With low tumor load before there has been replacement of a significant portion of the marrow content, the MR imaging appearance can be normal. In the leukemias, the diffuse MR imaging pattern of marrow involvement is typical but not specific for the disease. In patients with acute myeloid leukemia, changes in posttreatment bulk T1 measurements show no significant differences in responding and nonresponding patients during and after the first induction course of treatment.[34] Although sequential quantitative assessment is not useful in assessing the effect of treatment in patients with acute myeloid leukemia, it seems to have value in predicting response in patients with acute lymphoid leukemia.[35] The higher sensitivity of MR imaging to detect residual disease in patients with acute lymphoid leukemia compared with patients with acute myeloid leukemia is based on inherent differences of lymphoid and myeloid cells.[9] One of the complications of acute leukemia is the development of chloromas, more frequently associated with acute myeloid leukemia. This tumor arises in the bone marrow and spreads to the extraosseous space. As in lymphomatous involvement of the bone marrow, extraosseous extension of tumor may occur without obvious bone destruction.[9]

Bone marrow necrosis is an unusual entity (0.3%–0.4% of marrow biopsies) that occurs in close association with malignancy, particularly

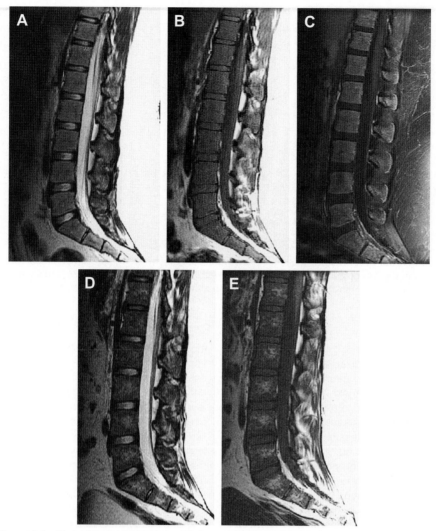

Fig. 7. Another child with leukemia presenting with leg weakness and incontinence illustrating the often subtle appearance of diffuse marrow involvement in the spine with increased signal on T2 frFSE (*A*) uniform reduced signal on T1 (*B*), and increased enhancement following contrast administration (*C*). Following treatment more heterogeneity within the vertebral bodies is evident on T2- (*D*) and T1-weighted sequences (*E*).

acute lymphocytic leukemia. Bone marrow necrosis is characterized by a loss of myeloid tissue and marrow fat without trabecular destruction, unlike avascular necrosis. MR imaging findings are similar to those of avascular necrosis, although bone marrow necrosis tends to be more diffuse, involving the axial skeleton without vertebral collapse.[18]

In lymphoproliferative disorders, infiltration of the bone marrow occurs in 5% to 15% of patients with Hodgkin's disease and in 25% to 45% of patients with non-Hodgkin's lymphoma,[9,18,36] and by definition indicates stage IV disease with both therapeutic and prognostic implications.[36] The diagnosis of bone marrow involvement is established with bone marrow biopsies, which are usually obtained from the posterior superior iliac crest. Because only a small volume of the bone is examined, sampling errors exist even with bilateral iliac crest biopsies.[36] In patients with lymphoma, MR imaging has been shown to be superior to bone marrow scintigraphy in the evaluation of bone marrow. The diagnostic yield of bone marrow biopsy can be increased if the biopsy site is selected with the aid of MR imaging.[9,36] MR imaging may be used to rule out bone marrow involvement, provided that its sensitivity is sufficiently high.[36] MR imaging can also direct harvest procedures for autologous bone marrow transplantation to sites of relatively uninvolved marrow.[9,37] On MR imaging, lymphomatous involvement of the bone marrow is seen as diffuse heterogeneous replacement of the marrow and less frequently as focal marrow lesions.[18] The ability to detect focal bone marrow involvement in patients with lymphoma has substantial consequences, because it is used to assess patient prognosis and select the specific type of therapy.[18] MR imaging cannot differentiate between the different histologic subtypes of lymphoma. Extraosseous tumor extension in patients with lymphoma often occurs without obvious destruction of the cortical bone, reflecting the permeative nature of the tumor. This characteristic appearance is not pathognomonic for this disease; however, its presence may raise the possibility of lymphoma and direct the appropriate work-up.[9]

MR imaging has been applied to the posttreatment follow-up of patients with lymphoma. Dynamic contrast-enhanced MR imaging may be useful to assess treatment response, because a decrease in degree of contrast enhancement has been shown to correlate with a good response or remission.[18] Quantitative MR imaging with serial measurements of T1 relaxation times showed a decrease in the latter in patients who responded to treatment.[9,38]

Bone marrow metastases may arise in any of the solid tumors but are most commonly seen in neuroblastoma (**Figs. 8** and **9**) and the primary bone and soft tissue sarcomas including Ewing's and rhabdomyosarcoma (**Fig. 10**). Bone marrow metastases are usually focal or multifocal and more commonly seen in red marrow, but can be seen anywhere in the marrow. The MR imaging appearances of metastases vary depending on the tumor and the response of the host bone; metastases can be osteolytic, osteoblastic, or mixed. Some tumors grow between trabeculae within marrow without causing gross trabecular or cortical destruction, and similar growth may occur in the earliest stages of tumor extension within marrow. MR imaging is superior to radiographs and bone scan in detecting such intratrabecular tumor deposits.[18] In osteosarcoma, MR imaging demonstrates the extent of spread of the tumor in the bone marrow, not visible with plain film radiograph.[33] Diffuse marrow involvement by tumor can be seen in neuroblastoma and rhabdomyosarcoma, which can simulate leukemia.

POSTTREATMENT CHANGES

MR imaging is a useful method in the evaluation of posttreatment changes in tumors. Patients undergoing chemotherapy show fatty transformation of the bone marrow. Several drugs used in oncology patients can cause side effects in the immature skeleton, some of which can be misdiagnosed as neoplastic involvement on MR imaging.[18] Osteopenia, fractures, osteonecrosis, and avascular necrosis are well-known complications of prolonged administration of steroids in patients of all ages (**Fig. 11**). In children, methotrexate can cause osteopenia; severe bone pain; and metaphyseal insufficiency fractures (described as methotrexate osteopathy).[18] The administration of hematopoietic growth factors may delay the fatty transformation of marrow or may cause reconversion of fatty to hematopoietic marrow and simulate persistent or relapsing disease.[18,39]

Radiation therapy kills the hematopoietic cells and destroys the vascular sinusoids, causing conversion of hematopoietic into fatty bone marrow.[2] The initial marrow response to irradiation consists of a short period of cellular depletion, vascular congestion, edema, and hemorrhage.[18] STIR MR images may detect this effect of radiotherapy within a few hours or days after treatment, which peaks approximately 9 days after radiation therapy.[11] After this acute period there is a chronic phase with fatty marrow transformation, which is sharply limited to the radiation portals. Fatty marrow replacement progresses rapidly during the first 6 weeks of therapy and then continues at a much slower rate (**Fig. 12**).[11] The two most important factors affecting the ability of marrow to regenerate are patient age and radiation dose.[18] Younger patients had superior marrow recovery, with full marrow regeneration occurring in patients younger than 18 years of age, independent of radiation dose.[18] Fatty marrow

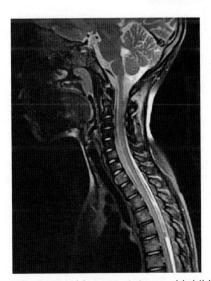

Fig. 8. Stage 4 neuroblastoma. A 4-year-old child with multifocal vertebral involvement showing high signal intensity on T2-weighted sagittal image.

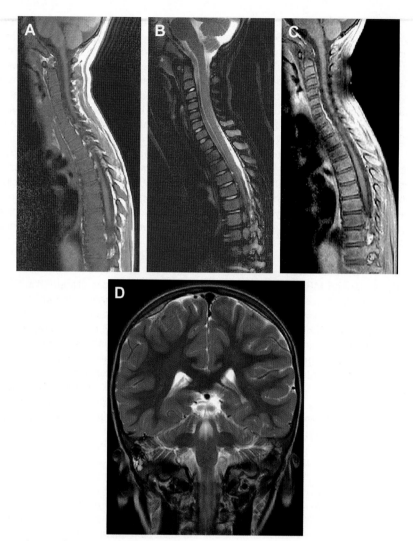

Fig. 9. Another patient with neuroblastoma and diffuse marrow involvement. There is diffuse low signal within the visualized spine on T1-weighted image (*A*), which increases in signal on T2-weighted sequence (*B*) and following contrast (*C*). Note the calvarial extradural metastases (*D, arrowheads*).

replacement is nonreversible for doses equal to or higher than 30 to 40 Gy, because destruction of vascular sinusoids does not permit the migration of hematopoietic cells into the radiation field from adjacent nonirradiated areas.[9] For doses less than 30 Gy, regeneration of the bone marrow may occur by 1 year after radiation therapy. After radiation therapy MR imaging is particularly helpful, because irradiated lesions are easily distinguishable from new lesions.[2] Radiation-induced complications in the marrow include osteonecrosis, avascular necrosis, fractures, and radiation-induced neoplasm.[18]

Dynamic-enhanced MR imaging may be helpful in the differentiation of regenerating hematopoietic marrow from relapse of the disease. Fibrotic changes in the bone marrow that may develop

after treatment may also enhance, as may reactive peritumoral changes. Dynamic images showing early enhancement and early washout of contrast suggest the presence of residual viable tumor, whereas delayed and more prolonged patterns of enhancement suggest reactive changes[9] or nonviable tumor.[40] Further studies are needed to evaluate the efficacy of dynamic MR imaging in the detection of minimal residual disease or early relapse in patients with hematologic malignancies.

INFILTRATIVE DISORDERS

In increased marrow-iron stores from hemosiderosis or hemochromatosis, or in markedly hypercellular marrow, as can be seen in sickle cell disease with reconversion, the marrow signal

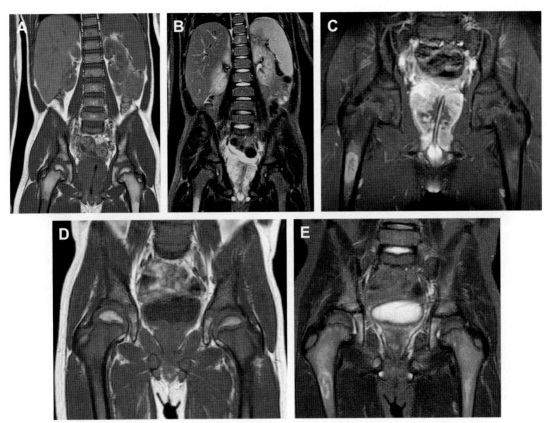

Fig. 10. Patient with metastatic rhabdomyosarcoma. Note the primary involving the bladder base and large focal metastasis within the proximal right femur and smaller, more subtle vertebral involvement (*A–C*). Following therapy with granulocyte colony–stimulating factor note the reduced marrow signal on T1 (*D*) and increased signal on T2 (*E*).

intensity is lower than that of muscle or nondegenerated intervertebral disks.[20] By MR imaging criteria, iron overload may be present if bone marrow signal intensity is less than that of muscles on T1- and T2-weighted images.[3] Normal signal intensity on T1-weighted images does not exclude iron overload because T2-weighted and especially T2* images are more sensitive to iron overload. The transverse relaxation rate (1/T2) of the bone marrow water fraction has a positive correlation with the serum ferritin in normal individuals, as measured in the lumbar spine with chemical-shift misregistration.[41] Knowledge of the patient's transfusion history is very important for the interpretation of the MR imaging findings of bone marrow.

Gaucher disease is the most common of the lysosomal storage disorders, and is an inherited disorder in which glucocerebroside accumulates in the reticuloendothelial system. Glucocerebroside accumulation in the lysosomes of various cell types is responsible for the clinical manifestations of Gaucher disease, which may include

hepatomegaly, splenomegaly, anemia, thrombocytopenia, and bone marrow infiltration by lipid-engorged "Gaucher cells".[42] Replacement of bone marrow by Gaucher cells produces low signal intensity lesions on both T1- and T2-weighted images. Occasional high signal intensity is observed on fluid-sensitive sequences, which can be caused by infection or osteonecrosis (**Fig. 13**). Both homogeneous and inhomogeneous patterns of altered signal intensity have been described. Marrow involvement generally follows the distribution of red marrow and progresses from a proximal to distal direction in the appendicular skeleton. With more advanced disease, epiphyseal involvement and secondary osteonecrosis may develop. Dixon quantitative chemical shift imaging and bone marrow burden scores have been used to quantify the marrow involvement in Gaucher disease.[11] The bone marrow burden scoring method is preferred over the other available scoring systems because it includes measurements of both lumbar spine and femur, key

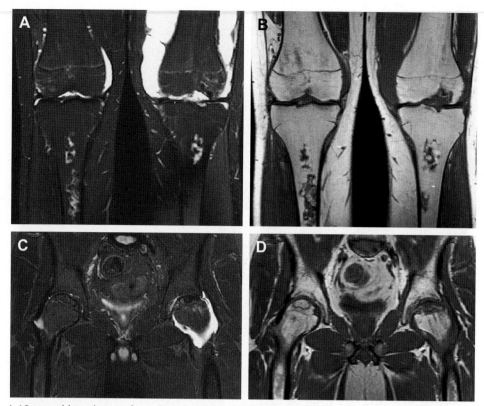

Fig. 11. A 16-year-old on therapy for acute myeloid leukemia with knee pain. There is a huge left knee effusion, and extensive areas of osteonecrosis involving the tibial shafts bilaterally with serpiginous high signal regions on fat-sat T2-weighted image (*A*) and heterogeneous low signal intensity on T1 (*B*). Focal subchondral involvement of the distal left femur is also present. Another example illustrating the typical appearance of avascular necrosis of the hips in a child with acute lymphoid leukemia on fat-sat T2-weighted sequence (*C*) and T1-weighted sequence (*D*).

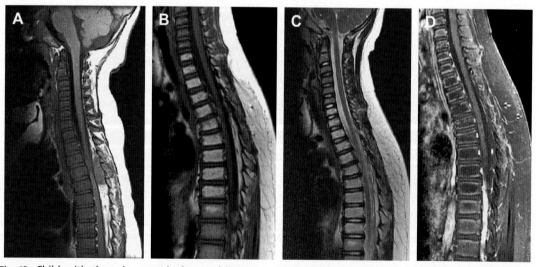

Fig. 12. Child with thoracic paraspinal neuroblastoma with initial intraspinal soft tissue mass and vertebral involvement illustrating the changes in the vertebral marrow following radiation. (*A*) Initial T1-weighted image. (*B*) T1-weighted image 5 years later with fatty marrow replacement of hematopoietic marrow and tumor region. Corresponding T2-weighted (*C*) and post–contrast-enhanced images (*D*).

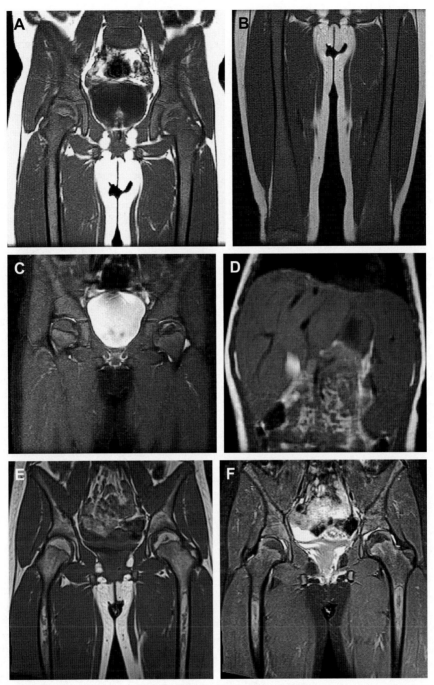

Fig. 13. A 6-year-old child with Gaucher disease. (*A, B*) Diffuse marrow infiltration is present within the pelvis and proximal femora. (*B, C*) Note the Erlenmeyer flask deformity of the distal femora and the avascular necrosis of the left hip. (*D*) Marked hepatosplenomegaly was present. (*E, F*) Follow-up at 14 years of age shows significant improvement with minimal marrow heterogeneity.

anatomic sites for Gaucher cell infiltration, and has been validated against other methods and applied in multiple studies.[42]

In myelofibrosis the bone marrow may be hypercellular or depleted of hematopoietic elements.

Fibrotic marrow is visualized as foci of markedly low signal intensity on all MR imaging sequences. A pattern of low signal intensity on both T1- and T2-weighted images, similar to that in Gaucher disease, with loss of the signal intensity of fat in the epiphyses and apophyses, may also be seen in myelofibrosis.[11]

The infantile form of osteopetrosis is the most severe and is characterized by a complete lack of signal intensity on both T1- and T2-weighted MR images, resulting in "black bones" (**Box 1, Fig. 14**).[11]

MARROW APLASIA AND MYELODYSPLASTIC DISORDERS

In aplastic anemia (idiopathic or secondary to drugs, toxic substances, ionizing radiation, or viral infections) MR imaging demonstrates fatty replacement of the bone marrow,[33] caused by the absence of cellular elements. On T1-weighted images the bone marrow may be entirely fatty or predominantly fatty with small hypointense nodules (**Fig. 15**).[32] The detection of either focal or diffuse hypointense nodules in the bone marrow of patients with aplastic anemia, in the absence of hemosiderosis, may provide evidence of underlying myelodysplastic disorders or evidence of marrow regeneration in patients with aplastic anemia who respond to treatment.[9]

In patients with myelodysplastic disorders an increase in the extent of marrow involvement and in its signal intensity on STIR images indicates progression of the disease. MR imaging can help increase the positive yield of marrow biopsies by guiding marrow sampling procedures to sites of hypercellular marrow.

ISCHEMIA

Marrow blood supply is derived from two major sources: the nutrient artery, which supplies most of the marrow blood flow; and smaller periosteal arteries, which directly penetrate the bone.[1,4] Within the marrow cavity, blood flows from trans-osteal vessels into a highly branched network of medullary venous sinuses.[5] These sinuses form an extensive anastomosis of thin-walled, relatively large vascular channels that drain into a large central sinus before entering the systemic venous circulation.[5] The vascular supply in the red marrow is typically rich and arborized, whereas fatty marrow has a much sparser vascularity supply.[5,7] Osteonecrosis predominates in the fatty marrow.[11] Most nonepiphyseal infarcts in the long tubular bones occur in the metadiaphyses, probably because of the poor collateral circulation in this region.

The initial ischemic insult is followed by cellular loss. Hematopoietic cells die within the first 6 to 12 hours of anoxia. Osteocytes, osteoblasts, and osteoclasts begin to show evidence of cellular death after 48 hours. The adipocytes are most resistant and survive for 2 to 5 days. MR imaging is a very sensitive method for detecting osteonecrosis. At a very early stage, osteonecrosis produces a nonspecific pattern of poorly defined regions identical to findings of bone marrow edema. Once the ischemic process has passed the acute phase, the typical low signal intensity margins of reactive bone can be identified with MR imaging, with the double-line sign believed to be particularly characteristic of osteonecrosis.[11]

MR imaging has also been used to evaluate bone infarcts in patients with sickle cell anemia, and characterize acute and remote foci of osteonecrosis. In patients with normal hemoglobin, infarction occurs predominantly in fatty marrow, whereas in patients with sickle cell anemia infarction occurs in both hematopoietic and fatty marrow (**Fig. 16**).[11]

MISCELLANEOUS MARROW ABNORMALITIES
Fractures

Bone marrow edema may be observed in fractures and bone bruises including adjacent to stress fractures or occult fractures. In these cases a dark linear band, representing the fractures line, is usually seen on both T1- and T2-weighted sequences. When the edema is extensive, the fractures line may be obscured, particularly in T1-weighted sequences.[11]

Bone marrow edema is particularly important in case of stress fractures and stress related-response, because it may be the only MR imaging finding and can be quite prominent.

Arthritis

In arthritis, MR imaging can directly visualize both the soft tissue and osseous inflammatory and destructive aspects. It is more sensitive than radiographic examination for detection of inflammatory soft tissue and bone changes including

Box 1
Low signal intensity marrow on both T1- and T2-weighted imaging
Focal
Benign bone islands
Sclerotic metastases
Diffuse
Myelofibrosis
Osteopetrosis
Iron overload
Gaucher disease

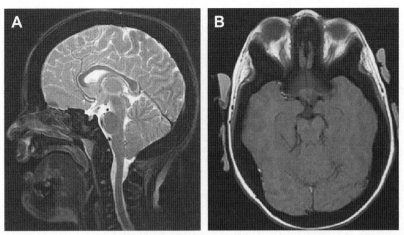

Fig.14. (*A, B*) Child with known osteopetrosis showing marked low signal intensity on T2- and T1-weighted image of the calvarium.

bone marrow edema and inflammatory infiltrates.[43]

In patients with spondyloarthropathy, MR imaging can be used if necessary to diagnose sacroileitis or other focal or multifocal bone marrow infiltrates earlier than is possible radiologically.[43]

New techniques are under evaluation for better and earlier assessment of synovial, cartilaginous, or osseous abnormalities. Diffusion-weighted imaging demonstrates the normal translational movement (Brownian motion) of water molecules that occurs in all tissues. Alteration of normal

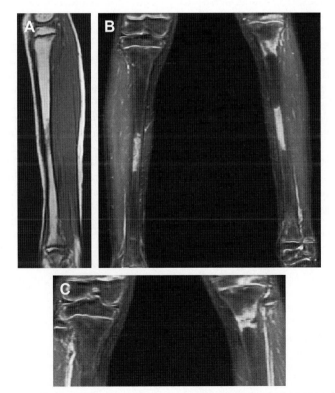

Fig. 15. Child with known aplastic anemia and leg pain. Sagittal T1-weighted image of the right calf shows abnormal marrow signal within diaphyses (*A*), confirmed on coronal fast inversion recovery image (*B*). Note stress fracture with edema and low signal intensity line within proximal left tibia (*C*).

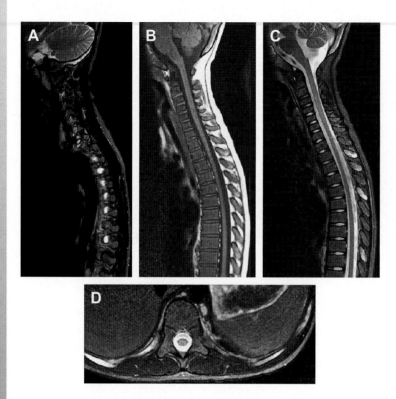

Fig. 16. Child with known sickle cell disease. Blood culture positive for gram-positive bacilli. (*A–C*) Multifocal areas of bone infarction or osteomyelitis are noted involving multiple ribs and vertebra with abnormal increased signal intensity within several spinous processes and ribs on T2-weighted images. (*D*) Note the low signal intensity spleen, which may be secondary to iron overload.

diffusion can occur in pathologic events with a loss of tissue integrity, making this technique very promising for evaluating ischemic tissues and functional changes associated with osteoporosis. Perfusion imaging assesses blood flow using intravenously administered paramagnetic contrast and may be helpful in characterizing ischemic or hyperemic areas, with potential uses in recognition of epiphyseal ischemia, quantification and monitoring of synovial inflammation, and directing therapeutic scheduling for rheumatoid arthritis according to enhancement patterns.[43]

RECENT DEVELOPMENTS AND NEW IMAGING TECHNIQUES IN MR IMAGING

Ultrasmall superparamagnetic iron oxide particles have been developed for the potential MR imaging evaluation of the phagocytic activity of bone marrow. Sufficient ultrasmall particles are taken up by the reticuloendothelial system of the bone marrow to reduce the T1 and T2 signal.[30] The decrease in signal seems to be more marked on gradient echo and T2-weighted images. Phagocytic activity is a marker of normal red marrow being typically absent or significantly reduced in bone tumors, improving tumor–normal marrow contrast.[30]

In recent years whole-body MR imaging primarily with STIR imaging has been introduced as a method that allows surveying the entire

body and bone marrow in cases of suspected neoplasia. The development and improvement of whole-body MR imaging techniques has impacted the field of oncologic imaging, as an adjunct or alternative technique to established multimodality approaches (eg, radiographs, multislice CT, ultrasound, scintigraphy) for initial tumor staging or screening for tumor recurrence after curative therapy.[2] Promising results have been reported for the detection of distant metastatic disease. In particular, pediatric patients benefit from a whole-body MR imaging examination, because bone marrow metastases in the peripheral skeleton are more common in children than in adults.[36] Recently, the use of whole-body MR imaging has been widened to include histiocytosis, osteomyelitis, suspected child abuse, and systemic muscle diseases.[44–47] By assessing a large volume of bone marrow noninvasively and relatively quickly, whole-body MR imaging shows the exact location of foci of marrow involvement in diseases with focal patterns of infiltration and can increase the rate of successful bone marrow biopsies. Prior technical challenges including long examination times and need for time-consuming patient and coil repositioning have been overcome with the introduction of multichannel MR imaging scanners using a system of multiple phased-array coils covering the whole body. Imaging the total skeletal system without compromise in spatial resolution has become possible. In particular, the combination of free table movement with parallel imaging acquisition techniques, and the use of such sequences as breath-hold gradient echo and whole-body turbo STIR, has resulted in substantially shorter room time.[2,18] Additionally, new three-dimensional pulse sequences have been introduced, which may improve spatial resolution and allow better reformations of flat bones including ribs.[29]

Although studies are limited to date, fluorodeoxyglucose positron emission tomography may show a higher sensitivity for detection of bone metastasis than whole-body MR imaging in children and young adults. Fluorodeoxyglucose positron emission tomography may, however, demonstrate a higher number of false-positive lesions.[29] Fluorodeoxyglucose positron emission tomography requires complimentary CT or MR imaging to localize an area of increased glucose metabolism. Another problem with fluorodeoxyglucose positron emission tomography is the identification of skull metastases, because normal brain exhibits a high glucose metabolism, which may obscure metastases.[48] Recent development of positron emission tomography–MR imaging theoretically improves the sensitivity and specificity for the detection of bone marrow metastases.

High resolution diffusion-weighted MR imaging with the STIR echo planar imaging sequence and free breathing scanning, can be used to create optimum three-dimensional display. Three-dimensional diffusion-weighted MR imaging has great potential as a novel tool for evaluating pathologic lesions including malignancy, although its use in pediatrics has been limited.[49]

SUMMARY

MR imaging is an excellent noninvasive modality for evaluating bone marrow and detecting marrow lesions. It plays an integral role in the detection and characterization of bone marrow lesions, guiding biopsy, staging, treatment planning, and in following therapy-related changes. To evaluate findings in pediatric bone marrow MR imaging evaluation, it is essential to be aware of the changing pattern of the bone marrow that occurs with age.

MR imaging of the bone marrow is increasingly successfully applied, because MR imaging depicts bone marrow pathologies with high resolution and excellent tissue contrast representing an effective method for analyzing many of these disorders. Although MR imaging is more sensitive than specific in detecting marrow changes, clinical and radiologic correlation often leads to the appropriate clinical interpretation.

REFERENCES

1. Abboud C, Lichtman M, et al. Structure of the bone marrow. In: Beutler E, Lichtman M, Coller B, editors. Williams hematology. 5th edition. New York: McGraw-Hill; 1995. p. 25–38.
2. Schmidt G, Reiser M, Baur-Melnyk A. Whole-body imaging of the musculoskeletal system: the value of MR imaging. Skeletal Radiol 2007; 36:1109–19.
3. Babyn P, Ranson M, McCarville E. Normal bone marrow: signal characteristics and fatty conversion. Magn Reson Imaging Clin N Am 1998;6: 473–95.
4. Weiss L. Bone marrow. In: Weiss L, editor. Cell and tissue biology: a textbook of histology. Baltimore: Urban and Schwarzenberg; 1988.
5. Trubowitz S, Davis S. The bone marrow matrix. The human bone marrow: anatomy, physiology, and pathophysiology. Boca Raton (FL): CRC Press; 1982. p. 43–75.
6. Steiner RM, Mitchell DG, Rao VM, et al. Magnetic resonance imaging of diffuse bone marrow disease. Radiol Clin North Am 1993;31: 383–409.
7. Vogler JBD, Murphy WA. Bone marrow imaging. Radiology 1988;168:679–93.
8. Moore SG. Pediatric musculoskeletal magnetic resonance. In: Pediatric imaging: update 91. International Pediatric Radiology; 1991. p. 217–23.
9. Moulopoulos L, Dimopoulos M. Magnetic resonance imaging of the bone marrow in hematologic malignancies. Blood 1997;90:2127–47.
10. Hwang S, Panicek D. Magnetic resonance imaging of bone marrow in oncology, Part 1. Skeletal Radiol 2007;36:913–20.
11. Resnick D, Sik Kang H, Pretterklieber M. Bone and bone marrow: anatomy and pathophysiology. In: Resnick D, Sik Kang H, Pretterklieber M, editors. Internal derangements of joints, 2nd edition, vol. 1. Saunders Elsevier; 2007. p. 231–57.
12. Caldmeyer K, Smith R, Harris A, et al. Hematopoietic bone marrow hyperplasia: correlation of spinal MRI findings, hematologic parameters, and bone mineral density in endurance athletes. Radiology 1996;198: 503–8.
13. Pui M, Chang S. Comparison of inversion recovery fast spin-echo (FSE) with T2-weighted fat-saturated FSE and T1-weighted MR imaging in bone marrow lesion detection. Skeletal Radiol 1996;25:149–52.
14. Sebag G, Moore S. Effect of trabecular bone on the appearance of marrow in gradient-echo imaging of the appendicular skeleton. Radiology 1990;174: 855–9.
15. Vanel D, Dromain C, Tardivon A. MRI of bone marrow disorders. Eur Radiol 2000;10:224–9.

16. Baur A, Staebler A, Bartl R, et al. MRI gadolinium enhancement of bone marrow: age-related changes in normals and diffuse neoplastic infiltration. Skeletal Radiol 1997;26:414–8.

17. Moulopoulos L, Varma D, Dimopoulos M, et al. Multiple myeloma: spinal MR imaging in patients with untreated newly diagnosed disease. Radiology 1992;185:833–40.

18. Hwang S, Panicek D. Magnetic resonance imaging of bone marrow in oncology, part 2. Skeletal Radiol 2007;36:1017–27.

19. Siegel M, Luker G. Bone marrow imaging in children. Magn Reson Imaging Clin N Am 1996;4:771–96.

20. Carroll K, Feller J, Tirman P. Useful internal standards for distinguishing infiltrative marrow. J Magn Reson Imaging 1997;7:394–8.

21. Vande Berg BC, Lecouvet FE, Galant C, et al. Normal variants and frequent marrow alterations that simulate bone marrow lesions at MR imaging. Radiol Clin North Am 2005;43:761–70.

22. Rosen B, Fleming D, Kushner D, et al. Hematologic bone marrow disorders: quantitative chemical shift MR imaging. Radiology 1988;169:799–804.

23. Disler DG, McCauley TR, Ratner LM, et al. In-phase and out-of-phase MR imaging of bone marrow: prediction of neoplasia based on the detection of coexistent fat and water. Am J Roentgenol 1997;169:1439–47.

24. Zajick DC Jr, Morrison WB, Schweitzer ME, et al. Benign and malignant processes: normal values and differentiation with chemical shift MR imaging in vertebral marrow. Radiology 2005;237:590–6.

25. Mirowitz SA, Apicella P, Reinus WR, et al. MR imaging of bone marrow lesions: relative conspicuousness on T1- weighted, fat-suppressed T2-weighted, and STIR images. AJR Am J Roentgenol 1994;162:215–21.

26. Flickinger F, Salahattin S. Bone marrow MRI: techniques and accuracy for detecting breast cancer metastases. Magn Reson Imaging 1994;12:829–35.

27. Frank JA, Ling A, Patronas NJ, et al. Detection of malignant bone tumors: MR imaging vs scintigraphy. AJR Am J Roentgenol 1990;155:1043–8.

28. Eustace S, Tello R, DeCarvalho V, et al. A comparison of whole-body turbo STIR MR imaging and planar 99m Tc-methylene diphosphonate scintigraphy in the examination of patients with suspected skeletal metastases. AJR Am J Roentgenol 1997;169:1655–61.

29. Daldrup-Link H, Franzius C, Link T, et al. Whole-body MR imaging for detection of bone metastases in children and young adults: comparison with skeletal scintigraphy and FDG PET. AJR Am J Roentgenol 2001;177:229–36.

30. Seneterre E, Weissleder R, Jaramillo D, et al. Bone marrow: ultrasmall superparamagnetic iron oxide for MR imaging. Radiology 1991;179:529–33.

31. Daldrup HE, Link TM, Blasius S, et al. Monitoring radiation-induced changes in bone marrow histopathology with ultra-small superparamagnetic iron oxide (USPIO)-enhanced MRI. J Magn Reson Imaging 1999;9:643–52.

32. Imamura F, Kuriyama K, Seto T, et al. Detection of bone marrow metastases of small cell lung cancer with magnetic resonance imaging: early diagnosis before destruction of osseous structure and implications for staging. Lung Cancer 2000;27:189–97.

33. Cohen M, Klatte E, Baehner R, et al. Magnetic resonance imaging of bone marrow disease in children. Radiology 1984;151:715–8.

34. Vande Berg B, Schmitz P, Scheiff J, et al. Acute myeloid leukemia: lack of predictive value of sequential quantitative MR imaging during treatment. Radiology 1995;197:301–5.

35. Vande Berg B, Michaux L, Scheiff J, et al. Sequential quantitative MR analysis of the bone marrow: differences during treatment of lymphoid versus myeloid leukemia. Radiology 1996;201:519–23.

36. Kwee T, Kwee R, Verdonck L, et al. Magnetic resonance imaging for the detection of bone marrow involvement in malignant lymphoma. Br J Haematol 2008;141:60–8.

37. Smith R, Schilder K, Shaer A, et al. Lymphoma staging with bone marrow MRI. Proc Am Soc Clin Oncol 1995;14:390–2.

38. Smith S, Williams C, Edwards R, et al. Quantitative magnetic resonance studies of lumbar vertebral marrow in patients with refractory or relapsed Hodgkin's disease. Ann Oncol 1991;2:39–42.

39. Fletcher B, Wall J, Hanna S. Effect of hematopoietic growth factors on MR images of bone marrow in children undergoing chemotherapy. Radiology 1993;189:745–51.

40. Van der Woude H, Bloem J, Verstraete K, et al. Osteosarcoma and Ewing's sarcoma after neoadjuvant chemotherapy: value of dynamic MR imaging in detecting viable tumor before surgery. AJR Am J Roentgenol 1995;165:593–8.

41. Ishijima H, Ishizaka H, Aoki J, et al. T2 relaxation time of bone marrow water and lipid: correlation with serum ferritin in normal individuals. J Comput Assist Tomogr 1997;21:506–8.

42. Maas M, Hangartner T, Mariani G, et al. Recommendations for the assessment and monitoring of skeletal manifestations in children with Gaucher disease. Skeletal Radiol 2007;37:185–8.

43. Babyn P, Doria A. Radiologic investigation of rheumatic diseases. Rheum Dis Clin North Am 2007;33:403–40.

44. Ghanem N, Lohrmann C, Engelhardt M, et al. Whole-body MRI in the detection of bone marrow infiltration in patients with plasma cell neoplasm in comparison to the radiological skeletal survey. Eur Radiol 2006;16:1005–14.

45. Buhmann S, Schoenberg S, Becker CR, et al. Whole-body imaging approach of patients with

multiple myeloma: comparing MR imaging with MD-CT. Eur Radiol 2006;16(Suppl 1):B-003.

46. O'Connell MJ, Powell T, Brennan D, et al. Whole-body MR imaging in diagnosis of polymyositis. AJR Am J Roentgenol 2002;179:967–71.

47. Lenk S, Fischer S, Kotter I, et al. Possibilities of whole-body MRI for investigating musculoskeletal diseases. Radiology 2004;44:844–53.

48. Hoh K, Glaspy J, Rosen P, et al. Whole-body FDG PET imaging for staging of Hodgkin's disease and lymphoma. J Nucl Med 1997;38:343–8.

49. Takahara T, Imai Y, Yamashita T, et al. Diffusion weighted whole body imaging with background body signal suppression (DWIBS): technical improvement using free breathing, STIR and high resolution 3D display. Radiat Med 2004;22(4):275–82.

The Growing Skeleton: MR Imaging Appearances of Developing Cartilage

Paritosh C. Khanna, MD, DMRE*, Mahesh M. Thapa, MD

KEYWORDS
- Hyaline cartilage • Articular cartilage
- Epiphyseal cartilage • Physeal cartilage
- MR imaging • Advanced cartilage imaging

Hyaline cartilage at developing ends of long bones is comprised of three distinct histological types: (1) epiphyseal, (2) physeal, and (3) articular. The epiphyseal and physeal components are responsible for longitudinal growth of long bones by endochondral ossification and demonstrate a distinct laminar pattern at histology. At very high and sometimes, at clinical field-strength MR imaging, this laminar pattern can be discerned. Articular cartilage protects and nourishes subchondral bone at joint surfaces and is itself nourished by joint fluid and synovium. It transmits and buffers physiologic and abnormal forces across joints, particularly at weight-bearing sites, playing a part in maintaining the integrity of joint surfaces. Articular cartilage also demonstrates a laminar pattern on sequences specific to its imaging.

Various imaging techniques for the evaluation of these cartilaginous components have evolved over the years. Sequences have been developed at various field strengths to accentuate the contrast between joint fluid and articular cartilage. Techniques developed increase the conspicuity of epiphyseal and physeal cartilage and differentiate one from the other and from subjacent normal and abnormal osseous structures. Low field strength open magnets do not provide good articular cartilage-joint fluid and epiphyseal-physeal-osseous

contrast and extensive research has led to the development of techniques with closed-bore 1.5-Tesla (T) and 3.0-T magnets. A host of spin echo and gradient recalled echo (GRE) sequences have been developed with and without fat suppression.

Considerable work has been done with contrast-enhanced MR imaging, particularly for epiphyseal and physeal cartilage, and with MR arthrography for articular cartilage, because the latter helps distend the joint, in addition to providing excellent contrast between joint fluid and articular surfaces. Advanced imaging techniques have been developed for molecular and functional imaging of cartilage. These include proton density (PD) imaging for water content; T2 mapping for collagen ultrastructure; sodium imaging; delayed gadolinium-enhanced MR imaging of cartilage (an indirect contrast-enhanced technique) for glycosaminoglycans; T2; magnetization transfer T1rho and diffusion imaging to study the macromolecular state of cartilage.

All these techniques have been used for the study of normal-developing cartilage, to define normal variants, and to segregate them from and evaluate abnormal cartilage. These techniques facilitate early intervention, preoperative and postoperative evaluation, and eventual rehabilitation.

Department of Radiology, Seattle Children's Hospital, University of Washington School of Medicine, 4800 Sand Point Way NE, M/S-5417, Seattle, WA 98105, USA
* Corresponding author.
E-mail address: pkhanna@u.washington.edu (P.C. Khanna).

Magn Reson Imaging Clin N Am 17 (2009) 411–421
doi:10.1016/j.mric.2009.03.012

STRUCTURE OF DEVELOPING CARTILAGE
Biochemical Composition

Hyaline cartilage consists mainly of chondrocytes embedded in a matrix of water, collagen, noncollagenous glycoproteins, and proteoglycan monomers that consist of glycosaminoglycans (chondroitin sulfate and keratan sulfate) that bind to hyaluronic acid. Water is the most abundant component of hyaline cartilage; a fraction of water is free, the remainder being bound to collagen fibrils. Physeal and epiphyseal collagen is continuous, unlike articular cartilage where collagen fibers are oriented differently in different layers.[1–3]

Histology

Histology reveals three hyaline cartilaginous components: (1) the epiphyseal cartilage; (2) the physeal cartilage, composed of a columnar array of chondrocytes that proliferate and hypertrophy; and (3) the articular cartilage. Endochondral ossification plays two important roles: mineralization at the zones of provisional calcification (ZPC) and development and growth of the secondary ossification center within the epiphyseal cartilage.[1,2]

Immediately surrounding the secondary ossification center, there is a ZPC (the secondary ZPC). This is surrounded by a layer of cartilage known as the secondary physis, which is structured much like the growth plate (also known as the primary physis). The secondary physis is in turn surrounded by the epiphyseal cartilage.

The growth plate or primary physis is along the metaphyseal aspect of the epiphyseal cartilage. From its epiphyseal to metaphyseal aspects, the primary physis is subdivided into the germinal, proliferating, and hypertrophic zones. The hypertrophic zone is further subdivided into zones, and another zone of provisional calcification, the primary ZPC, is located just adjacent to the primary spongiosa of the metaphysis. Endochondral ossification results in deposition of osseous mineral within the primary ZPC, which unites with recently formed new bone at the juxtaphyseal metaphysis.

With advancing maturity, the epiphysis assumes a more hemispheric contour, and the secondary physis and epiphyseal cartilage become thinner.[1,2] The primary physis becomes progressively more undulating but retains a fairly constant thickness until skeletal maturity is attained.[4]

Multiple vascular channels (containing arterioles, capillaries, and a venous plexus) exist within the epiphysis and initially are nonanastomotic and randomly configured or parallel to one another. They induce and facilitate ossification. At a later stage, these vessels begin to converge toward the developing secondary ossification center and decrease in number. Others originate at the secondary ossification center and diverge from it in a radial pattern.[1,2,5,6] Based on the stage of development, Barnewolt and colleagues[5] have classified epiphyses into five types. Very immature physeal cartilage is also supplied by nonanastomotic vascular channels that provide nutrients.[5,6]

Articular cartilage at the joint surface merges with epiphyseal cartilage during childhood and is separated from underlying subchondral bone by a thin zone of calcified cartilage when skeletal maturity is reached.[4] Articular cartilage is divided into four zones: (1) superficial or tangential, (2) transitional or middle, (3) deep or radial, and (4) calcified. This normal stratification can sometimes be perceived in older children and adolescents with appropriate cartilage-sensitive MR imaging sequences.[3] Articular cartilage volume demonstrates normal diurnal variations, variations caused by physical exercise, and disease states.

Apophyses also have recognizable physes that contribute little to longitudinal growth and are relatively weak.[4] These have similar structures and imaging features as those of primary physes at the end of long bones.

MR Imaging Characteristics of Developing Cartilage

The T1 and T2 characteristics of cartilage are dependent on its water content because a fraction of water is bound to solid components of cartilage, such as proteoglycans and collagen macromolecules. This shortens the T1 and T2 relaxation times of cartilage compared with free water. Collagen binding and chondrocytes themselves result in magnetization transfer that decreases MR imaging signal intensity.[2,4] Orientation of collagen fibers influences tissue anisotropy and cartilage signal. Physis has about 70% water content and has signal intensity closer to water than epiphyseal or articular cartilage. Signal differences in physeal and epiphyseal cartilage are likely from differences in noncollagenous matrix contents, because collagen has similar arrangement in both types of cartilage. Water is less tightly bound in physeal cartilage, presumably the reason for longer T2 values. Mineralization and vascularity contribute less to the imaging features of cartilage.[4]

In children, a variety of MR imaging sequences can bring out the differences between the various components of hyaline cartilage in developing bones and also surrounding structures. It has been demonstrated in newborn lambs and piglets that, in the epiphysis-physis complex, five regions of distinct signal intensities are discernable on modern 1.5-T and 3-T systems, between the marrow of the secondary ossification center and metaphysis. From the secondary ossification center to metaphysis these are as follows: secondary ZPC, secondary physis, epiphyseal cartilage, primary physis, and primary ZPC. In children, and especially in neonates, these layers are readily defined with T2-weighted images but less so using T1. T1 images should be obtained with larger number of averages in young patients. The bilaminar appearance of secondary ZPC and physis is less well defined than the primary ZPC and physis. T2 signal intensity and relaxation time are greater in physeal than in epiphyseal cartilage. Again, these are not as well differentiated on T1 and GRE sequences (**Fig. 1**).[7] Further, the two physes and ZPCs demonstrate similar MR imaging signal characteristics. Both physes have longer T1 and T2 relaxation times than epiphyseal cartilage. In children, the ZPC is hypointense to adjacent metaphysis on T1, unless there is abundant hematopoietic marrow. The thickness of all these layers on MR imaging correlates with that of histologic zones.[1]

In neonates, epiphyseal signal intensity is generally homogeneous and always exceeds metaphyseal signal intensity.[1,2,8] As a child matures, areas within the epiphyseal cartilage that are about to form bone can demonstrate increased T2 signal. This is particularly evident in the trochlea of the elbow and the posterior aspect of the distal femoral condyle (**Fig. 2**). With growth and development, decreased signal intensity develops in weight-bearing cartilage. This is readily seen in the distal and proximal femur and acetabulum (**Fig. 3**).[4] Also, with skeletal maturity, the physis becomes thinner with areas of increased undulations (**Fig. 4**). The progressively thinning epiphyses and secondary physes demonstrate decreasing T2 signal with advanced maturity and weight-bearing, until these two layers become indistinguishable and epiphyseal cartilage develops a homogeneous appearance.[1,2,9]

Epiphyseal vascular channels are best delineated with intravenous contrast administration. Cartilaginous epiphyses appear homogeneous on unenhanced T1 sequences and have linear or punctate areas of high signal intensity with contrast administration as a result of vascular enhancement (**Fig. 5**). Some canals extend from the metaphysis to the epiphysis, across the physis in younger infants. Epiphyseal vascular canals increase in diameter with increasing maturity. The primary and secondary physes demonstrate uniform, bright enhancement that decreases with increasing maturity and disappears with fusion of the epiphysis and metaphysis.[1,2,5,6] These vascular channels can become conspicuous in

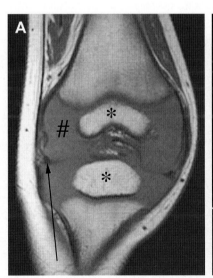
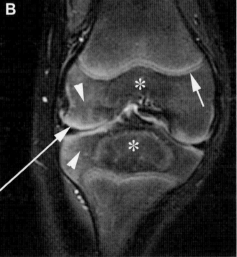

Fig. 1. (*A*) Normal coronal T1 image of the knee in a 22-month-old girl. All hyaline cartilage (epiphysis, physis, and articular cartilage), designated by #, demonstrates uniform intermediate signal. Fibrocartilaginous structures, such as menisci (*arrow*), are low in signal. (*B*) Normal coronal T2 fat-saturated image at the same location as Fig. 1A. The physis (*short arrow*) and the articular cartilage (*long arrow*) demonstrate higher T2 signal than epiphyseal cartilage (*arrowheads*). On the metaphyseal side, the thin layer of low signal immediately adjacent to the high T2 signal of the physis represents the ZPC; the second thin line of high T2 signal on the metaphyseal side of the ZPC represents the primary spongiosa. Fat-filled marrow of the epiphyseal secondary ossification center is also seen (**in A and B*).

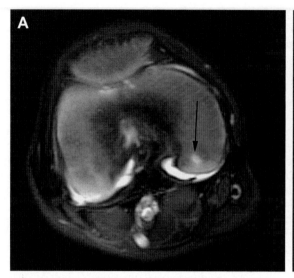
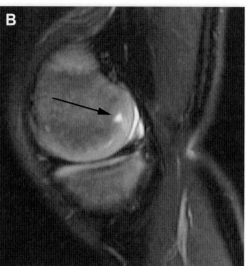

Fig. 2. Normal axial (*A*) and sagittal (*B*) T2 fat-saturated images from a 2-year-old girl demonstrate a small focus of high signal in the posterior epiphyseal cartilage of the medial femoral condyle (*arrow*), representing a "preossification" center, an area about to form bone.

inflammatory and infective states. The degree of epiphyseal enhancement is always less than the metaphysis, which demonstrates a prominent juxtaphyseal enhancing zone called the "metaphyseal stripe," which represents enhancement in the primary spongiosa of the metaphysis and should be differentiated from the physis itself.[8,9]

Pediatric articular cartilage has characteristics similar to physeal cartilage.[7] It is of intermediate signal intensity on conventional and fast spin echo techniques and appears as a rim of high signal on water-sensitive sequences (see **Fig. 1**). For effective imaging, articular cartilage specific sequences should provide good differential contrast from synovial fluid, other hyaline cartilage components (epiphysis, physis), fibrocartilage (meniscus, labrum), combined with relatively high in-plane and slice resolution.[3] Bilaminar or trilaminar appearance of articular cartilage may be noted with appropriate pulse sequences on clinical MR imaging systems and should not be mistaken for abnormality. The superficial zone is thin and hypointense, the transitional zone appears hyperintense, and the deepest radial zone also appears hypointense. These differences are accentuated with increasing echo time (TE). In most cases, however, current scanners do not have sufficient resolution to image the thinnest superficial layer.[3]

COMPONENTS OF PEDIATRIC CARTILAGE MR IMAGING PROTOCOLS

Optimal evaluation of developing pediatric cartilage and remaining elements of the musculoskeletal system in the same study requires a combination of imaging sequences. Physeal signal is homogeneous and very high on PD and spoiled gradient-recalled echo (SPGR) images, high on T2-weighted images, and intermediate on T1-weighted images. Carey and colleagues[10] described the use of fast field echo with off-resonance magnetization transfer for evaluation of cartilage in some of their patients. Susceptibility effects, however, limited concomitant evaluation

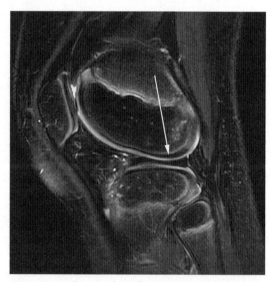

Fig. 3. Normal sagittal T2 fat-saturated image of the knee in an ambulating 6-year-old girl. Note the areas of low signal in the weight-bearing epiphyseal cartilage of lateral femoral condyle (*arrow*). This is thought to be caused by extrusion of water from the epiphyseal cartilage.

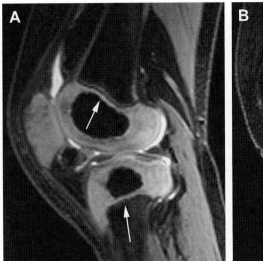
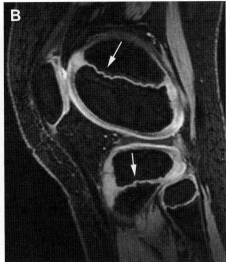

Fig. 4. Sagittal double-echo steady-state (DESS) image of a normal 22-month-old girl's knee (*A*) and 9-year-old boy's (*B*). Note the changes in the physes. In the younger child, the physis is thicker with fewer undulations. In the older child, the physis is thinner with more undulations (*arrows*, compare corresponding physes in *A* and *B*). Eventually, the high signal physis fuses and disappears altogether.

of bone. In other patients, they used T1 and PD spin echo sequences.

A complete evaluation of the physeal plate begins with coronal and sagittal T1 sequences. Maximal physeal conspicuity can be achieved by suppressing the signal from adjacent bone either by fat suppression (for fast spin echo PD, T2, and SPGR images) or with the phase direction perpendicular to the physis to prevent degradation of physeal signal by chemical shift artifact. Physeal conspicuity is also enhanced with GRE sequences

or by acquiring out-of-phase images (when water and fat are out-of-phase). Gadolinium-enhanced T1-weighted images provide additional information by demonstrating physeal vascularity. Physeal closure generally occurs from center to periphery and is well evaluated with GRE, SPGR, and PD images.[4,7] In the distal tibial metaphysis, closure starts anteromedially at "Kump's bump" and progresses posterolaterally.[4,7]

Epiphyseal cartilage is of low signal intensity on T2 and short tau inversion recovery (STIR) images

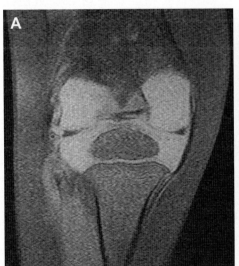
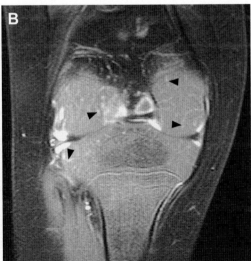

Fig. 5. Epiphyseal vascular channels. (*A*) Unenhanced coronal T1 fat-saturated image of a 1-year-old girl demonstrates homogenous cartilage signal. (*B*) Following administration of IV gadolinium, cor T1 fat-saturated image through the same location demonstrates linear and punctate enhancing vascular channels.

and of high signal intensity on PD and SPGR (or fast low-angle shot) sequences in the infant and young child. Magic angle artifact is noted when collagen fibers in hyaline cartilage are oriented at an angle of 55° to the main magnetic field (B_0) of the MR scanner. At this angle, dipole interactions between water molecules and collagen fibers approach zero resulting in lengthened T2 relaxation times and increased signal of otherwise hypointense structures. This is especially evident on low TE sequences (such as T1, PD, and some GRE sequences) and disappears on T2 sequences.

Fat-suppressed SPGR was commonly used for evaluation of articular cartilage in the past; however, surrounding structures are not well depicted. Potter and colleagues[11] have described the use of long TE sequences, such as the multiplanar high-resolution fast spin echo PD sequence in the accurate assessment of articular cartilage injury. This has been validated for use in the pediatric population by Oeppen and colleagues[12] because it produces good contrast between lower-intensity articular cartilage and higher-intensity joint fluid. Fast spin echo sequences provide high in-plane resolution and make partial thickness lesions more conspicuous. Use of wider receiver bandwidth minimizes chemical shift misregistration and reduces interecho spacing that in turn reduces edge-blurring. Fast spin echo sequences also do not suffer from susceptibility artifact as do GRE sequences. T2 fat-suppressed sequences have been used additionally for evaluation of subchondral bone. Good correlation with arthroscopy has been shown with the use of this combination.[12] By changing the flip angle with GRE sequences, tissue contrast between articular cartilage and adjacent joint fluid can be altered. Decreasing the flip angle to about 20 degrees increases the T2 weighting, with increased contrast between lower-intensity cartilage and higher-intensity joint fluid. Increasing the flip angle to 45 degrees or more increases the T1 weighting, with higher signal intensity from cartilage compared with adjacent joint fluid. This T1 contrast is further accentuated by adding fat-suppression.[9]

Newer gradient echo techniques to image pediatric hyaline and in particular articular cartilage include the steady-state sequences, such as double-echo steady state, refocused steady-state free precession (also known as FIESTA, Tru-FISP, and balanced fast-field echo), and WS-b steady-state free precession.[3] The authors routinely use the double-echo steady-state sequence, which combines two gradient echoes, provides high T2 contrast, and depicts joint morphology well. This may be combined with fat

suppression, but at the expense of signal-to-noise. Driven equilibrium Fourier transform, multiple echo techniques, and short echo time projection reconstruction imaging are other newer gradient sequences.[3]

Pediatric cartilage imaging protocols should be designed to include fat-suppressed and non–fat-suppressed sequences. Fat suppression may be accomplished by one of four methods. (1) Spectral presaturation produces good fat suppression that frequently is suboptimal along areas of curved or uneven body contours and large fields of view. Use of saline bags containing bismuth subsalicylate helps even out contours and improves fat suppression. (2) Inversion recovery (eg, STIR) sequences produce good fat suppression at the expense of some signal-to-noise. These should not be used after administration of gadolinium because contrast-enhancing areas are also likely to get suppressed. (3) With the Dixon method, both in-phase and opposed-phase images are summed[13] to produce a pure water image. This requires a minimum of two data acquisitions and is susceptible to static field inhomogeneities and is rarely used. (4) Opposed phase imaging relies on sampling of water and fat spins when they are in an opposed-phase state by selecting the appropriate echo time. In general, this technique is applicable only to gradient-echo sequences and is best suited to suppressing the signal from tissues that contain similar amounts of lipid and water. This technique is not useful for suppression of marrow fat adjacent to physes.[13,14] Anatomic detail is lost if fat-suppression is too robust (also with heavy T2 weighting). When using spectral presaturation, it is useful to produce incomplete fat saturation and when using STIR, an inversion time (TI) of 140 to 150 milliseconds is preferable.[9]

CONTRAST-ENHANCED MR IMAGING AND MR ARTHROGRAPHY

Besides adding to cost, contrast administration, both intravenous and intra-articular, converts an otherwise noninvasive examination into an invasive one. These techniques include standard gadolinium-enhanced T1 fat-suppressed techniques, delayed gadolinium-enhanced MR imaging of cartilage, and MR arthrography.

Epiphyseal and physeal characteristics on standard gadolinium-enhanced MR imaging in normal and disease states have been discussed elsewhere in this article. Delayed gadolinium-enhanced MR imaging of cartilage is a newer technique that involves an indirect T1 shortening effect produced following the intravenous injection of gadopentate dimeglumine, and mild exercise for about 10 minutes. This is followed by an 80-minute wait period, and a series of T1 fast-inversion recovery images are acquired. This creates an index of relative glycosaminoglycan distribution known as the "T1$_{Gd}$ index" and is used for disorders of articular cartilage.[3]

Direct MR arthrography is an imaging examination that combines the fluoroscopy-guided injection of a saline or dilute gadolinium solution into joint, followed by MR imaging of the joint. By distending the joint, intra-articular structures are optimally visualized and capsular integrity can be assessed by noting the distribution of fluid within the joint. Although this imaging technique has been increasingly used to evaluate pathology in several articulations, it is the shoulder joint and knee that have been most frequently interrogated by MR arthrography. The main indications for MR arthrography include the evaluation of articular cartilage surfaces and the diagnosis and characterization of osteochondral lesions. Although arthrography introduces an invasive component to the MR imaging evaluation of the joint, it is an established method for optimizing diagnostic accuracy and in pretreatment planning.[15] For MR arthrography the authors use a cocktail comprised of the following components: 10 mL normal saline, 5 mL 1% lidocaine, 5 mL Optiray 320, and 0.1 mL gadolinium. This solution is injected under fluoroscopic guidance. The loversol injection is used to verify proper placement of cocktail within the joint.

IMPACT OF FIELD STRENGTH

As familiarity with the use of 3-T clinical systems grows, a multitude of benefits have become apparent in the imaging of the musculoskeletal system. Besides the obvious increase in signal-to-noise and contrast-to-noise ratios, pediatric musculoskeletal MR imaging studies can be performed faster, decreasing effects of motion artifact in sedated and nonsedated patients. This results in improved cartilage evaluation and accurate lesion detection.

With 3-T, T1 and T2 relaxation times of tissues are different compared with 1.5-T systems. There is a decrease in T2 relaxation time by about 10% and an increase in T1 relaxation time by about 20%. So as to maintain similar contrast parameters compared with 1.5-T systems, repetition time (TR) needs to be increased to about 800 milliseconds and for PD and T2 sequences the echo time (TE) needs to be shortened slightly. Because T2 effects are greater on 3-T GRE sequences,

contrast similar to 1.5-T requires a decrease in flip angle and TE.[13]

MR IMAGING APPEARANCES OF ABNORMAL DEVELOPING CARTILAGE

The ability to image different layers of epiphyseal and physeal cartilage lends itself to practical applications in the characterization of hemimelias and other malformations of cartilage. Skeletal dysplasias reveal disruption of normal zonal arrangement of cartilage.[1,2] The ability to differentiate physis from epiphysis based on the pattern of enhancement may help in the evaluation of extent of cartilage injury, infection, and for the estimation of growth disturbances. Neonates with cartilage abnormalities, such as achondrogenesis and type II hypochondrogenesis, have been shown to have a significant increase in number and size of epiphyseal vascular channels (**Fig. 6**).[6,16] Metabolic disturbances, such as rickets and scurvy, rarely result in abnormal epiphyseal cartilage development.

The physis is a relatively weak region of bone and is easily damaged by trauma, infection, tumor invasion, ischemia, radiation, metabolic and hematologic disorders, electrical and thermal burns, and frostbite.[1,2,4,7,17–20] Traumatic physeal injuries result from many of the Salter-Harris type of fractures[21] and may be direct or indirect,

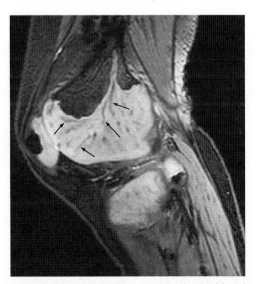

Fig. 6. Cartilage dysplasia. Sagittal double-echo steady-state sequence through this 1-year-old child's knee with a yet undetermined type of cartilage dysplasia demonstrates increase in size and number of vascular channels through the epiphyseal cartilage (*arrows*). Compare to appearance of normal cartilage in **Fig. 5B.**

through injury to the epiphysis or metaphysis. Generally, the frequency of growth arrest increases with increasing Salter number.[7] Transverse physeal fractures through the ZPC frequently heal without complication but those involving the proliferating and germinal physeal layers are susceptible to growth disturbance and arrest. Because Salter I and II injuries tend to spare these physeal layers, the incidence of growth disturbance is lower. An exception to this is the knee joint.[7] Because of the greater remaining growth potential, likelihood of growth disturbance is higher in patients who are more skeletally immature. Besides growth arrest, angular deformity, altered joint mechanics, leg length discrepancy, and long-term disability can result from injury of physes at weight-bearing sites, such as the knees.[4,7] A good example of focal physeal damage presumably from repetitive stress and altered dynamics is Blount disease, which results in tibia vara (**Fig. 7**). Physeal fractures are effectively imaged using spin echo T2 GRE and STIR sequences.[4]

Vertical physeal fractures permit transphyseal vascular communication and tend to result in formation of bony bridges or bars that frequently occur in areas of normal physeal closure and undulation (eg, physes around knee joint that are relatively infrequently injured but account for the highest proportion of bony bridge formation) (**Fig. 8**). Rarely, these bridges heal spontaneously. Peripheral bridges (Ogden type I) predispose to

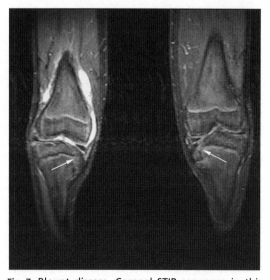

Fig. 7. Blount disease. Coronal STIR sequence in this 8-year-old child demonstrates bilateral medial metaphyseal fragmentation and tibia vara. Note the disruption of the zones of provisional calcification bilaterally (*arrows*). There is also a small right knee effusion.

angular deformities as a result of focal growth arrest; central bridges (Ogden type III) have a larger effect on longitudinal growth and result in leg length discrepancies. Together, these two types account for 89% of all physeal bridges. Linear central bridges (Ogden type II) account for the remainder.[4,17,18] In the distal tibial metaphysis, the anteromedial Kump's bump is the most common site of traumatic physeal closure.[4] It should be noted that small areas of bony bridging may be seen in a normal physis and should not be mistaken for physeal bars or early closure. Further, maximum intensity projection maps show low-intensity bony ridges, known as "mamillary processes," which are also normal.[7]

Physeal bridges are well imaged using thin-slice (less than 1-mm sections) three-dimensional fat-suppressed SPGR acquired perpendicular to the physeal plate in the sagittal or coronal plane.[4,7,17] These can be used to generate multiplanar reformats and axial maximum intensity projection maps of the physeal plate, all of which demonstrate high-intensity cartilage interrupted by the low-intensity physeal bridge. Manual image reconstruction algorithms have been used to generate three-dimensional models of the physeal plate that can be used for surgical planning.[17] Because larger bridges have a prominent marrow space, they appear bright on T1 sequences with smaller bridges appearing dark. PD, STIR, and T2 fat-saturated images help evaluate surrounding tissues. MR imaging reveals bony bridge formation earlier than radiographs.[4] PD and T1 sequences, in conjunction with radiographs, are used to evaluate Park-Harris growth recovery lines that are formed after recovery from a period of arrested bone growth. These lines are seen in the metaphysis, are hypointense on PD and T1, and are parallel to the physis. In areas of physeal injury, they appear bowed toward the injured portion of the physis.[4,7] Outcome of surgical resection is good with physeal bars that involve less than 50% of the physis. If greater than 50%, epiphysiodesis of the injured physis or of the contralateral or companion bone or an osteotomy may be required.

Disruption of epiphyseal vascularity may also result in focal ischemia of the proliferating and germinal physeal layers with resultant physeal disorganization, growth disturbance, or even bony bar formation. Metaphyseal vascular disruption causes endochondral ossification arrest with thickening of injured physes, as in gymnasts, and tongue-like cartilaginous physeal remnants in the metaphysis.[4]

In patients with open physes, chondral and osteochondral injuries predominate.[4,12] Articular

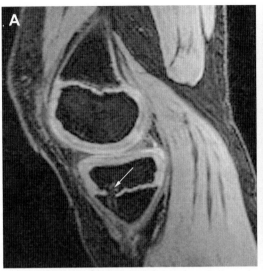
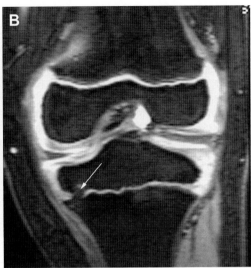

Fig. 8. Bony bridge formation. Sagittal (A) and coronal (B) double-echo steady-state images of an 8-year-old child with remote history of medial tibial fracture demonstrate a bony bridge through the medial physis (arrow).

cartilage and osteochondral injuries have been subdivided using the Outerbridge classification:[11,22]

Grade 0: Intact articular cartilage
Grade 1: Articular cartilage thickening with abnormal signal
Grade 2: Superficial ulceration or fissuring
Grade 3: Deep ulceration or fissuring
Grade 4: Full-thickness chondral injury with bruising of subchondral bone
Grade 5: Osteochondral injury with separation of osteochondral fragment

Osteochondritis dissecans frequently affects the femoral condyles, talar dome, and capitellum. MR imaging demonstrates flattening, increased T2 signal, irregularity, and even discontinuity of the articular cartilage of the osteochondritis dissecans itself. There may be distortion or loss of the laminar appearance of the articular cartilage involved in the osteochondritis dissecans fragment. Subchondral edema and necrosis are often seen. Fluid separating the osteochondral fragment from parent bone signifies instability of the fragment. Loose bodies are often noted (**Fig. 9**).[4]

Hyaline cartilage damage can also ensue following inflammatory injury, such as from juvenile idiopathic arthritis. Total articular and epiphyseal cartilage thickness has been shown to decrease. Other findings include contour irregularity and signal heterogeneity. These findings are best imaged using fast spin echo PD and three-dimensional SPGR sequences. All these features can be verified at arthroscopy; additionally, arthroscopy shows pitting and superficial and deep fissuring.

As expected, T1 fat-saturated postcontrast sequence demonstrates hyperemia with prominent radial, "spoke-wheel" enhancement of epiphyseal cartilage in some patients. This may result in epiphyseal enlargement, increased maturation, premature physeal closure, and growth disturbance. Because of the increased vascularity and

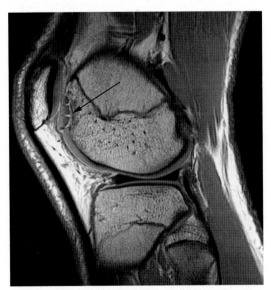

Fig. 9. Osteochondritis desiccans. Sagittal proton density image of a 15-year-old boy demonstrates injury to the cartilage and underlying bone of the anterior lateral femoral condyle at the patellofemoral joint. Note the high signal separating the injured fragment from the underlying bone, indicating instability (arrow).

increased turnover, erosive changes are fewer in the pediatric population compared with adults.[22]

Apart from diagnosis and follow-up of traumatic and inflammatory conditions of articular cartilage, MR imaging is also used in the imaging of cartilage repair procedures,[3,23] such as microfracture, osteochondral autografts and allografts, and autologous chondrocyte implantation, some of which are performed in the pediatric population.

ADVANCED IMAGING TECHNIQUES

Connolly and colleagues[24] have worked with fetal pig specimens and have shown good correlation between fetal MR imaging and histology that may prove useful in prenatal diagnosis of skeletal abnormalities facilitating early prognostication and therapy planning. This is likely to impact generalized diseases, such as skeletal dysplasias, and focal abnormalities, such as clubfoot and developmental hip dysplasia.

Newer developments in coil technology permit faster imaging, an essential requisite for pediatric musculoskeletal imaging. At the expense of signal-to-noise, such techniques as parallel imaging reduce the number of phase-encoding steps by using multichannel coils. This has been overcome by the use of multiple phased-array surface coil elements, multiple independent receiver channels, and integrated parallel acquisition, a strategy that provides high-resolution images in addition to decreasing imaging time.[9]

Multiple newer techniques[3,25] have been developed and are being researched for the noninvasive molecular or biochemical and functional imaging of hyaline cartilage. These include the following:

1. PD for the imaging "measurement" of water content of cartilage. PD can directly measure water density and is a specific but less sensitive method.
2. Collagen ultrastructure imaging or "T2 mapping" by measuring the angular dependence or anisotropy of T2 images (magic angle imaging). It is this effect that is responsible for the multilaminar appearance of developing hyaline cartilage. Collagen orientation is responsible for the orientation of water dipoles bound to it in cartilage matrix and this is accomplished by measuring T2 at various angles.
3. Measurement of glycosaminoglycans. This is done using two methods: sodium imaging and delayed gadolinium-enhanced MR imaging of cartilage. Both methods assess the fixed charge in the cartilage macromolecule. Most of this fixed charge derives from glycosaminoglycans bound within the macromolecule. In

disease states, glycosaminoglycans decrease and so does the fixed charge.

4. T2 to measure tissue composition. In contrast to measuring T2 at various angles for measuring collagen orientation, information about tissue composition can be obtained by measuring T2 at arbitrary angles. Tissue hydration, collagen content, glycosaminoglycans, and solid volume fraction can potentially be measured based on their T2 attributes.
5. Magnetization transfer to evaluate macromolecular state of cartilage. This is based on the fact that the magnetization transfer effect is dominated by the collagen component and structure of cartilage.
6. T1rho imaging to evaluate macromolecular state of cartilage. T1rho imaging has been shown to be dependent on glycosaminoglycans and to a lesser extent collagen.

SUMMARY

Pediatric musculoskeletal MR imaging has the potential to provide substantial information about developing normal and abnormal hyaline cartilage. In the appropriate clinical setting, MR imaging protocols may include fat-suppressed and non–fat-suppressed cartilage-specific sequences that provide reasonable information about surrounding osseous and soft tissue structures. High-resolution spin-echo T1, PD, and T2, various gradient echo and T1 fat-suppressed, contrast-enhanced sequences have been used for routine cartilage imaging. It is important to recognize normal appearances with these imaging techniques, so as to differentiate them from abnormal cartilage. Physeal injury caused by a multitude of reasons probably has the largest impact on longitudinal growth and the development of growth disturbances. Finally, research efforts have led to the development of many newer techniques, some of which provide information about the biochemical, molecular, and functional state of cartilage.

REFERENCES

1. Jaramillo D, Connoly SA, Mulkern RV, et al. Developing epiphysis: MR imaging characteristics and histologic correlation in the newborn lamb. Radiology 1998;207:637–45.
2. Li X, Wang R, Li Y, et al. MRI characteristics and transverse relaxation time measurements in normal growing cartilage. J Huazhong Univ Sci Technolog Med Sci 2004;24:411–3.
3. Potter HG, Foo LF. Articular cartilage. In: Stoller DW, Beltran S, Li AE, et al, editors. Magnetic resonance imaging in orthopedics and sports medicine. 3rd

edition. Philadelphia: Lippincott, Williams and Wilkins; 2006. p. 1099–129.

4. Oeppen RS, Jaramillo D. Sports injuries in the young athlete. Top Magn Reson Imaging 2003;14: 199–208.

5. Barnewolt CE, Shapiro F, Jaramillo D. Normal gadolinium-enhanced MR images of the developing appendicular skeleton: part I. Cartilaginous epiphysis and physis. AJR Am J Roentgenol 1997;169:183–9.

6. Cairns R. Magnetic resonance imaging of the growth plate: pictorial essay. JACR 2003;54:234–42.

7. Li X, Wang R, Li Y, et al. Epiphyseal and physeal cartilage: normal gadolinium-enhanced MR imaging. J Huazhong Univ Sci Technolog Med Sci 2005;25:209–11.

8. Dwek J, Shapiro F, Laor T, et al. Normal gadolinium-enhanced MR images of the developing appendicular skeleton: part II. Epiphyseal and metaphyseal marrow. AJR Am J Roentgenol 1997; 169:191–6.

9. Jaramillo D, Laor T. Pediatric musculoskeletal MRI: basic principles to optimize success. Pediatr Radiol 2008;38:379–91.

10. Carey J, Spence L, Blickman H, et al. MRI of pediatric growth plate injury: correlation with plain film radiographs and clinical outcome. Skeletal Radiol 1998;27:250–5.

11. Potter H, Linklater J, Allen A, et al. Magnetic resonance imaging of articular cartilage in the knee: an evaluation with the use of fast spin echo imaging. J Bone Joint Surg Am 1998;80:1276–84.

12. Oeppen R, Connolly S, Bencardino J, et al. Acute injury of the articular cartilage and subchondral bone: a common but unrecognized lesion in the immature knee. AJR Am J Roentgenol 2004;182:111–7.

13. Dixon WT. Simple proton spectroscopic imaging. Radiology 1984;153:189–94.

14. Delfaut EM, Beltran J, Johnson G, et al. Fat Suppression in MR imaging: techniques and pitfalls. Radiographics 1999;19:373–82.

15. Chung CB, Isaza IL, Angulo M, et al. MR arthrography of the knee: how, why, when. Radiol Clin North Am 2005;43:733–46.

16. Gruber H, Lachman R, Rimoin D. Quantitative histology of cartilage vascular canals in the human rib: findings in normal neonates and children, and in achondrogenesis II-hypochondrogenesis. J Anat 1990;173:69–75.

17. Sailhan F, Chotel F, Gybal AL, et al. 3-Dimensional MR imaging in the assessment of physeal growth arrest. Eur Radiol 2004;14:1600–8.

18. Ogden JA. The evaluation and treatment of partial physeal arrest. J Bone Joint Surg Am 1987;69: 1297–301.

19. Peterson HA. Partial growth plate arrest and its treatment. J Pediatr Orthop 1984;4:246–58.

20. Ogden JA. Injury to the growth mechanisms. In: Ogden JA, editor. Skeletal injury in the child. 2nd edition. Philadelphia: WB Saunders; 1990. p. 97–173.

21. Salter R, Harris W. Injuries involving the epiphyseal plate. J Bone Joint Surg Am 1963;45:587–622.

22. Gylys-Morin V, Graham T, Blebea J, et al. Knee in early juvenile rheumatoid arthritis: MR imaging findings. Radiology 2001;220:696–706.

23. Recht M, Goodwin D, Winalski C, et al. MRI of articular cartilage: revisiting current status and future directions. AJR Am J Roentgenol 2005;185:899–914.

24. Connolly S, Jaramillo D, Hong J, et al. Skeletal development in fetal pig specimens: MR imaging of femur with histologic comparison. Radiology 2004;233:505–14.

25. Gray M, Burstein D. Molecular (and functional) imaging of articular cartilage. J Musculoskel Neuronal Interact 2004;4:365–8.

Infectious and Inflammatory Disorders

Sumit Pruthi, MD, Mahesh M. Thapa, MD*

KEYWORDS

- Pediatric • MR Imaging • Infection • Inflammation
- Osteomyelitis • Juvenile idiopathic arthritis

Musculoskeletal infections and inflammatory disorders in the pediatric population are commonly encountered, and they affect the bones, cartilage, muscle, soft tissues, and joints. Imaging plays a key role in the evaluation of patients with known or suspected musculoskeletal infection or inflammation. After thorough clinical examination and biochemical assessment, the imaging evaluation traditionally begins with plain radiography. Although neither specific nor sensitive, plain films still play a crucial role in narrowing the differential diagnosis and helping us to select the next most appropriate imaging study. They also are readily available and relatively inexpensive to perform. Additional imaging studies include ultrasound (US), CT, nuclear medicine, and MR imaging. Arguably, MR imaging is often the best imaging modality to diagnose early and chronic infectious/inflammatory conditions.

OSTEOMYELITIS

Osteomyelitis is infection of cortical bone and bone marrow and can further be subclassified into various groups depending on the age of presentation, route of infection, onset of the disease, and causative organisms involved.[1,2] The route of infection is typically hematogenous in children, with direct inoculation or spread from contiguous structures seen occasionally.[1] Hematogenous infection usually begins at the metaphysis secondary to its abundant blood supply coupled with slow, sluggish flow within the venous channels along the metaphyseal side of the growth cartilage. There is also decreased phagocytic activity around the metaphysis, which further predisposes to infection.[3] Subsequent pattern of spread of infection changes with various age groups secondary to different microanatomy of the vascular supply. In infants younger than 1 year, infection can spread easily to the epiphysis and joint cavity secondary to transphyseal bridging vessels extending from metaphysis to epiphysis. After 1 year of age, joint involvement is seen uncommonly because the blood supply between the metaphysis and epiphysis is severed. After physeal closure occurs and the vascular connection is restored, however, the joint cavity becomes susceptible to infection again.[1,2]

Acute infection results in extensive inflammatory response and leads to exudate formation, increased intraosseous pressure, blood stasis, thrombosis, and subsequent bone necrosis.[2,4] There is associated cortical destruction, periosteal elevation, and spread of infection into the contiguous soft tissues. Subacute infection, on the other hand, remains localized either by the low virulence of the organism or increased host resistance.[2] Chronic infection generally results either from untreated acute infection or ongoing low-grade infection, manifesting as extensive bony sclerosis or resulting in formation of sequestrum (necrotic bone), involucrum (thick periosteal bone formation surrounding a sequestrum), and cloaca (connection between marrow and periosteum) or sinus (connection between marrow and skin) formation.[4] Sequestrum or devitalized bone formation is seen less commonly in neonates because of rapid decompression of the exudate. On the other hand, periosteal elevation is more pronounced compared with adults because of loose attachment of the periosteum to bone.[4,5]

Department of Radiology, Seattle Children's Hospital, University of Washington School of Medicine, 4800 Sand Point Way NE M/S-5417, Seattle, WA 98105, USA
* Corresponding author.
E-mail address: thapamd@u.washington.edu (M.M. Thapa).

Magn Reson Imaging Clin N Am 17 (2009) 423–438
doi:10.1016/j.mric.2009.03.006
1064-9689/09/$ – see front matter © 2009 Elsevier Inc. All rights reserved.

Apart from these differences, certain other unique features of pediatric osteomyelitis pose a separate set of diagnostic and therapeutic challenges.[6] As opposed to the adult population, infection in infants and neonates can be clinically silent during the initial course of the disease.[7] Clinical presentation can be nonspecific. A child may refuse to bear weight or may limp. Infection can mimic other pathologies, such as lumbar disc disease, and changes in neurologic status may indicate infection involving the vertebra or spinal canal.[6] This manifestation is in contrast to classic signs and presentations of local infection in the form of pain, swelling, tenderness, erythema, and fever. Classic presentation may still be seen in the pediatric population with abnormal biochemical markers such as elevated erythrocyte sedimentation rate and leukocytosis. Early detection facilitates prompt and proper treatment and avoids undesirable consequences of sepsis, chronic infection, and growth arrest.[8]

Generally, hematogenous infections are primarily bacterial in origin, with *Staphylococcus aureus* being the most common organism, followed by *Streptococcus* species, *Pneumococcus* species, *Haemophilus influenzae* (decreased in incidence after widespread immunization), *Escherichia coli*, and *Pseudomonas aeruginosa*.[1,2,4,9] Although still prominent in third world nations, tuberculosis is rarely seen in North America or other developed countries. Infrequently, one might encounter fungal osteomyelitis in immunocompromised children, with Aspergillus being the most common offending organism.[2] The most commonly involved sites include the metaphysis of the distal femur (**Fig. 1**) and proximal tibia, followed by the distal humerus, distal radius, proximal femur, and proximal humerus.[1,10] Of course, any bone can be involved.

The role of imaging in acute osteomyelitis is multifold. First, imaging may be performed to confirm a clinical suspicion of infection. Once confirmed and localized, the next step is to assess its extent and associated complications. Imaging also can be useful for guiding drainage/biopsy for diagnostic and therapeutic purposes. Finally, imaging can be used to assess response to therapy.

Plain Film

Plain film is generally the first imaging modality (**Fig. 1**). Not surprisingly, initial plain film results are often negative; however, they may provide guidance for further imaging and exclude other pathologic conditions, such as fractures or tumors. If positive, plain film findings of infection/inflammation include loss of soft tissue planes and soft tissue swelling in the early stages with eventual bony cortical destruction and periosteal elevation. Loss of approximately 30% to 50% of bone mineralization is required for changes to be apparent on plain films, which usually occurs after approximately 7 to 10 days after the onset of disease.[4,6] The sensitivity and specificity for plain film radiography range from 43% to 75% and 75% to 83%, respectively.[4,11]

Ultrasound

Because it is readily available, inexpensive, and nonionizing, there have been attempts to diagnose osteomyelitis with US. Findings may include visualization of elevated periosteum with associated soft tissue swelling, fluid, or abscess. In our experience, however, the main use of US is to help guide percutaneous drainage of the fluid collections associated with infection for diagnostic and therapeutic purposes.

Scintigraphy

The relative merit of performing scintigraphy after plain radiographs, as opposed to MR imaging, is still debatable. Some argue that scintigraphy is less expensive and rarely requires sedation.[6] Imaging also can be performed more than once with the potential of performing delayed imaging (24 hours after the injection) in difficult cases to improve detection of subtle lesions. Scintigraphy also has the added advantage of detecting multiple foci of disease, which is not infrequent, ranging from 7% in children[12] to 22% in neonates.[7] The capacity to image the entire skeleton can be crucial in infants and neonates, in whom localizing signs are generally poor and often nonspecific.[6] If results are abnormal, three-phase ^{99m}Tc-methylene diphosphonate demonstrates relatively elevated blood flow and abnormal increased deposition of tracer at the site of infection. Despite their advantages, bone scintigraphy findings are nonspecific and may not be able to confidently discern among infection, neoplasm, and trauma. There also can be initial false-negative results secondary to relative ischemia from vascular compression and thrombosis and obscuration of subtle abnormal uptake at the metaphysis from normal high physeal uptake.[1,13] For the reasons listed previously and scintigraphy's lack of fine anatomic detail often required for therapeutic purposes, we consider MR imaging to be superior when evaluating for osteomyelitis.

CT

With the advent of multidetector scanners, its high spatial resolution capability, and ability to perform

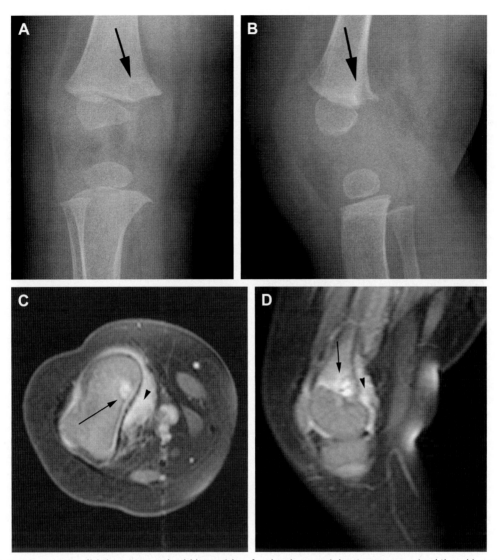

Fig. 1. Acute osteomyelitis in a 14-month-old boy with refusal to bear weight. Anteroposterior (A) and lateral (B) views of the right knee demonstrate a relatively well-defined lucency in the distal medial femoral metaphysis (*arrow*). Axial (C) and sagittal (D) T1 fat-saturated postcontrast image through the same area reveals enhancing osteomyelitis (*arrow*) with extension to the adjacent periosteum and soft tissues (*arrowhead*).

isovolumetric multiplanar reconstruction, CT scan can provide excellent cross-section cortical bony detail. It is the best method for detecting small foci of intraosseous gas, areas of cortical erosion or destruction, tiny foreign bodies, and involucrum and sequestration formation seen in chronic cases.[4] Contrast administration can help delineate the presence and extent of associated soft tissue abscesses. CT scan also can help guide bone biopsies and drain deep-seated intrapelvic abscesses. The biggest disadvantage of CT is the associated radiation dose, especially in children. It should be

used sparingly and its protocol tailored to answer specific clinical questions.

MR imaging

Although it often requires sedation and is relatively expensive to perform, in our experience, MR imaging is still the best imaging tool to diagnose, assess response to therapy, and follow-up cases of suspected or known osteomyelitis (**Fig. 1**). MR imaging also can reliably differentiate acute from chronic infection and has excellent soft tissue contrast and inherent multiplanar capabilities. The basic imaging protocol consists of T1 and fluid-sensitive sequences, including T2 with chemical fat suppression and short tau inversion recovery (STIR) performed in orthogonal planes. T1-weighted images are useful in assessing the normal anatomy and the marrow. Fluid-sensitive sequences help delineate contrast between normal and abnormal tissue. Although the use of intravenous gadolinium in MR imaging for osteomyelitis is still a contentious topic, use of fat-suppressed, contrast-enhanced, T1-weighted images has become a routine part of the diagnostic evaluation for osteomyelitis at various institutes, including ours. Various studies have shown the efficacy of fat-suppressed, contrast-enhanced, T1-weighted sequences in osteomyelitis with increased sensitivity and specificity, compared with three-phase bone scan and noncontrast MR imaging. Contrast can help delineate the extent of marrow abnormality, differentiate devitalized from vascularized bone, and demonstrate the extent of soft tissue abscesses and sinus tracts.[1,14,15] Intravenous contrast use, however, may not be helpful in differentiating infections from noninfectious inflammatory conditions.

Imaging features generally parallel the ongoing pathologic process.[1] In early cases, marrow demonstrates low signal intensity on T1-weighted images and high signal intensity on T2-weighted and STIR images, indicating underlying marrow edema and inflammatory infiltrate. It is important, however, to recall the variability in marrow appearance in children with ongoing conversion of hematopoietic marrow to fatty marrow, which may create a confusing appearance.[1,4,16] Use of fluid-sensitive sequences alone can be misleading; marrow signal may be diffusely hyperintense because fluid and fat may both appear bright. T1-weighted imaging is the ideal sequence for assessing marrow because it better delineates normal marrow morphology.[17]

Subsequently, there may be spread of infection with cortical destruction, periosteal elevation, and spread of infection into contiguous soft tissue structures. Arguably, it may be difficult to see cortical destruction or periosteal elevation on MR imaging in a few cases, but MR imaging easily can demonstrate accompanying cellulitis, myositis, phlegmon, soft tissue abscesses, and associated sinus tracts. Periosteal reaction, sequestra, or involucrum can be identified on MR imaging as focal hypointense regions on all imaging sequences, however.[17,18] Gradient echo sequences can be helpful in these circumstances because susceptibility artifact from mineralization is exaggerated. Contrast enhancement not only helps delineate normal from abnormal

marrow but also allows us to define the extent of soft tissue abscesses and differentiate viable from nonviable tissue. In our experience, obtaining pre- and postcontrast fat-suppressed T1-weighted images is crucial to avoid misinterpretations. For example, if an area of apparent enhancement is noted on the T1 postcontrast, fat-suppressed sequence, it is paramount to compare it to the non-enhanced T1 fat-saturated sequence to ensure that the area of apparent enhancement was dark on the precontrast sequence.

To summarize, MR imaging features of osteomyelitis generally include the following:

1. Marrow edema with or without associated contrast enhancement at early stages
2. Focal cortical destruction and associated periosteal elevation
3. Associated intraosseous or juxtacortical soft tissue abscesses or edema
4. Cloaca (marrow to periosteum) or sinus tract formation
5. Sequestrum or involucrum formation

SUBACUTE OSTEOMYELITIS

Subacute osteomyelitis is one of the many clinical presentations of hematogenous osteomyelitis. Factors that may influence the behavior of a septic process in bone may relate to host resistance, virulence of the infecting organism, and adequacy of antibiotic therapy.[19] Subacute osteomyelitis seems to depend on the interplay between the infecting bacteria and the immune mechanism of the host, representing a favorable host-pathogen response. The initial attack is presumably controlled and results in central area of suppurative necrosis contained by dense fibrous reaction or granulation tissue.[2] Pain is the most consistent presenting feature with insidious onset of disease.[19]

Typical radiographic features consist of a localized destructive lesion of bone with surrounding variable rim of sclerosis usually within metaphysis, classically known as a Brodie abscess.[4] Considered as a subacute and chronic form of infection, Brodie abscess is more commonly seen in boys and is mainly caused by S aureus. It most commonly occurs within the tibial metaphysis.[4] On MR imaging, Brodie abscess has a characteristic layered or target appearance with four distinct layers identified. Centrally there is an abscess cavity that is low on T1-weighted images and high on T2-weighted or STIR images. A layer of granulation tissue, which appears isointense on T1- and hyperintense on T2- weighted images, surrounds the abscess cavity. This layer is best appreciated on postcontrast images because of the associated enhancement of the granulation tissue. Next is a fibrous layer that demonstrates low signal on all sequences. The outermost layer is comprised of a peripheral rim of endosteal reaction that is hypointense on T1-weighted images.[20]

A characteristic but not pathognomonic MR imaging finding that favors subacute infection rather than tumor is the penumbra sign. Reported by Gray and colleagues,[21] it has 75% sensitivity, 99% specificity, and 99% accuracy. It is characteristically identified on T1-weighted sequences and is caused by a thick layer of highly vascularized granulation tissue. It is a discrete peripheral zone of marginally higher signal intensity than the abscess cavity and surrounding marrow edema/sclerosis and lower signal intensity than the fatty bone marrow. The hyperintensity may be caused by the high protein content of the granulation tissue. A similar appearance has been described in the wall of brain abscesses.

Although fairly typical and easily recognizable, there are many other protean forms of subacute osteomyelitis apart from Brodie abscess. Various types of radiologic classifications based on imaging pattern exist, but they are beyond the scope of this article. Fortunately rare, other forms can be misleading and can present as solely lucent lesions, aggressive lesions with associated cortical break, or diaphyseal lesions with varying degrees of cortical hyperostosis or various forms of periosteal new bone formation.[22,23]

CHRONIC OSTEOMYELITIS

Chronic osteomyelitis can result from ongoing acute infection or a low-grade continuous infection (**Fig. 2**). If it results from inadequately treated or nontreated acute infection, the radiographic features include sequestrum formation with multiple draining sinus tracts from the involucrum and abscess cavities. Alternatively, if it is a low-grade process, then the main imaging features include bony sclerosis with some associated underlying bony resorption and cystic changes.[2] Because of its insidious onset, mild symptoms, lack of systemic reaction, and inconsistent supportive laboratory data, subacute or chronic osteomyelitis may mimic various benign and malignant conditions, resulting in delayed diagnosis and treatment. Distinguishing subacute or chronic osteomyelitis from primary tumor of bone—particularly Ewing's sarcoma—or entities such as eosinophilic granuloma or osteoid osteoma sometimes may be diagnostically challenging.[17]

In the absence of recent pathologic fracture, untreated primary tumors of bone usually do not have loculated fluid collections. Cortical destruction in tumors tends to be diffuse, rather than focal. The degree of surrounding edema related to primary tumors of bone is significantly less compared with mass-like edema related to granulation tissue from osteomyelitis.[17] It is important to correlate MR imaging findings with plain radiographic or CT findings because it may help to

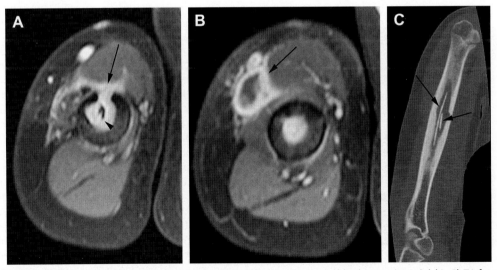

Fig. 2. Chronic osteomyelitis in a 12-year-old boy with arm pain, fever, and leukocytosis. Axial (*A, B*) T1 fat-saturated postcontrast images through the proximal right humerus demonstrate low signal sequestrum in the medullary cavity (*arrowhead*) and extension of infection through a bony defect into the adjacent soft tissue (*arrow*) with abscess formation just below the skin (*arrow*). Coronal CT reconstruction (*C*) through the same humerus defines the intramedullary bony destruction and contained sequestra (*arrows*).

differentiate osteomyelitis from other entities. Relying on MR imaging alone may be misleading.

SPECIAL CIRCUMSTANCES
Epiphyseal Osteomyelitis

Epiphyseal osteomyelitis is generally seen in infants younger than 1 year of age or as part of the unique condition of neonatal osteomyelitis. Susceptibility of the epiphysis to infection is secondary to trans-physeal vascular channels extending from the metaphysis across the physis and into the epiphysis. These vessels generally disappear by 15 months of age, with the growth plate subsequently acting as a barrier to infection. Although rare, epiphyseal osteomyelitis is also seen in older children.[24] The most commonly affected site is the epiphyses at the knee. The reason for this predilection is not well established. Considerations include the fact that the most rapid and extensive bone growth occurs in this area and trauma occurs with a greater frequency around the knees.[24] MR imaging can help identify classic imaging features of osteomyelitis and differentiate it from other epiphyseal entities such as chondroblastoma, osteoid osteoma, and eosinophilic granuloma.[1]

Metaphyseal-equivalent Infections

As opposed to the usual metaphysis of the long bones, approximately 30% of cases of hematogenous osteomyelitis in childhood are encountered at other sites (**Fig. 3**).[24] Initially described by Nixon,[25] these cases are seen adjacent to cartilage with a vascular arrangement analogous to the metaphysis, known as "metaphyseal-equivalent" sites. Awareness and knowledge of these sites can be crucial for early and more accurate identification of osteomyelitis. Some consider epiphysis a part of "metaphyseal-equivalent" sites, which explains the occurrence of epiphyseal osteomyelitis in older children.[24] "Metaphyseal-equivalent" sites include the acetabulum, sacroiliac joint, ischiopubic synchondrosis, pubic bones, vertebrae, calcaneus, greater trochanter, ischium, tibial tubercle, scapula, and talus.[1] Hematogenous osteomyelitis should be an important consideration in a flat or irregular bone lesion in a subchondral site. Although presence of a lesion at these locations does not exclude a neoplasm, origin or predominant involvement in a diaphyseal-equivalent area essentially excludes the diagnostic of hematogenous osteomyelitis.[25] Contrast-enhanced MR imaging can help reveal marrow edema and inflammation as early as 24 to 48 hours after symptom onset.[6] Most of the "metaphyseal-equivalent" sites are clustered around the pelvis, with a higher occurrence of abscesses associated with acute pelvic hematogenous osteomyelitis.[26] The relatively high prevalence of associated fluid collections and abscesses in pelvic osteomyelitis favors the use of MR imaging. Pelvic acute hematogenous osteomyelitis also can be difficult to differentiate clinically from septic arthritis, pyomyositis, and infections of the pelvic organs (eg, appendicitis and tubo-ovarian abscesses) or may mimic lumbar disc disease, again emphasizing of the importance of using MR imaging to evaluate these conditions.[26]

Vertebral Osteomyelitis

Discitis and vertebral osteomyelitis seem to be at the ends of the same disease spectrum, but differentiation is necessary for initiation of appropriate therapy (**Fig. 4**). Children with discitis are generally younger and less likely to be ill appearing or febrile, with more frequent involvement of lumbar spine.[27] Delayed clearance of micro-organisms or entrapped emboli within the vascular channels and abundant intraosseous arterial anastomoses commonly seen within the cartilaginous portion of the disc seem to be the plausible cause of discitis. These channels disappear as a child grows older, which explains the low incidence of discitis later in life.[28] In contrast, vertebral osteomyelitis is considered a "metaphyseal-equivalent" area infection. Micro-organisms lodge in the low-flow, end-organ vasculature adjacent to the subchondral plate region.[27] The most frequent finding in discitis is decreased height of the disk space and erosion of adjacent vertebral endplates. Spine radiographs

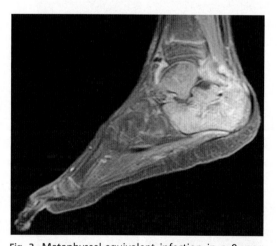

Fig. 3. Metaphyseal-equivalent infection in a 9-year-old boy with ankle pain and fever. Sagittal T1 fat-saturated postcontrast image of the ankle demonstrates extensive enhancement of the calcaneus and, to a lesser extent, the talus, with adjacent synovitis and retrocalcaneal bursitis.

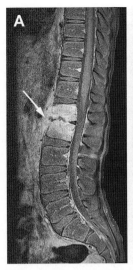
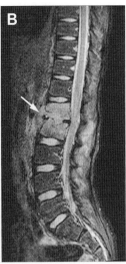

Fig. 4. Discitis and vertebral osteomyelitis in a 15-year-old boy with back pain and fever. Sagittal T1 fat-saturated postcontrast (A) and STIR (B) images of the thoracolumbar spine demonstrate abnormal signal and enhancement in L1-2 vertebral bodies with endplate irregularity, slight height loss, and intervertebral disc desiccation. Also note the extension of the inflammation/infection into the anterior prevertebral space (arrows).

should be obtained in all children with suspected discitis; if they demonstrate characteristic findings of discitis, the diagnosis is established.[27]

MR imaging is the imaging study of choice to evaluate children with clinically suspected vertebral osteomyelitis and normal results on plain radiography. Edema and purulent material in the marrow or disk space appear as a dark signal on T1-weighted images and bright signal on T2-weighted images with associated loss of vertebral or disc height. Contrast-enhanced MR imaging is generally performed for equivocal results or assessment of adjacent soft tissues. MR imaging is substantially more sensitive and specific than nuclear bone scan or routine roentgrams.[29] MR imaging is a rapid, accurate, and noninvasive method that can distinguish disk inflammation from pyogenic bone involvement. It also provides detail about the extent of soft tissue involvement, presence of epidural abscesses, and possible spinal cord involvement. *M tuberculosis* infection, although rare in North America, is notorious for sparing the disc initially with extensive associated abscess early in the course of disease that can track along muscle planes.[2]

Sickle Cell Disease

Patients who have sickle cell hemoglobinopathy are more susceptible to osteomyelitis than normal people, secondary to multiple factors, including functional asplenia, defective opsonins, and tissue infarction (**Fig. 5**).[4,30] There are some unique features of osteomyelitis in patients who have sickle cell disease, including involvement of diaphysis, multifocal and extensive areas of involvement, and worse prognosis. Debate exists about which are the most common causative organisms, *Staphylococcus* or *Salmonella* species.[4,30] Whatever the organism, the most important distinction to make is osteomyelitis versus vasocclusive crisis with bone infarction, with the latter being more common. Clinical presentation can be similar for both forms, with bone pain and fever being two common complaints. Infection is favored if the symptoms persists despite adequate medical management or there is sudden onset of unifocal bone pain.[4] Radionuclide scans, when used in a timely fashion, can assist in the diagnosis. Normal or increased radiotracer uptake at a suspicious site virtually excludes the possibility of infarction.[2] Radionuclide scans also can identify multifocal areas of involvement and evaluate the extent of disease. MR imaging reveals classic findings of osteomyelitis.

Septic Arthritis

Septic arthritis, frequently encountered in neonates, is generally seen in children younger

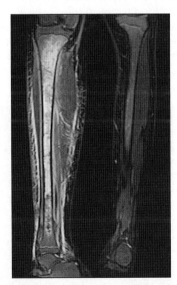

Fig. 5. Osteomyelitis in a 15-year-old girl who has sickle cell disease and presented with right leg pain and fever. Coronal STIR sequence demonstrates extensive signal abnormality almost throughout the entire length of the right tibia. Osteomyelitis in patients who have sickle cell disease often involves the diaphysis and tends to be more extensive than osteomyelitis in patients who do not have sickle cell disease.

than 3 years (**Fig. 6**).[4] The hip joint is the most commonly affected joint, followed by the shoulder, knee, elbow, and ankle. Commonly caused by *S aureus*, plain radiographic results initially may be negative with subsequent findings of joint space widening (effusion), periarticular osteopenia, and apparent joint dislocation.[31] US is sensitive in detecting joint effusion; however, it is difficult to differentiate infection from clear effusion based on the size and relative echogenicity of the joint fluid.[31] This determination can be crucial in differentiating other causes of joint effusion, including toxic synovitis, limiting the role of US in septic arthritis. US, however, is the imaging modality of choice for guiding aspirations. MR imaging is sensitive to small joint effusions.[4] Findings of joint effusion coupled with thick enhancement of the synovium on MR imaging can be seen in toxic synovitis and septic joint. Detection of adjacent bone marrow abnormalities on MR imaging helps differentiate septic arthritis (with possible osteomyelitis) from toxic synovitis.[4]

SOFT TISSUES INFECTION
Cellulitis

Characterized by diffuse inflammation of skin and underlying subcutaneous soft tissues, cellulitis is generally caused by gram-positive cocci.[4] Generally a clinical diagnosis, the role of MR imaging in investigating cellulitis is to evaluate cases that do not respond to therapy and evaluate for possible pyomyositis, soft tissue abscess, and osteomyelitis. On MR imaging, cellulitis appears as strands of low signal intensity on T1-weighted images and appears bright on T2-weighted images,

extending to varying degrees into muscles or fascial planes with associated mild diffuse enhancement without any associated rim-enhancing fluid collections or underlying bony or marrow abnormality.[1] If the cellulitis is extensive, however, abnormalities of marrow signal are not uncommon. Marrow edema and enhancement in the context of deep cellulitis may reflect either reactive marrow edema or true osteomyelitis. More specific signs that favor the diagnosis of osteomyelitis include focal bone destruction, periosteal reaction, and sequestra. Necrotizing fasciitis is a rare, fulminant, and rapidly progressive infection of the skin and underlying fascial planes. Imaging features may be indistinguishable from cellulitis.[4] Finding foci of gas, seen especially well on plain radiography or CT scan, may be the most helpful imaging clue for diagnosing necrotizing fasciitis.

Soft Tissue Abscess

Soft tissue abscesses appear as areas of low signal intensity on T1-weighted images and appear bright on T2-weighted images, with an enhancing rim of tissue of variable thickness and surrounding soft tissue edema.

Pyomyositis

Pyomyositis is defined as suppurative infection of the striated muscle, generally caused by muscle trauma with underlying degree of immunosuppression in the setting of bacteremia (**Fig. 7**).[32] In early stages, MR imaging reveals muscle enlargement and high signal on T2-weighted images, which makes it difficult to differentiate from myositis.

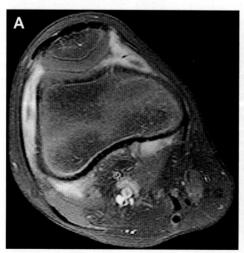
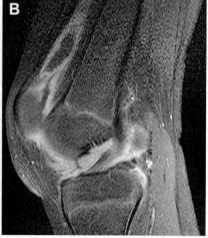

Fig. 6. Septic arthritis in a 7-year-old girl with knee pain. Axial (*A*) and sagittal (*B*) T1 fat-saturated postcontrast images of the knee demonstrate extensive synovial thickening and enhancement with an accompanying moderate joint effusion, which is characteristic of septic arthritis.

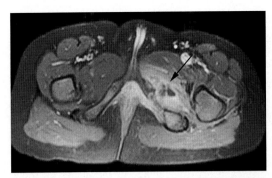

Fig. 7. Pyomyositis in a 7-year-old boy with left pelvic pain and fever. Axial T1 fat-saturated postcontrast image through the inferior ramus of the obturator ring demonstrates multiloculated, rim-enhancing fluid collections in the adductor muscles (*arrow*), which is characteristic of pyomyositis.

Subsequently, pyomyositis develops into a rim-enhancing abscess with central fluid/pus collection and variable amount of adjacent edema. MR imaging also can assess associated cellulitis, osteomyelitis, and septic arthritis if present.[4] Intramuscular hematoma and pyomyositis with abscess may have similar imaging features, and at times it may be difficult to differentiate the two. An important concept to keep in mind is that hematomas related to muscle tears generally occur at the weakest point, which is the myotendinous junction. If multicompartmental myositis is present and there is a strong clinical suspicion for infection, abscess should be favored over trauma.[17]

Musculoskeletal Inflammatory Conditions

Several pediatric musculoskeletal inflammatory disorders can affect the joint/synovium, tendons/bursa, muscles, and soft tissues. Most of these conditions are chronic and tend to evolve over time, with rheumatologic disorders constituting most of the conditions. After clinical assessment, imaging evaluation should begin with plain radiographs to exclude noninflammatory etiologies, including—but not limited to—trauma and tumor. Subsequently, additional imaging is usually performed to further characterize the disease process, help arrive at a definite diagnosis, and customize therapy.

Chronic Recurrent Multifocal Osteomyelitis

A rare inflammatory disorder of unknown origin, chronic recurrent multifocal osteomyelitis is noninfectious and clinically distinct from bacterial osteomyelitis (**Fig. 8**).[33] Seen primarily in the pediatric population, it has a strong female predominance.[34] Clinically, this entity usually presents with painful bony lesions at several sites in the

body, usually waxing and waning in severity over time. Tubular bones are most commonly affected, with the spine, clavicle, and pelvis less commonly affected. Multifocal disease is the norm, although in rare cases, a single site may be involved.[35]

Clinically there is pain, swelling, and erythema over the affected region, and skin lesions such as marked acne, psoriasis, and palmoplantar pustulosis may be present.[36] As a result, this entity may represent a variant of SAPHO syndrome (synovitis, acne, pustulosis, hyperostosis, and osteitis), a disease traditionally thought of as exclusively an adult entity, consisting of inflammatory bony lesions and skin eruptions. There is still a contentious issue as to whether it is a separate entity or two different points of the same continuum. Although often seen in association with other autoimmune disorders, serologic test results for rheumatoid factor, antinuclear antibodies, and HLA-B27 are usually negative. Histopathologic results, laboratory findings, and bacterial culture results are also usually negative or nonconclusive.[33,35,37] As a result, the diagnosis is one of exclusion after more common entities such as infection and tumor have been ruled out.

As a diagnosis of exclusion, the following criteria were recommended in a study by King and colleagues[38] before a diagnosis of chronic recurrent multifocal osteomyelitis should be made: (1) multifocal (two or more) bone lesions, clinically or radiographically diagnosed, (2) a prolonged course (> 6 months) characterized by varying activity of disease, with most patients being healthy between recurrent attacks of pain, swelling, and tenderness, (3) lack of response to antimicrobial therapy given for at least 1 month, (4) typical radiographic lytic regions surrounded by sclerosis with increased uptake on bone scan, and (5) lack of an identifiable organism. Jurik and Egund[35] subsequently added other criteria: (6) no abscess, fistula, or sequestra formation, (7) atypical site for classical bacterial osteomyelitis such as clavicles and multiple sites, (8) nonspecific histopathologic findings and laboratory results compatible with osteomyelitis, and (9) sometimes acne and palmoplantar pustulosis. Symmetry of the lesions also has been reported as a helpful feature.[36]

Imaging can play an important role in helping to establish the diagnosis, assess extent and the distribution of lesions, document response to treatment, and assess long-term follow-up. Lesions that affect the tubular bones have a characteristic appearance on plain radiographs, highlighting the importance of plain radiography in this entity.[33,35] Lesions appear as areas of lytic destruction adjacent to the growth plate, with

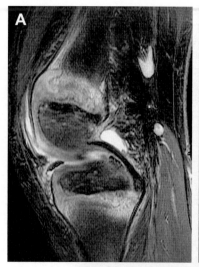
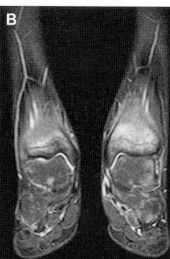
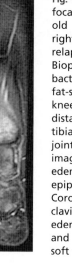
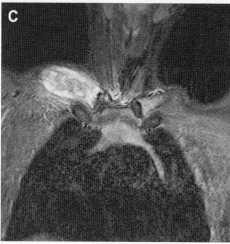

Fig. 8. Chronic recurrent multifocal osteomyelitis in a 9-year-old boy with ankle, knee, and right clavicular pain that relapsed over several months. Biopsy showed no evidence of bacterial infection. Sagittal T2 fat-saturated image of the knee (*A*) shows edema in the distal femoral and proximal tibial metaphysis with a small joint effusion. Coronal STIR image of the ankles (*B*) shows edema in the metaphysis and epiphysis of both distal tibias. Coronal STIR image of the right clavicle (*C*) shows extensive edema of the medial clavicle and surrounding periosteum/soft tissue.

a defined sclerotic rim demarcating it from normal bone. There is usually no associated periosteal reaction or soft tissue swelling, and a sequestrum is not a typical feature. MR imaging also can be a valuable tool, usually revealing more extensive bone marrow involvement than can be seen with conventional radiography.[35] Abscess and sinus tract formation commonly seen in chronic infectious osteomyelitis are not present in chronic recurrent multifocal osteomyelitis and can be easily excluded with MR imaging. MR imaging can be useful for follow-up after therapy and to guide biopsy. Bone scintigraphy can be helpful to identify nonsymptomatic sites, which are not uncommon, and stage to the full extent of this multifocal disease.

Lesions on MR imaging appear as eccentric areas of low T1 and bright STIR signal abnormality involving the metaphysis and extending to the growth plate. Other classic features of infection are not usually present. Epiphyseal involvement

is generally not seen, although signal abnormality can rarely spread to the diaphysis.[33,35] These lesions evolve in appearance and heal over time, with sclerosis and resolution of abnormal STIR signal. After multiple episodes, the end result can be a fairly well-defined area of metaphyseal sclerosis, which can be difficult to differentiate from subacute osteomyelitis or Brodie abscess.[39]

In some cases, spinal involvement may present with features similar to discitis or partial vertebral collapse. Again, MR imaging can help identify areas of disease activity and differentiate these lesions from bacterial osteomyelitis. The lytic phase demonstrates decreased signal intensity on T1-weighted images and increased signal intensity on T2-weighted images, with endplate erosion and either no disc involvement or partial disc involvement.[40,41] This eventually evolves into a more chronic, sclerotic phase, with decreased signal intensity on both T1- and T2-weighted images. The early lytic phase usually demonstrates avid enhancement, which usually resolves in the chronic sclerotic phase. Unlike with pyogenic osteomyelitis and discitis, there is typically no abscess formation or soft tissue involvement. Multifocal involvement of the spine usually skips vertebral bodies, with predominantly anterior vertebral involvement, and the pathology does not cross the intervertebral disc. Occasionally, there can be complete collapse of a vertebral body (ie, vertebra plana), making it difficult to differentiate this entity from Langerhans cell histiocytosis or other tumors.[36,40]

Imaging appearance of the clavicular lesion, although generally nonspecific, can be dramatic. The initial phase reveals a lytic medullary lesion within medial aspect of the clavicle with associated laminated periosteal reaction evident as homogenous low signal intensity on T1-weighted images with associated bony expansion and abnormal bright signal on STIR images. The abnormal signal on STIR sequence also extends and involves the surrounding soft tissues. There is associated contrast enhancement within the clavicle and surrounding tissue without any associated fluid collection or abscess formation. Based on imaging alone, the radiographic features are difficult to differentiate from chronic infection or malignancy. The lesion eventually heals after recurrent bouts of inflammation, leading to hyperostosis and a sclerotic clavicle.

Juvenile Idiopathic Arthritis

Juvenile idiopathic arthritis (JIA) is the most common chronic rheumatic disease of childhood (**Fig. 9**). Characterized by clinical manifestations systemically and in multiple organ systems, this disorder classically features chronic involvement of one or more joints, lasting at least 6 weeks in a patient younger than age 16. Most frequent in girls, the knee is the most commonly affected joint in the body.[42] The term JIA has replaced previously used terms such as "juvenile chronic arthritis" or "juvenile rheumatoid arthritis," to more accurately identify homogenous groups of children with distinct clinical features. The International League of Associations for Rheumatology currently identified seven subtypes of JIA in their most recent classification, with specific exclusion and inclusion criteria.[43]

Pathologically, there is typically an initial synovitis, which then progresses to synovial hyperplasia and formation of a highly cellular inflammatory pannus. This pannus eventually erodes into the overlying cartilage and bone, resulting in articular destruction and ankylosis. Because JIA is an important cause of short- and

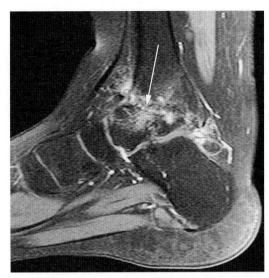

Fig. 9. Advanced JIA in a 15-year-old girl with a long history of polyarticular JIA. Sagittal T1 fat-saturated postcontrast image of the ankle demonstrates extensive destruction at the tibiotalar joint with synovitis (*arrow*).

long-term disability, timely diagnosis can facilitate treatment earlier in the course of this potentially debilitating disease, resulting in better clinical outcomes and less long-term disability.[42] In the active phase of the disease, articular synovitis generally can be adequately evaluated with clinical examination. Initial radiographs serve an important purpose, however, because they allow exclusion of other causes of pain and establish a radiographic baseline.[44] Unfortunately, radiographs cannot depict early synovial and cartilaginous involvement and generally do not show abnormal results until the disease reaches an advanced stage, with bony erosions, joint space narrowing, ankylosis, and growth disturbances. Numerous attempts have been made to develop radiographic scoring systems, none of which have been widely accepted.[44,45]

US and MR imaging have been used for early assessment of the disease process. Sonography can be effective in depicting the severity of the disease by allowing assessment of joint effusions, synovial thickening, cartilage destruction/thinning, and associated synovial cysts. Synovial proliferation appears as hypoechoic, irregular synovial membrane thickening and is easily distinguishable from joint fluid. Cartilaginous involvement is evident in the form of alteration of the normal smooth contour of the cartilage, with blurring and obliteration of the typically sharp margins. Activity of the disease can be assessed when the vascular pannus is demonstrated by power Doppler. Serial US is also useful in monitoring disease activity and following response to therapy, because there is typically a decrease in the thickness and vascularity of the synovium and a decrease in joint fluid.[46] Despite these advantages, US is still an operator-dependent modality, with only limited visualization of some joints. The acoustic window can be narrow, which precludes complete assessment of the entire joint. The efficacy of US can be limited further by the difficulty in positioning active children with swollen, painful joints.

Although US can be somewhat useful, MR imaging is the ideal modality to assess joint disease in cases of JIA. MR imaging is superior to US in depicting early inflammatory change and synovitis and evaluating cartilage. MR imaging accurately evaluates the late manifestations of the disease, including erosions, joint space loss, and ligamentous involvement.[44,46]

Synovial involvement

Acute synovitis is the initial presentation of the disease process. Abnormal synovium appears as a thickened, irregular, wavy layer of low T1 and high T2 signal abnormality. It can present difficulty in reliably differentiating thickened synovium from joint fluid on conventional spin echo images, because both have similar imaging features. Heavily T2-weighted images or the use of fast spin echo technique can highlight the difference between more hyperintense joint fluid and the relatively hypointense synovium, however. Intra-articular loose bodies are also easily evident on heavily T2-weighted images, which can be of clinical importance because it precludes the use of intra-articular steroids. Although some normal enhancement can be seen within the synovium, demonstration of abnormal contrast enhancement on fat-saturated, postgadolinium T1-weighted images unequivocally confirms the presence of synovitis, differentiating it from a simple joint effusion. Enhanced MR imaging not only establishes the diagnosis of synovitis but also helps distinguish active hypervascular synovium from fibrotic inactive synovium.[44–46] Although not routinely used in standard clinical practice, studies have demonstrated that the rate of contrast enhancement and dynamic contrast enhancement measurements of the synovium can be used to assess the degree of inflammatory response. Quantitative MR assessment of the synovial volumes can be obtained to determine response.[47,48]

Cartilage

MR imaging is the most sensitive modality to detect alterations in the articular cartilage. Fat-suppressed, T1-weighted three-dimensional gradient echo techniques can reliably assess cartilage loss with relatively high sensitivity and specificity. Normal cartilage is of high signal intensity against a background of low signal intensity, with focal defects appearing as low intensity areas. Subtle irregularities, cystic changes, and underlying desiccation can be visualized easily. Three-dimensional data can be further analyzed, with quantitative assessment of cartilage volume and thickness and contour mapping, which may be of potential value in assessing response to treatment and establishing long-term prognosis.[44] Newer gradient echo techniques for imaging pediatric hyaline, particularly articular cartilage, include the steady state sequences such as double echo steady state, refocused steady state free precession (SSFP, also known as FIESTA, Tru-FISP, and balanced fast field echo or BFFE), and WS-bSSFP. At our institution, we routinely use the double echo steady state sequence, which combines two gradient echoes, provides high T2 contrast, and depicts joint morphology well. New sequences that assess biochemical and biophysical changes within the cartilage are under development, perhaps allowing earlier diagnosis.[49]

Other changes

Soft tissue edema, an early feature of the disease, can be easily appreciated on STIR images. Marrow edema that reflects underlying osteitis, a marker of subsequent erosive changes, also can be demonstrated easily as high STIR signal abnormality in the marrow. Although CT and plain radiography classically have been used to assess for erosions, MR imaging has been shown to be sensitive for depicting erosions, evident as well-circumscribed low T1 and high T2 lesions with marked contrast enhancement.[44] MR imaging also allows assessment of tenosynovitis and enthesitis and may be of some value in subclinical tendon rupture.

Additional applications include assessment and screening of ischemic necrosis before and after intra-articular steroid injections and assessment of joint deformities and growth disturbances. Growth disturbances are a unique feature of pediatric JIA, generally resulting in premature fusion of the physis, growth stunting, and limb length discrepancies. The mandible is commonly affected in a significant number of these patients with growth disturbances. The use of dedicated coils with open and closed mouth dynamic assessment allows the depiction of abnormal joint motion, disc abnormality, and growth disturbances. Common findings include shortening of the body and ramus, flattening of the condyle, widening of the intercondylar joint, joint space loss, and concave abnormality of the undersurface of the mandibular body, known as antegonial notching.[44,46]

SERONEGATIVE SPONDYLOARTHROPATHIES

The juvenile seronegative spondyloarthropathies include four main entities that can be diagnosed before the age of 16: juvenile ankylosing spondylitis, juvenile psoriatic arthritis, inflammatory bowel disease–associated arthropathy, and Reiter's syndrome. These four disorders are generally grouped together because they share several common clinical and radiologic features and often can be difficult to distinguish one from another.[50] Classically, there is involvement of the spine (with sacroiliitis and spondylitis particularly common), large joints, and tendons. In addition to the musculoskeletal system, there can be involvement of the eyes, heart, lung, skin, and gastrointestinal tract. Despite the fact that the list of affected organ systems superficially resembles the adult form of these disease, symptoms such as inflammatory back pain and classic radiographic changes commonly seen in adults are rare in the childhood form of these diseases, especially before age 9.[51] Rather, monoarticular or asymmetric arthritis associated with enthesitis is the more common presentation in the pediatric population, which makes the diagnoses of these entities much more challenging.

JUVENILE ANKYLOSING SPONDYLITIS

Most commonly seen in male patients in late adolescence, this entity typically presents with early extra-axial involvement and a higher frequency of peripheral arthritis and enthesitis. The hips, knees, and shoulders are the most frequently involved, whereas there is relative sparing of the more peripheral joints.[50,52,53] Common radiographic findings include joint space narrowing and erosions, which, unlike the adult population, do not typically evolve into severe joint destruction. Enthesitis, a common element of seronegative arthropathies, can present as a bony erosion, lucency, or spur (particularly in the calcanei, the insertion of Achilles tendon, or the insertion of the plantar aponeurosis). Not uncommonly, periostitis can be present along the hand and, in certain cases, along other bones.

Radiographic abnormalities in the axial skeleton take much longer to appear than those in the peripheral skeleton, however, and radiographic demonstration of sacroiliac arthritis often is seen only after the clinical symptoms have progressed to an advanced stage. Bilateral asymmetric involvement is the most common pattern, although occasionally, unilateral involvement can mimic tuberculosis and subacute septic arthritis. Unlike juvenile rheumatoid arthritis, cervical spine involvement is rare. Syndesmophyte formation is rarely seen in children, and the "bamboo spine" seen in adults is typically not seen in the early phases of the disease. Sacroiliac arthritis is almost always seen well before any radiographic abnormality of the spine.[50,52,53]

PSORIASIS

Typically seen in female children around 11 to 12 years of age, pediatric psoriatic arthritis is rare compared with the adult form of the disease.[54] Unlike the adult form, musculoskeletal symptoms can precede the skin manifestations, often delaying diagnosis or leading to misdiagnosis. A family history of psoriasis is present in almost half of all cases and can be critical in making this diagnosis in a timely fashion.[50,54] Making this diagnosis even more difficult in children are radiographs that usually appear normal at presentation. Common radiographic features include soft tissue swelling, periarticular osteoporosis, joint space narrowing, erosions associated with enthesitis, and periostitis.[50] As in adults, the hands are involved more than the feet, typically with asymmetric distal interphalangeal joint involvement. Destructive disease is rare but possible in any joint, especially with hip involvement. Periostitis with associated radiotracer uptake on bone scan is another characteristic feature of juvenile psoriatic arthritis, as is tendon sheath involvement of a finger or a toe, leading to the classic "sausage digit pattern."[50,55]

With early clinical or radiologic findings often unhelpful, MR imaging can be of great diagnostic utility; once the diagnosis is made, MR imaging can help assess disease activity and extent and complications of the disease to plan appropriate therapy. Various studies have shown that synovial abnormality is the most common MR imaging finding in children with juvenile psoriatic arthropathy, which manifests as synovial thickening or enhancement or both. As opposed to adults, articular abnormality is much less commonly seen in children. Small joint effusions and multifocal bone marrow edema associated with enhancement at nonarticular sites are also possible findings on MR imaging in children with juvenile psoriatic arthropathy.[54,56]

ARTHRITIS ASSOCIATED WITH INFLAMMATORY BOWEL DISEASE

Arthritis is the most common manifestation of inflammatory bowel disease outside of the

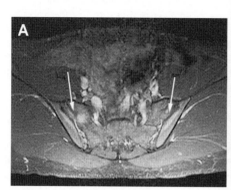
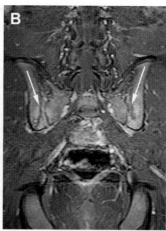

Fig. 10. Ulcerative colitis in a 16-year-old girl with ulcerative colitis and new back pain. Axial (*A*) and sagittal (*B*) images through the pelvis demonstrate bilateral enhancement around the sacroiliac joints (*arrows*), which indicates sacroiliitis.

gastrointestinal tract, more commonly seen with ulcerative colitis than with Crohn's disease. Joint manifestations of the two diseases, however, are indistinguishable (**Fig. 10**). Two different types of arthritis can occur: (1) a peripheral form with no preference for either sex and (2) a less common form seen predominantly in males that primarily affects the sacroiliac joints and spine and is virtually indistinguishable from ankylosing spondylitis.[50]

REITER'S SYNDROME

Reiter's syndrome is a reactive arthritis associated with a classic triad of symptoms (arthritis, conjunctivitis, and urethritis) that occurs either at the same time or sequentially. Although classically related to urogenital infection, the disease in children more often is the sequela of a gastrointestinal tract infection, such as Yersinia, Salmonella, or Shigella.[50] More commonly seen in male patients, this entity is rarely seen in the pediatric population. In rare instances in which a pediatric case is encountered, MR imaging can delineate the extent

of the process: the presence of synovitis, bursitis, and tenosynovitis, especially in the peroneal, anterior tibial, and posterior tibial tendons, and other associated findings, such as synovial cysts. Erosive arthritis and synovitis also may develop in the hands and wrists.[57]

IDIOPATHIC INFLAMMATORY MYOPATHIES

Idiopathic inflammatory myopathies are a heterogeneous group of disorders with autoimmune inflammatory process that affects muscle, skin, and internal systems to varying degrees (**Fig. 11**). Juvenile dermatomyositis is the most common of these entities in children.[58] Clinically manifesting as symmetric proximal muscle weakness, the basic pathologic process is the infiltration of various muscle groups by inflammatory cells. Along with clinical assessment, MR imaging is an excellent method to easily depict inflammation within various muscle groups. MR imaging is also useful in assessing the disease activity and identifying long-term sequela associated with it.

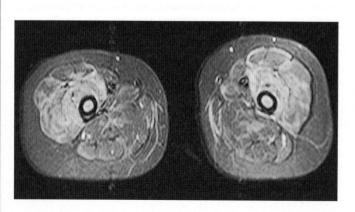

Fig. 11. Dermatomyositis in a 16-year-old girl with proximal muscle weakness. Axial T1 fat-saturated postcontrast image demonstrates bilateral, symmetric abnormal enhancement in the extensor muscles of the proximal anterior thigh and their surrounding fascia.

Although not specific, findings in the acute/active stages typically consist of increased signal intensity on T2 or STIR images within and around the muscles groups corresponding to inflammatory edema. This helps delineate involved muscles from normal muscles. Involvement is generally patchy, both within the muscle itself and between muscle groups and the extent of involvement differs in different patients.[58,59]

Other findings during the acute stage consist of perimuscular edema, enhanced chemical-shift artifact, and changes in the subcutaneous fat.[60] Various attempts have been made to assess disease activity on MR imaging. A study by Maillard and colleagues[59] showed that measuring MR imaging T2 relaxation time is a reliable measure of inflammation and disease activity within muscles in children with juvenile dermatomyositis. They concluded that a score of more than 86 ms indicates acute inflammation. MR imaging is also useful in following up these patients and assessing response to treatment because muscle edema detected by MR image improves with therapy, without concomitant change in histologic score. MR imaging can assess for fatty infiltration or fatty atrophy in these cases. Finally, MR imaging can help guide biopsy.

REFERENCES

1. Gylys-Morin VM. MR imaging of pediatric musculo-skeletal inflammatory and infectious disorders. Magn Reson Imaging Clin N Am 1998;6(3):537–59.

2. Schmit P, Glorion C. Osteomyelitis in infant and children. Eur Radiol 2004;14:L44–54.

3. Green NE, Edwards K. Bone and joint infection in children. Orthop Clin North Am 1987;18:555–75.

4. Kothari NA, Pelchovitz DJ, Meyer JS. Imaging of musculoskeletal infections. Radiol Clin North Am 2001;4:112–7.

5. Willis RB, Rozencwaig R. Pediatric osteomyelitis masquerading as skeletal neoplasia. Orthop Clin North Am 1996;27:625–34.

6. Jaramillo D, Treves ST, Kasser JR, et al. Osteomyelitis and septic arthritis in children: appropriate use of imaging to guide treatment. Am J Roentgenol 1995;165(2):399–403.

7. Asmar BI. Osteomyelitis in the neonate. Infect Dis Clin North Am 1992;6:117–32.

8. Morrisy RT. Bone and joint infections. In: Morrisy RT, editor. Pediatric orthopaedics. Philadelphia: JB Lippincott; 1990. p. 539–61.

9. Resnick D. Osteomyelitis, septic arthritis and soft tissue infections: organisms. In: Resnick D, editor. Bone and joint disorders. Philadelphia: WB Saunders; 2002. p. 2510–24.

10. Tachdjian MO. Orthopedics problems in childhood. In: Rudolph AM, Hoffman J, Axelrod S, editors. Pediatrics. 17th edition. Norfolk (CT): Appleton-Century-Crofts; 1982. p. 2421–56.

11. Boutin R, Brossmann J, Sartoris D, et al. Update on imaging of orthopedic infections. Orthop Clin North Am 1998;29:41–66.

12. Nelson JD. Acute osteomyelitis in children. Infect Dis Clin North Am 1990;4:513–22.

13. Tuscon CE, Hoffman EB, Mann MD. Isotope bone scanning for acute osteomyelitis and septic arthritis in children. J Bone Joint Surg 1994;76: 306–10.

14. Hopkins KL, Li KSP, Bergman G. Gadolinium-DTPA-enhanced magnetic resonance imaging of musculo-skeletal inefctious processes. Skeletal Radiol 1995; 24:325–30.

15. Morrison WB, Schweitzer ME, Bock GW, et al. Diagnosis of osteomyelitis: utility of fat-suppressed contrast-enhanced MR imaging. Radiology 1993; 189:251–7.

16. Erdman W, Tamburro F, Jayson H, et al. Osteomyelitis: characteristics and pitfalls of diagnosis with MR imaging. Radiology 1991;180:533–9.

17. Kan JH. Major pitfalls in musculoskeletal imaging: MR. Pediatr Radiol 2008;38(Suppl 2):S251–5.

18. Marin C, Sanchez-Alegre ML, Gallego C, et al. Magnetic resonance imaging of osteoarticular infections in children. Curr Probl Diagn Radiol 2004;33: 43–59.

19. Khoshhal K, Letts RM. Subacute osteomyelits (Brodie's abscess). Available at: www.emedicine.com/orthoped/topic27.htm. Accessed February 4, 2009.

20. Marti-Bonmati L, Aparisi F, Poyatos C, et al. Brodie abscess: MR imaging appearance in 10 patients. J Magn Reson Imaging 1993;3:543–6.

21. Grey AC, Davies AM, Mangham DC, et al. The "penumbra sign" on T1-weighted MR imaging in subacute osteomyelitis: frequency, cause and significance. Clin Radiol 1998;53(8):587–92.

22. Gledhill RB. Subacute osteomyelitis in children. Clin Orthop Relat Res 1973;96:57–69.

23. Roberts JM, Drummond DS, Breed AL, et al. Subacute hematogenous osteomyelitis in children: a retrospective study. J Pediatr Orthop 1982;2(3):249–54.

24. Rosenbaum DM, Blumhagen JD. Acute epiphyseal osteomyelitis in children. Radiology 1985;156:89–92.

25. Nixon GW. Hematogenous osteomyelitis of metaphyseal-equivalent locations. AJR Am J Roentgenol 1978;130:123–9.

26. Connolly SA, Connolly LP, Druback LA, et al. MRI for detection of abscess in acute osteomyelitis of the pelvis in children. AJR Am J Roentgenol 2007;189: 867–72.

27. Fernandez M, Carrol CL, Baker JC. Discitis and vertebral osteomyelitis in children: an 18-year review. Pediatrics 2000;105(6):1299–304.

28. Cushing AH. Diskitis in children. Clin Infect Dis 1993; 17:1–6.

29. Modic MT, Feiglin DH, Piraino DW. Vertebral osteomyelitis: assessment using MR. Radiology 1985; 157:157–66.

30. Epps C, Bryant D, Coles M, et al. Osteomyelitis in patients who have sickle cell disease. J Bone Joint Surg Am 1991;73:1281–94.

31. Blickman JG, van Die CE, de Rooy JWJ. Current imaging concepts in pediatric osteomyelitis. Eur Radiol 2004;14:L55–64.

32. Rodgers WB, Yodlowski ML, Mintzer CM. Pyomyositis in patients who have the human immunodeficiency virus. J Bone Joint Surg Am 1993;75:588–92.

33. Jurik AG. Chronic recurrent multifocal osteomyelitis. Semin Musculoskelet Radiol 2004;8(3):243–53.

34. Huber AM, Lam PY, Duffy CM, et al. Chronic recurrent multifocal osteomyelitis: clinical outcomes after more than five years of follow-up. J Pediatr 2002; 141(2):198–203.

35. Jurik AG, Egund N. MRI in chronic recurrent multifocal osteomyelitis. Skeletal Radiol 1997;26:230–8.

36. Anderson SE, Heini P, Sauvain MJ, et al. Imaging of chronic recurrent multifocal osteomyelitis of childhood first presenting with isolated primary spinal involvement. Skeletal Radiol 2003;32:328–36.

37. Jurriaans E, Singh NP, Finlay K, et al. Imaging of chronic recurrent multifocal osteomyelitis. Radiol Clin North Am 2001;39:305–27.

38. King SM, Laxer RM, Manson D, et al. Chronic recurrent multifocal osteomyelitis: a non-infectious inflammatory process. Pediatr Infect Dis 1987;6:907–11.

39. Jurik AG, Helmig O, Ternowitz T, et al. Chronic recurrent multifocal osteomyelitis: a follow-up study. J Pediatr Orthop 1988;8:49–58.

40. Yu L, Kasser JR, O'Rourke E, et al. Chronic recurrent osteomyelitis: association with vertebra plana. J Bone Joint Surg Am 1989;71:105–12.

41. Jurik AG, Møller BN. Chronic sclerosing osteomyelitis of the clavicle: a manifestation of chronic recurrent multifocal osteomyelitis. Arch Orthop Trauma Surg 1987;106:144–51.

42. Jordan A, McDonagh JE. Juvenile idiopathic arthritis: the paediatric perspective. Pediatr Radiol 2006;36(8):734–42.

43. Hashkes PJ, Laxer RM. Medical treatment of juvenile idiopathic arthritis. JAMA 2005;294(13):1671–84.

44. Johnson K. Imaging of juvenile idiopathic arthritis. Pediatr Radiol 2006;36:743–58.

45. Pettersson H, Rydolm U. Radiographic classification of knee joint destruction in juvenile chronic arthritis. Pediatr Radiol 1984;14:419–21.

46. Lamer S, Sebag GH. MRI and ultrasound in children with juvenile chronic arthritis. Eur J Radiol 2000;33: 85–93.

47. Ostergaard M, Ejbjerg B. Magnetic resonance imaging of the synovium in rheumatoid arthritis. Semin Musculoskelet Radiol 2004;8:287–99.

48. Workie DW, Dardzinski B, Graham TB, et al. Quantification of dynamic contrast enhanced MR-imaging of the knee in children with juvenile rheumatoid arthritis based on pharmacokinetic modelling. Magn Reson Imaging 2004;22:1201–10.

49. Mosher TJ, Dardzinski BJ. Cartilage MRI T2 relaxation time mapping: overview and applications. Semin Musculoskelet Radiol 2004;8:355–68.

50. Azouz EM, Levesque RY. Radiologic findings in children with seronegative spondyloarthropathies. Can Fam Physician 1992;38:1857–67.

51. Akin E. Juvenile spondyloarthropathies inflammation in disguise. Available at: http://www.gillettechildrens. org/default.cfm/PID=1.7.8.1. Accessed February 4, 2009.

52. Schaller J, Bitnum S, Wedgwood RJ. Ankylosing spondylitis with childhood onset. J Pediatr 1969; 74:505–16.

53. Ladd JR, Cassidy JT, Martel W. Juvenile ankylosing spondylitis. Arthritis Rheum 1971;14:579–90.

54. Lee EY, Sundel RP, Kim S, et al. MRI findings of juvenile psoriatic arthritis. Skeletal Radiol 2008;37: 987–96.

55. Petty RE, Malleson P. Spondyloarthropathies of childhood. Pediatr Clin North Am 1986;33:1079–96.

56. Offidani A, Cellini A, Valeri G, et al. Subclinical joint involvement in psoriasis: magnetic resonance imaging and X-ray findings. Acta Derm Venereol 1998;78:463–5.

57. Aribandi AK, Demuren OA. Reactive arthritis: musculoskeletal. Available at: http://emedicine.medscape. com/article/395020-overview. Accessed February 4, 2009.

58. Millard SM, Jones R, Owens C, et al. Quantitative assessment of MRI T2 relaxation time of thigh muscles in juvenile dermatomyositis. Rheumatology 2004;43:603–8.

59. Studynkova JT, Charvat F, Jarosova K, et al. The role of MRI in the assessment of polymyositis and dermatomyositis. Rheumatology 2007;46(7): 1174–9.

60. Hernandez RJ, Sullivan DB, Chenevert TL. MR imaging in children with dermatomyositis: musculoskeletal findings and correlation with clinical and laboratory findings. AJR Am J Roentgenol 1993; 161:359–66.

MR Imaging of PediatricTrauma

Thomas Ray S. Sanchez, MD[a],*, Siddharth P. Jadhav, MD[b],
Leonard E. Swischuk, MD[b]

KEYWORDS

- Musculoskeletal trauma • Occult fractures
- Stress fractures • Avulsion injury
- Osteochondritis dissecans

Trauma continues to be one of the most significant causes of mortality and lifelong morbidity in pediatric patients. Osseous trauma in particular can result in severe disabilities if not properly treated. Hence, it is important to diagnose and define injuries early on to treat and prevent further damage. In this regard, plain radiography has proved the most appropriate and cost-effective imaging modality for screening osseous injury. In the absence of any plain films findings, however, and to further characterize injury to radiolucent structures, such as developing cartilage and ligaments, MR imaging in the past several decades has emerged as an important adjunct and, in most cases, a primary tool in musculoskeletal imaging.

More than a decade ago, the term, *pediatric fracture without radiographic abnormality*, was used, because of the expanding use of MR imaging and increasing number of occult traumatic injuries identified.[1] Most of the children initially described had physeal fractures not seen on plain films. Several studies later demonstrated the unique ability and high sensitivity of MR imaging to define these types of injuries involving the immature skeleton.[2,3]

GROWTH PLATE INJURY

The epiphyses and the growth plate are the main contributors to bone growth. Injury to these structures can have lasting and devastating effects on the potential growth and can lead to limb shortening and deformity. The zone of provisional calcification is the transition between physeal cartilage and bone and is the weakest part of the epiphyseal unit. It is substantially weaker than the supporting ligaments and adjacent bone, hence bears the brunt of any trauma to this region.[2] The growing skeleton, especially during active pubertal growth, thus is more prone to injury. This observation led to the original classification of epiphyseal injuries by Salter and Harris, published in 1963, describing the plain film findings of physeal injuries with varying involvement of the metaphysis or epiphysis.[4] Since then, this classification has expanded but the original classification still serves as the basis for categorizing the severity of physeal injuries and their risk for subsequent growth complications. Most of the time, plain radiographs suffice in identifying a fracture and categorizing its type. Recent data, however, have confirmed that Salter-Harris fractures probably are underreported because a significant number of normal radiographs turned out to have physeal fractures after undergoing MR imaging and such identification led to a significant change in the clinical management of these patients.[3,5] In the authors' experience, a proton density image or T2-weighted fat-saturated sequence in coronal and sagittal views are important for evaluating for physeal widening and demonstrating any associated fracture line (**Figs. 1–3**). The adjacent marrow edema and bone contusion and the presence of joint fluid also are exquisitely demonstrated using short tau inversion recovery sequence (STIR) (**Fig. 4**).

[a] Division of Pediatric Radiology, Department of Radiology, University of California, Davis Medical Center and UC Davis Children's Hospital, 4860 Y Street, Suite 3100, Sacramento, CA 95817, USA
[b] Department of Radiology, University of Texas Medical Branch, 301 University Boulevard, Route 0709, Galveston, TX 77555, USA
* Corresponding author.
E-mail address: thomas.sanchez@ucdmc.ucdavis.edu (T.R.S. Sanchez).

Magn Reson Imaging Clin N Am 17 (2009) 439–450
doi:10.1016/j.mric.2009.03.007
1064-9689/09/$ – see front matter. Published by Elsevier Inc.

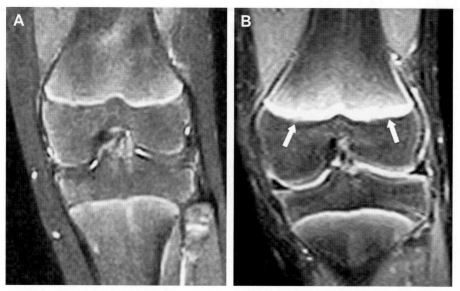

Fig. 1. Coronal STIR MR images of two different patients of compatible age. (*A*) Normal configuration and width of the physes of the distal femur and proximal tibia; (*B*) widening of the distal femoral physis (*arrows*) compatible with a nondisplaced Salter-Harris I fracture, which was not evident on the plain films. Note that even though it is the distal femoral physis that closes later and hence might appear wider in comparison to the tibial physis, the normal physeal high signal should not "bleed" into the metaphysis.

Growth arrest and angular deformity are the feared complications of physeal injuries and are secondary to the development of bone bridges. Most often they are posttraumatic and more commonly involve the distal ends of the femur and tibia.[6] It has been estimated that as many as 15% of physeal injuries lead to this complication.[7] MR imaging is valuable in evaluating the size and location of the bone bridge and helps guide clinicians in surgical planning. Bridges less than 50% of the physeal area carry a better prognosis after surgical resection.[8] The location of the bridge is

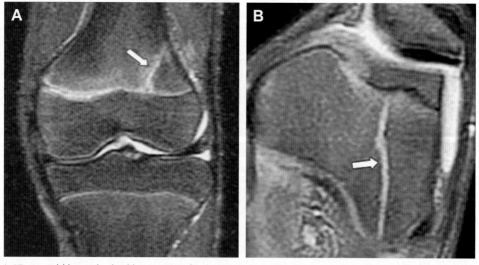

Fig. 2. A 15-year-old boy who had knee pain after sports injury with no evidence of fracture on plain films clearly demonstrates (*A*) the fracture line (*arrow*) through the lateral metaphysis with slight widening of the medial physis of the distal femur on the coronal STIR MR imaging sequence consistent with a Salter-Harris II fracture. (*B*) Fat-saturated T2-weighted axial image again shows the fluid-filled fracture line (*arrow*) through the metaphysis of the distal femur.

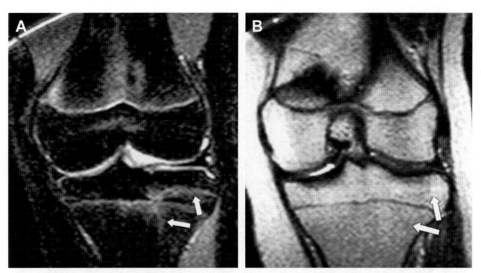

Fig. 3. A 15-year-old athlete who sustained a knee injury underwent a MR imaging scan after negative radiographs. (*A*) Coronal STIR shows a faint fracture line (*arrows*) through the epiphysis, physis, and metaphysis of the proximal tibia compatible with a nondisplaced Salter-Harris IV fracture. (*B*) The fracture line is so faint (*arrows*) that it is difficult to clearly identify it on the coronal proton density image. This highlights the importance of STIR sequences in making marrow edema more conspicuous, thus alerting to possible underlying fractures in subtle cases.

also a factor in predicting the ensuing complication. Central bridges cause growth stunting and eventual limb length discrepancy whereas peripherally located bridges cause partial tethering of bone development and result in angular deformity (**Fig. 5**).

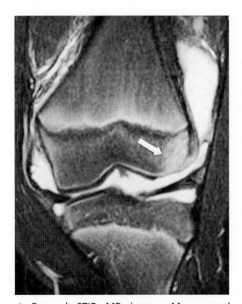

Fig. 4. Coronal STIR MR image. Marrow edema (*arrow*), joint fluid, and most soft tissue injuries are likewise very bright on STIR images, which often are used as a road map in the assessment of musculoskeletal trauma.

Slipped capital femoral epiphysis is a variant of Salter-Harris I fracture and as expected also occurs during the accelerated growth phase of adolescence. The underlying problem is attributed to chronic subclinical shearing stress to the epiphyseal-metaphyseal junction. It is classically more common in obese or heavyset boys and usually unilateral. However, 20% have synchronous or metachronous slippage within 2 years.[9] Plain radiography remains the mainstay of initial diagnosis and earliest findings include smoothness and sclerosis of the zone of provisional calcification and increased lucency and width of the growth plate. In the absence of subtle and early plain film findings, however, MR imaging potentially can diagnose preslip condition by demonstrating an increased physeal signal intensity or adjacent bone marrow edema, minimal joint effusion, and periarticular soft tissue edema (**Figs. 6** and **7**).[10] Contrast-enhanced MR imaging also has potential in evaluating vascularity of the femoral head and possible operative complications, such as avascular necrosis before and after surgery.[11]

OCCULT AND STRESS FRACTURES

Competitive sports coupled with the earlier age of rigorous training have produced a rise in pediatric musculoskeletal injuries. Youth participation in organized athletics is estimated at around 45 million in the United States alone.[12] Stress fracture is caused by chronic and repetitive microtrauma to

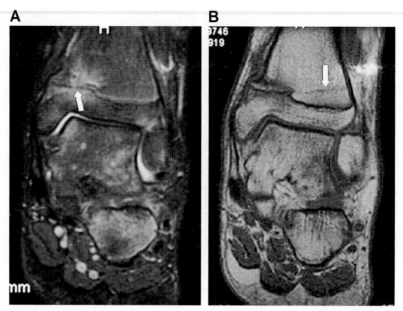

Fig. 5. A 13-year-old boy who had a previous Salter-Harris III fracture of the distal tibia. (*A*) Coronal STIR shows that a small bone bridge (*arrow*) has developed obliterating the low-signal physis of the medial portion of the distal tibia. (*B*) The growth recovery line (*arrow*) has migrated laterally but is tethered medially due to the absence of bone growth secondary to the bone bridge at this region. The bone bridge is small and less than 50% of the physis, and can be a candidate for surgical resection.

bone. It can be classified further as insufficiency fracture (application of normal stress to an abnormal bone) and fatigue fracture (excessive stress on normal bone). Most sports injuries in children are of the latter type. One study reported that as many as 20% of all sports medicine clinic injuries are secondary to stress fractures with runners and track and field athletes accounting

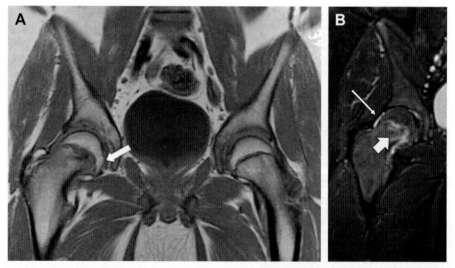

Fig. 6. A 13-year-old boy complained of 6 months of pelvic pain with previously normal radiographs, prompting the clinician to request a MR image, which showed (*A*) slipped capital femoral epiphysis on the right with medial and posterior tilting of the epiphysis (*arrow*) on the coronal T1-weighted image. (*B*) Coronal, T2-weighted, fat-saturated image demonstrates the high-signal marrow edema (*thick arrow*) in the proximal femoral metaphysis due to the buttressing of the slipped epiphysis. The minimal joint effusion (*thin arrow*) also is partially visualized on this image. Although the epiphysis has already slipped in this case, the presence of increased physeal signal, marrow edema, and joint fluid can potentially detect a preslip condition if the radiographs are negative.

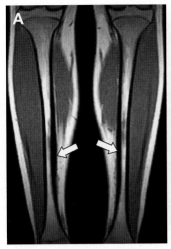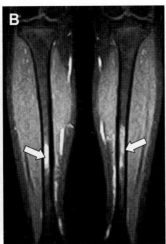

Fig. 7. An athletic 16-year-old male with persistent bilateral leg pain and negative radiographs. Non-contrast MR images of both legs were obtained. (*A*) Coronal T1-weighted MR images shows cortical thickening (*arrows*) with adjacent low signal in the marrow. (*B*) Coronal STIR MR image depicts the high signal marrow edema in both tibial mid-diaphyses. The clinical history, bilaterality and symmetry as well as the absence of aggressive periostitis and soft tissue component clearly indicates stress injury.

for the highest incidence of this type of injury. The tibia, metatarsals, and fibula were the most common sites of involvement.[13] Although radiographs can confidently diagnose the presence of stress fractures, its sensitivity can be as low as 15%, and even follow-up radiographs reveal helpful findings in only 50% of cases.[14] Also, at least 2 weeks or more are needed for follow-up radiographs to show changes of cortical thickening and sclerosis. Radionuclide scanning, alternatively, is sensitive but lacks the specificity to differentiate marrow changes of stress fractures from tumors and infection, which are known mimickers of stress injury. The importance of diagnosing stress fractures cannot be overly stated because it is critical in aiding clinicians institute necessary precautions to avoid further injury and prevent full-blown fractures. In this regard, recent studies have concluded that MR imaging is the single best technique in the prompt and early diagnosis of stress fractures with sensitivity, specificity, and negative predictive values all approaching 100%.[15,16] STIR and T2-weighted imaging with fat saturation are the best sequences for demonstrating the high-intensity signal of marrow edema surrounding the low-intensity fracture line (**Figs. 8–10**). Without the low-signal fracture line that is pathognomonic for a stress fracture, re-imaging after contrast administration with acquisition of fat-suppressed T1-weighted images might be helpful in differentiating marrow edema from tumor or infection.[8] Other MR imaging findings that point to stress injury include cortical abnormalities (such as striations and resorption cavities appearing as small high-signal foci within the uniformly dark cortex on T2-weighted sequences) and periosteal edema.[15] Clinical history greatly aids in confirming any suggestive findings on MR imaging.

AVULSION INJURIES

Although avulsion injuries occur in adult and pediatric populations, they are seen more commonly during puberty, when increasing muscular strength coupled with violent contraction creates greater stress to a developmentally weak and unfused apophysis.

Avulsion injuries often result before the ossification of the tendon and ligamentous attachments to bone. Although they can involve the ankle, foot, humerus, and elbow, they are more common particularly around the pelvis, femur, and knees (**Table 1**). Acute avulsion injuries can be diagnosed confidently using plain radiographs. Findings of fracture fragments, displacement of the

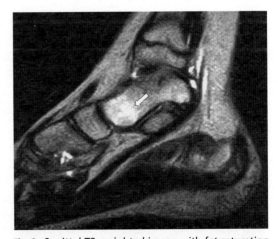

Fig. 8. Sagittal T2-weighted image with fat saturation in an 11-year-old boy who complained of foot pain, with normal radiographs showing the high-signal marrow edema in the anterior portion of the talus indicating a stress injury. A fracture line was not demonstrated.

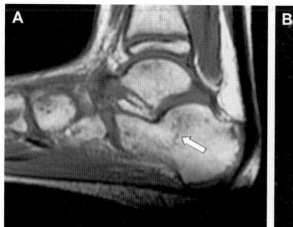
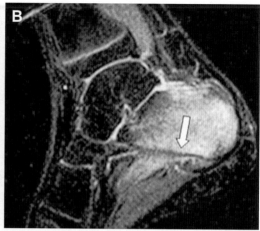

Fig. 9. Calcaneal stress fractures. (*A*) Sagittal proton density image through the calcaneus shows a faint fracture line with adjacent low-signal marrow edema. (*B*) In a different patient, the calcaneal marrow edema is more conspicuous on the STIR images, making the low-signal fracture line (*arrow*) stand out.

apophysis, and adjacent soft tissue swelling are straightforward and do not require additional imaging. In the absence of clear history of trauma and negative radiographs, however, the persistence of pain becomes a source of discomfort to patients and their parents. MR imaging then can be used in locating the cause of pain and extent of injury, whether or not it affects primarily the soft tissue or involves the osseous structures.

Familiarity with the musculotendinous anatomy and characteristic imaging features facilitates accurate recognition of avulsion injuries (see **Table 1**). Coronal and axial T2-weighted images,

including STIR sequence, demonstrate soft tissue and marrow edema and surrounding hematoma.[17] In the pelvis, the anterior superior iliac spine, anterior inferior iliac spine, and the ischial tuberosities are the most common sites of involvement (see **Fig. 10**). Osgood-Schlatter disease is a common injury in adolescents who are involved in activities that require jumping and running. Clinically, it manifests as pain below the patella with associated soft tissue swelling and tenderness (**Fig. 11**). Sinding-Larsen-Johansson disease (jumper's knee) is similar to Osgood-Schlatter disease but involves primarily the proximal

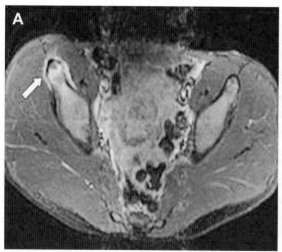
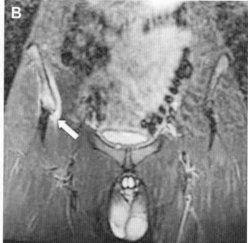

Fig. 10. A 16-year-old boy who complained of hip pain after kicking a soccer ball during play. (*A*) Axial, T2-weighted, fat-saturated sequence shows marrow edema and slight widening of the anterior inferior iliac spine apophysis (*arrow*) consistent with an avulsion injury. (*B*) The surrounding soft tissue edema (*arrow*) and marrow edema again are demonstrated on the coronal T2-weighted image.

Table 1
Common sites of avulsion injuries

Pelvis	Tendon/ligament
Anterior superior iliac spine	Sartorius/tensor fascia lata
Anterior inferior iliac spine	Rectus femoris
Ischial tuberosity	Hamstrings
Femur	
Greater trochanter	Gluteus medius and minimus
Lesser trochanter	Iliopsoas
Knee	
Inferior portion of patella	Patellar tendon (Sinding-Larsen disease)
Anterior tibial tuberosity	Patellar tendon (Osgood-Schlatter disease)

attachment of the patellar tendon, which can result in apophysitis and fragmentation of the distal pole of the patella (**Fig. 12**). Baseball elbow (medial epicondylitis) is another overuse injury caused by repetitive stress and excessive force applied to the growing skeleton (**Fig. 13**). Although the plain radiograph and MR imaging findings are often highly suggestive of acute avulsion injuries, subacute and healing injuries can be problematic and might mimic an aggressive bony lesion.[18] Biopsies are dangerous because any regions undergoing healing can have a high mitotic figure count and hence mimic a sarcoma, leading to unnecessary surgery.[19] Clinical correlation,

familiarity with characteristic location of avulsion injuries, comparison with previous radiographs, and follow-up plain film studies are helpful in these cases.

OSTEOCHONDRITIS DISSECANS

Osteochondritis dissecans (OCD) is a disease of the subchondral bone with involvement of the overlying articular cartilage, resulting in fragmentation and possibly intra-articular displacement of the bony or cartilaginous "loose body." The most plausible theory explaining the pathophysiology of OCD is mechanical-traumatic factors caused

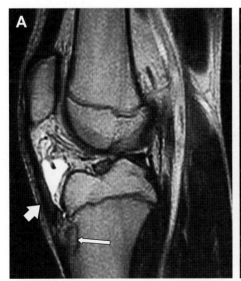 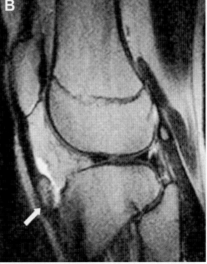

Fig. 11. Osgood-Schlatter disease. (*A*) Fragmentation of the anterior tibial tubercle (*long arrow*), thickened infrapatellar tendon with abnormal signal (*short arrow*), and edema/fluid in the Hoffa's fat pad on this sagittal, T2-weighted, FSE image indicate acute avulsion. (*B*) Sagittal T2-weighted image with fat saturation shows fragmentation of the anterior tibial tubercle (*arrow*) with minimal adjacent inflammation, more consistent with a chronic/healing avulsion injury.

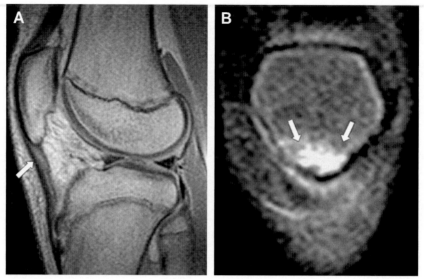

Fig. 12. Sinding-Larsen-Johansson disease (jumper's knee). (*A*) Sagittal proton density image shows a thickened patellar tendon with high signal at its proximal attachment. (*B*) The coronal STIR MR image clearly shows the high-signal marrow edema involving the inferior pole of the patella.

by repetitive microtraumas or overuse related to increased athletic activity.[20] Although relatively rare, OCD is considered an important cause of joint pain in active adolescents.[21] If not recognized early and treated accordingly, it can lead to disabling degenerative arthritis. Most OCD lesions affect the weight-bearing cartilage and frequently involve the medial femoral condyle, talar dome, and capitelum. Plain radiographs generally

establish the diagnosis of OCD and often can show if there is a displaced osseous fragment within the joint. They are unreliable, however, in evaluating the stability of the lesion. It is important for clinicians to fully evaluate the stability of the fragment to help guide patient management and possible surgical intervention. MR imaging findings that indicate OCD instability include (1) linear high signal between the fragment and parent

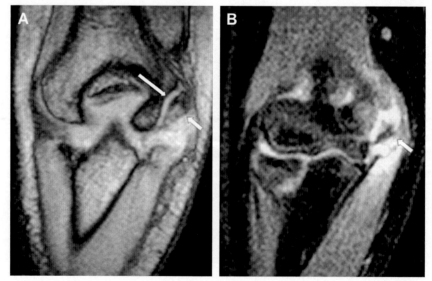

Fig. 13. A 10-year-old boy who had arm pain. (*A*) Coronal proton-density MR image shows widening of the physis (*long arrow*) with avulsion of the medial epicondyle (*short arrow*). (*B*) Coronal STIR image anterior to the MR image (*A*) shows the surrounding soft tissue edema and bone contusion and the completely torn flexor-pronator conjoined tendon (*arrow*).

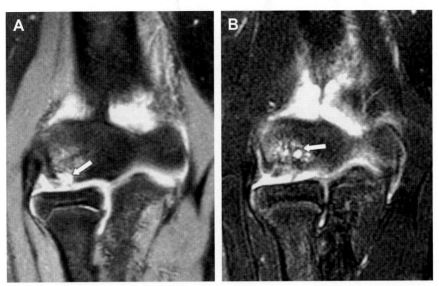

Fig. 14. MR imaging findings in unstable OCD in a 16-year-old boy. (*A*) Coronal T2-weighted image of the elbow with fat saturation shows a focal 8-mm fluid filled osteocartilaginous defect in the capitelum. (*B*) Coronal STIR of the same patient but imaged slightly more posteriorly demonstrates several cystic foci deep to the osteocartilagenous fragment with the largest measuring 6 mm.

bone, indicating synovial fluid surrounding the fragment; (2) 5-mm or larger cystic foci behind the fragment (3); high-signal linear focus in the overlying cartilage; and (4) focal fluid-filled cartilage defect larger than 5 mm.[22] These findings are better evaluated using STIR or T2-weighted fast spin-echo (FSE) sequences with fat saturation (**Figs. 14–16**). Recent data, however, indicate that the mere presence of high-signal line behind the fragment is not a definite sign of instability and

that it also may represent vascular granulation tissue of healing OCD.[23] Hence, a combination of two or more of the MR imaging findings (described previously) likely will improve specificity.

TRANSIENT PATELLAR DISLOCATION

Traumatic patellar dislocations are common injuries in children and most of the time are difficult to evaluate or even suspect on plain film. Often,

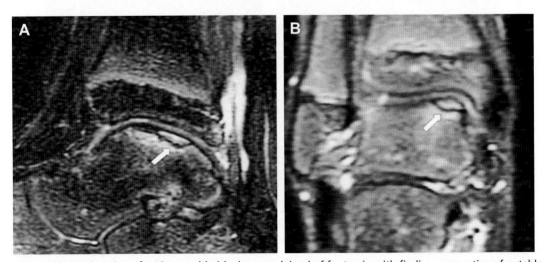

Fig. 15. Ankle MR imaging of a 10-year-old girl who complained of foot pain with findings suggestive of a stable osteochondritis dissecans. (*A*) Sagittal STIR MR image shows a well-defined osteocartilagenous fragment in the talar dome with a low-intensity fracture line (*arrow*) and no significant surrounding marrow edema or high signal adjacent to the fragment. (*B*) Coronal T2-weighted image of the talus again shows the well-defined and nondisplaced talar dome fragment (*arrow*).

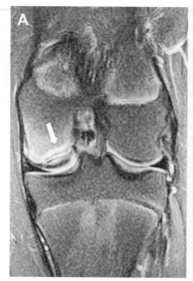
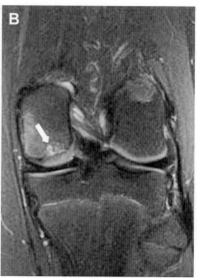

Fig. 16. A 16-year-old boy who had known case of bilateral OCD of the knee underwent MR imaging examination to evaluate for stability. Coronal proton-density MR image with fat saturation of the same patient shows (A) a linear high signal subjacent to the osteocartilagenous fragment of the medial femoral condyle (arrow) and (B) several adjacent 4- to 5-mm cysts (arrow), all of which indicate fragment instability.

the only finding on plain film is the presence of suprapatellar joint effusion. This is because most cases of patellar dislocations are transient and by the time patients are imaged, the patella is back in its normal position. Internal derangement usually is suspected because of the persistence of the pain, and invariably MR imaging is obtained. MR imaging can detect transient dislocation by the identification of the following: (1) bone contusion involving the inferomedial aspect of the patella and anterolateral aspect of the lateral femoral condyle as they collide when the patella

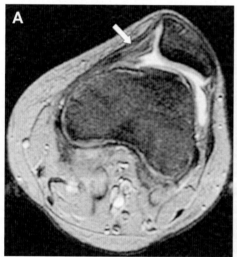
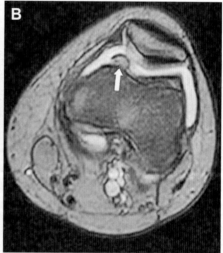

Fig. 17. (A) A 13-year-old girl who had "knee injury" with plain radiographs showing only a small suprapatellar joint effusion. Axial gradient MR image shows thickening and irregularity of the medial patellar retinaculum with abnormal signal within (arrow) indicating a grade 2 strain/partial tear. The patellar notch is shallow/dysplastic but there is no frank dislocation/subluxation although the patella is tilted laterally. These telltale signs point to a transient patellar dislocation. (B) A 16-year-old boy who had persistent knee pain and again showed only minimal suprapatellar joint fluid on plain radiographs. The axial gradient MR image shows a well-defined cartilage fragment displaced within the joint space (arrow) with the donor site in the medial portion of the patellar cartilage.

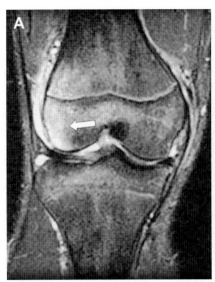
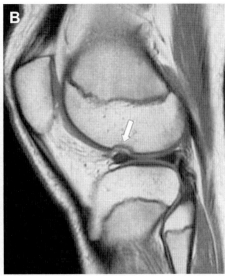

Fig. 18. Lateral femoral condyle injuries in patellar dislocation. (*A*) A male 18-year-old who had unremarkable knee radiographs after a sports injury showed bone contusion involving the epiphysis and metaphysis of the lateral femoral condyle in this coronal STIR MR image. There also is minimal joint effusion and grade 1 strain of the medial collateral ligament. (*B*) Sagittal proton density image in a 13-year-old girl who had patellar dislocation shows an osteochondral defect in the anterior portion of the lateral femoral condyle. Both injuries are the result of the patella's impact on the femoral condyle as it relocates.

relocates; (2) osteochondral defect or cartilage damage involving the same sites of bone contusion; (3) strain, partial tear, or complete disruption of the medial patellar retinaculum; (4) patellar tilting or subluxation with associated dysplasia or shallow trochlear notch; and (5) other findings, such as joint effusion and Hoffa's fat pad edema (**Figs. 17** and **18**).[24] Radiologists should be aware of the subtle combinations of these findings and convey to clinicians the possibility of transient patellar dislocation.

SOFT TISSUE INJURIES

Common tendon, ligamentous, and meniscal injuries seen in the adult population have basically the same imaging characteristics seen in children. A brief overview of muscular and musculotendinous trauma, however, is beneficial in evaluating these frequent injuries, which occur in isolation or in conjunction with other bone abnormalities. In terms of soft tissue injuries, muscle strain/tears are significantly more common that ligamentous tears in the pediatric population. Muscle strains or

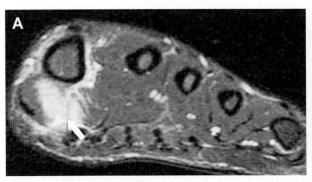
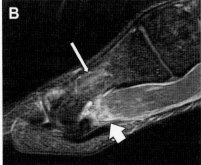

Fig. 19. A 17-year-old boy who had hyperextension injury to the great toe. (*A*) Axial proton density MR image with fat saturation shows high-signal edema and hematoma surrounding the flexor hallucis brevis muscle near its insertion at the base of the proximal phalanx (*arrow*). This is just a partial tear/grade 2 strain because more than half of the muscle fibers are still intact. (*B*) Sagittal STIR images again shows the high signal near the muscle insertion (*short arrow*). In addition, marrow edema is evident in the distal portion of the first metatarsal (*long arrow*).

tears can be partial or complete and are the result of sudden contraction or stretching of the muscle fibers. A grade 1 strain is a partial tear involving a few muscle fibers without loss of function; a grade 2 strain involves larger partial tears with some loss of muscle strength whereas a grade 3 sprain indicates complete rupture of the muscle with near total loss of function. MR imaging findings include increased interstitial signal (edema) for grade 1, thinning/thickening of the muscle tendon with surrounding hematoma and muscle laxity for grade 2, and signal gap/complete disruption or tendon-muscle discontinuity for grade 3 (**Fig. 19**).[25]

SUMMARY

Musculoskeletal injuries remain an important cause of morbidity in the pediatric population. Although plain radiography is still the primary imaging tool, MR imaging has evolved into an essential adjunct diagnostic tool for the prompt identification of occult musculoskeletal injuries. Growth plate injuries and their complications, osteochondritis dissecans, avulsion, stress fractures, and soft tissue injuries can be diagnosed early and confidently with MR imaging when other imaging modalities are equivocal. MR imaging, therefore, offers invaluable aid in clinical decisions regarding the timely institution of necessary management to help alleviate symptoms, promote healing, and, more importantly, prevent further complications, such as fractures, degenerative changes, malunion, and growth arrest.

REFERENCES

1. Naranja RJ, Gregg JR, Dromans JP, et al. Pediatric fracture without radiographic abnormality. Description and significance. Clin Orthop Relat Res 1997; 342:141–6.
2. Rogers LF, Poznanski AK. Imaging of the epiphyseal injuries. Radiology 1994;191:297–308.
3. Close BJ, Strouse PJ. MR of physeal fractures of the adolescent knee. Pediatr Radiol 2000;30:756–62.
4. Salter R, Harris W. Injuries involving the epiphyseal plate. J Bone Joint Surg Am 1963;45:587–622.
5. Smith BG, Rand F, Jaramillo D. Early MR imaging of lower extremity physeal fracture-separation: a preliminary report. J Pediatr Orthop 1994;14:526–33.
6. Ecklund K, Jaramillo D. Patterns of premature physeal arrest: MR experience in 111 children. AJR Am J Roentgenol 2002;178:967–72.
7. Peterson HA. Physeal and apophyseal injuries. Fractures in children. 3rd edition. Pennsylvania: Lippincott-Raven; 1996. p. 103–65.

8. Ecklund K. Magnetic resonance imaging of pediatraic musculoskeletal trauma. Top Magn Reson Imaging 2002;13(4):203–17.
9. Swischuk L. Imaging of the newborn, infant and young child. 5th edition. PA: Lippincott-Williams and Wilkins; 2004. p. 803–6.
10. Tins B, Cassar-Pulliciano V, McCall I. The role of pretreatment MRI in established cases of slipped capital femoral epiphysis. Eur J Radiol, in press.
11. Staatz G, Honnef D, Kochs A, et al. Evaluation of femoral head vascularization in slipped capital femoral epiphysis before and after cannulated screw fixation with use of contrast-enhanced MRI: initial results. Eur Radiol 2007;17(1):163–8.
12. Veigel JD, Pleacher MD. Injury prevention in youth sports. Curr Sports Med Rep 2008;7(6):348–52.
13. Fredericson M, Jennings F, Beaulieu C, et al. Stress fractures in athletes. Top Magn Reson Imaging 2006;17(5):309–25.
14. Anderson MW, Greenspan A. Stress fractures. Radiology 1996;199:1–12.
15. Gaeta M, Minutoli F, Scribano E, et al. CT and MR imaging findings in athletes with early tibial stress injuries: comparison with bone scintigraphy findings and emphasis on cortical abnormalities. Radiology 2005;235(2):553–61.
16. Kiuru MJ, Pihlajamaki HK, Hietanen HJ, et al. MR imaging, bone scintigraphy and radiography in bone stress injuries of the pelvis and lower extremity. Acta Radiol 2002;43(2):207–12.
17. Stevens MA, El-Khoury GY, Kathol MH, et al. Imaging features of avulsion injuries. Radiographics 1999;19(3):655–72.
18. Sanders TG, Zlatkin MB. Avulsion injuries of the pelvis. Semin Musculoskelet Radiol 2008;12(1):42–53.
19. Helms C. Fundamentals of skeletal radiology. 3rd edition. PA: Elsevier Saunders; 2005. p. 55.
20. Bohndorf K. Osteochondritis (osteochondrosis) dissecans: a review and new MRI classification. Eur Radiol 1998;8:103–12.
21. Obedian RS, Grelsamer RP. Osteochondritis dissecans of the distal femur and patella. Clin J Sport Med 1997;16(1):157–74.
22. De Smet AA, Fisher DR, Graf BK, et al. Osteochondritis dissecans of the knee: value of MR imaging in determining lesion stability and the presence of articular cartilage defects. AJR Am J Roentgenol 1990;155:549–53.
23. O'Connor MA, Palaniappan M, Khan N, et al. Osteochondritis dissecans of the knee in children. A comparison of MRI and arthroscopic findings. J Bone Joint Surg Br 2002;84(2):258–62.
24. Zaidi A, Babyn P, Astori I, et al. MRI of traumatic patellar dislocation in children. Pediatr Radiol 2006;36:1163–70.
25. Kaplan P, Helms C, Dussault R, et al. Musculoskeletal MRI. Pennsylvania: Saunders; 2001. p. 65–70.

MR Imaging of Pediatric Arthritis

Heike E. Daldrup-Link, MD*, Lynne Steinbach, MD

KEYWORDS

- Arthritis • MR imaging • Juvenile idiopathic arthritis
- Juvenile rheumatoid arthritis • Pediatric arthropathy

The role of MR imaging in pediatric arthritis is to detect early manifestations of arthritis, evaluate the extent of disease, and monitor disease activity during treatment. More specifically, MR imaging can characterize the pediatric arthropathy based on typical imaging findings, detect early signs of synovitis and erosions, stage the severity of joint involvement, demonstrate associated internal derangement, monitor disease progression or treatment response, and evaluate for complications. This article discusses MR imaging findings of juvenile idiopathic arthritis (JIA), enthesis-related arthritis, and juvenile psoriatic arthritis, and articular findings in collagen vascular diseases, septic arthritic, hemophilia, neuroarthropathy, and pseudoarthritides.

JUVENILE IDIOPATHIC ARTHRITIS: DEFINITION AND CLASSIFICATION

Juvenile idiopathic arthritis (JIA) encompasses a heterogenous group of arthropathies of childhood with an onset at less than 16 years of age and duration of symptoms for more than 6 weeks. JIA has been defined by the International League for Rheumatology and integrates criteria for juvenile rheumatoid arthritis, as defined by the American College of Radiology, and criteria for juvenile chronic arthritis, as defined by the European League of Associations for Rheumatology.[1] JIA has a prevalence of 57 to 113 per 100,000 children under 16 years of age, with currently about 30,000 to 50,000 affected patients in the United States.[1–3]

Different patterns of JIA include a classic systemic disease with little or no radiographic articular abnormalities, a polyarticular disease with less severe systemic manifestations, and an oligoarticular or monoarticular disease with infrequent systemic manifestations. Systemic JIA, also known as Still disease, involves about 10% of patients. The International League for Rheumatology classification of JIA is based on disease distribution and clinical criteria (**Table 1**).

The main clinical presentation of JIA is joint pain and swelling, most commonly affecting the knee, ankle, wrist, and small joints of the hands and feet. Radiographs may show periarticular soft tissue swelling with osteopenia, periostitis, and overgrown epiphyses, which may be prematurely fused. Joint involvement is bilateral if polyarticular and sporadic if oligoarticular or monoarticular. Other associated symptoms may include a symptomatic or asymptomatic chronic anterior uveitis and overall growth retardation. Affected joints may show a paradoxic overgrowth because of hyperemia of the growth plates. Late effects of JIA include joint space narrowing and erosions and joint contractures. Joints may become ankylosed, unlike adult rheumatoid arthritis.

INDICATION AND TECHNIQUES FOR MR IMAGING

MR imaging of large joints is indicated in children with persistent pain or swelling, or instability of knee, hip, or shoulder joints not associated with an injury and not responding to at least 3 weeks of conservative therapy. MR imaging of small joints is reserved for special cases. MR imaging should not replace, bypass, or precede clinical evaluation, radiographs, and ultrasound as primary diagnostic tools.

Department of Radiology and Biomedical Imaging, University of California, San Francisco, 512 Parnassus Avenue, San Francisco, CA 94143–0628, USA
* Corresponding author.
E-mail address: daldrup@radiology.ucsf.edzu (H.E. Daldrup-Link).

Magn Reson Imaging Clin N Am 17 (2009) 451–467
doi:10.1016/j.mric.2009.03.002

Table 1
Classification of juvenile idiopathic arthritis as defined by the International League for Rheumatology

Arthropathy	Distribution	Hand	Feet	Knees	Elbow	Shoulder	Hips	ISJ
Systemic arthritis	Symmetric	+++	+++	+++	++	+	++	+
Oligoarthritis, persistent and extended	Asymmetric or symmetric	++	++	+++				
Polyarthritis, RF positive	Symmetric	+++	+++	+++	++	+	++	+
Polyarthritis, RF negative	Symmetric	+++	+++	+++	++	+	++	+
Enthesitis-related arthritis	Asymmetric		+++	+++		++		+++
Psoriatic arthritis	Asymmetric	+++	+++	+++			++	++
Other								

Abbreviations: ISJ, iliosacral joints; RF, rheumatoid factor.

The role of MR imaging is to detect early manifestations of arthritis, differentiate JIA from other pathologies in case of equivocal clinical or conventional imaging studies, evaluate the extent of disease, and monitor disease activity during treatment. More specifically, MR imaging can characterize the arthropathy based on typical imaging findings, detect early signs of synovitis and erosions, stage the severity of joint involvement, demonstrate associated internal derangement, monitor disease progression or treatment response, and evaluate for complications.

The MR imaging technique and the choice of appropriate coils depend on the age and size of the child, the anatomic region of interest, and the clinical question. Practice guidelines from the American College of Radiology for the performance and interpretation of MR imaging studies in children can be found online: http://www.acr.org/Secondary MainMenuCategories/quality_safety/guidelines/dx/ mri_pediatric.aspx.

A variety of pulse sequences are available for assessment of different joint components. Short TI (inversion time) inversion recovery (STIR) or fat-saturated T2-weighted sequences can be used to detect pathology. Spoiled three-dimensional gradient echo sequences with fat saturation and fat-saturated proton density weighted spin echo sequences can help to evaluate for cartilage defects. T1-weighted images in the early phase (<5 minutes), after intravenous injection of gadolinium (Gd) chelates, can distinguish synovitis and effusion. Fat-saturated sequences after contrast medium administration are essential to differentiate contrast enhancement from fatty converted bone marrow and periarticular fat.

Several dedicated techniques are available for evaluation of articular cartilage. Standard sequences include proton density weighted fast spin echo, spoiled gradient echo, and dual echo steady-state sequences. T1-weighted sequences in the delayed phase after intravenous injection of Gd-based contrast agent can provide an indirect arthrogram, delineating ligamentous and cartilage injuries and areas of decreased glycosaminoglycan concentration, which represent early stages of cartilage defects. Cartilage mapping techniques and quantitative image processing techniques with three-dimensional reconstruction allow volumetric quantification of the entire cartilage or synovium.

Direct MR arthrography after intra-articular injection of dilute Gd-based contrast agent (typically 1:150-fold to 200-fold diluted [eg, stock solution of 0.3 mL of 0.1-M Gd-DTPA diluted in 50 mL NaCl]) can also delineate cartilage defects and fibrocartilage tears and detect tendon or ligament defects.

Time and expense are the main limiting factors for using MR imaging for the diagnosis and treatment monitoring of JIA. The use of sedation in younger children is also a limitation for those cases that are not absolutely indicated. In addition, MR imaging is limited to the evaluation of one or two target joints. New whole-body imaging techniques can be used to get an overview over the distribution of systemic JIA in special, clinically equivocal cases. Surface coils are needed to provide a detailed analysis of specific joint structures, however, thereby limiting a comprehensive MR imaging evaluation of polyarticular or systemic manifestations. Of note, MR imaging is not sensitive for the diagnosis of osteopenia or osteoporosis in JIA patients. Finally, surface coils limit functional assessments of joint motion. For example, MR imaging has a limited sensitivity for the detection of atlantoaxial subluxation in patients with JIA because these are often only apparent with neck flexion. These limitations have to be recognized when evaluating static MR imaging studies of one target joint in patients with polyarticular or systemic JIA.

GENERAL MR IMAGING FEATURES OF ARTHRITIS

When evaluating the joints for arthritis on MR images, it is helpful to use the "ABCDS": *Alignment*, *Bone* integrity, *Cartilage*-joint space, *Distribution*, and *Soft* tissue changes.

Alignment

JIA may be associated with joint subluxation or dislocation. Deviation of joints may be seen with JIA; collagen vascular disease; and Jaccoud's arthropathy (ulnar deviation of metacarpophalageal joints in patients with recurrent rheumatic fever or systemic lupus erythematosus).

Bone Integrity

One should look for erosions, new bone production, and subchondral cysts. Erosions are marginal and aggressive in patients with JIA and may be associated with new bone production. These manifest as whiskering, excrescences, periosteal reaction, and osseous ankylosis. Although osseous ankylosis now is rare in patients with JIA, it can still be seen in the large joints, wrists, and feet of patients with JIA and in the wrists of patients with hemophilia. In children and adolescents, subchondral cysts may be seen in JIA and hemophilia, pigmented villonodular synovitis, synovial chondromatosis, and trauma.

Cartilage and Joint Space

Uniform narrowing is present in joints affected by JIA. Hemophilia can have a variable appearance with uniform or nonuniform narrowing.

Distribution

The location of inflammatory joint disease can help to narrow down the differential. The radiocarpal joint is affected by JIA and hemophilia. The interphalangeal joints may be affected by JIA, psoriatic arthropathy, and multicentric reticulohistiocytosis. JIA can affect the distal interphalageal joints, which is rarely seen in adult rheumatoid arthritis.

Soft Tissue Changes

Using the joint as an epicenter, it is important to look for soft tissue swelling. If the swelling is fusiform with the joint at the epicenter, one would consider JIA. A diffuse swelling (sausage digit) is seen in rheumatoid variants, such as psoriatic arthritis. In children and adolescents, the lumpy bumpy asymmetric swelling is noted with sarcoid, amyloid, multicentric reticulohistiocytosis, and giant cell tumor of the tendon sheath.

MR IMAGING ASSESSMENT OF JUVENILE IDIOPATHIC ARTHRITIS

JIA excludes juvenile-onset spondyloarthropathies and psoriatic arthropathy.[1] It can present as an oligoarthritis, polyarthritis, or systemic arthritis. Clinical features of these three manifestations are shown in **Table 2**.

An oligoarthritis affects less than five joints. A polyarthritis is defined by involvement of five or more joints during the first 6 months of disease. Systemic arthritis (Still disease) is defined as arthritis, fever, and systemic manifestations. Initially, the patient may present with a rash, hepatosplenomegaly, lymphadenopathy, or serositis.

Table 2
Clinical characteristics of juvenile rheumatoid arthritis

	Oligoarthritis	Polyarthritis	Systemic Arthritis
Number of affected joints	<4	≥5	Variable
% Frequency	60	30	10
Male/female ratio	5:1	3:1	1:1
% Chronic uveitis	5%–15%	5%	Rare
% RF/ANA	Rare/80	10/50	Rare/10
Prognosis	Excellent	Moderate to good	Moderate to poor

Abbreviations: ANA, antinuclear antibody; RF, rheumatoid factor.
Data from Cassidy JT, Petty RE. Textbook of pediatric rheumatology. 5th edition. Philadelphia: WB Saunders; 2005.

A progressive polyarthritis develops over 2 to 3 years as systemic features slowly regress. Important complications of systemic arthritis include severe joint damage, growth delay, osteoporosis, macrophage activation syndrome, and amyloidosis. In general, MR imaging can help to detect various components of arthropathy. These include joint effusion, hemosiderin deposition, synovial inflammation and proliferation, cartilage and bone erosions, loose bodies, subtle osteophytes, subchondral cysts, reactive marrow changes, tenosynovitis, ligament and tendon tears, and soft tissue inflammation and masses. Visualizing these findings can aid in characterization and more specific diagnosis of an arthropathy.

Joint effusion is an early and nonspecific response to an articular insult. MR imaging is highly sensitive for the detection of effusions even smaller than 1 mL. A simple effusion shows a low T1-signal intensity and a high T2-signal intensity (**Fig. 1**). Paradoxically increased signal intensity on non–fat-suppressed T1-weighted images or areas of low signal intensity on T1- and T2-weighted MR images can indicate hemarthrosis. Of note, a joint effusion gradually enhances on postcontrast MR images, showing significant T1 shortening approximately 10 minutes after intravenous Gd-chelate injection.

Synovial inflammation represents the primary event of JIA, before radiographic abnormalities are apparent. A synovitis is characterized by a high signal intensity on STIR and fat-saturated T2-weighted images and a strong and early peak enhancement on postcontrast T1-weighted MR images (usually within 1 minute after intravenous injection of Gd-chelate) (**Fig. 2**). Of note, a synovitis is a nonspecific imaging finding, seen in a variety of joint disorders. With further progression of a JIA, synovial proliferation develops that is typically isointense or minimally hyperintense compared with joint effusion on T1-weighted MR images. Active pannus can be differentiated from joint fluid by rapid and strong enhancement on T1-weighted MR images. Postcontrast images should be obtained in the early phase (<5 min) after intravenous injection of Gd-chelates to provide an optimal discrimination between enhancing synovium and more slowly enhancing effusion. Normal synovium is usually not apparent on low-field MR imaging systems. High-field MR imaging scanners may delineate normal synovium on Gd-enhanced scans, however, thereby requiring additional criteria for the diagnosis of synovitis. A synovial thickness of 3 mm or more and a synovial volume of 3 mL or more have been proposed to define synovitis in the knee joint.[4] The quantity and rate of synovial Gd enhancement and the extent of synovial proliferation correlate with disease activity and can be used for monitoring of treatment response.

Progressive JIA can cause cartilage destruction, either because of degradation of cartilage on the joint surface by enzymes released from the inflamed synovium or because of subchondral resorption with the result of diffuse cartilage thinning.[4] Cartilage defects can present as areas of increased water content, contour abnormalities, defects, or thinning (**Fig. 3**). Cartilage defects are rarely seen in very young JIA patients. The increased thickness and blood supply of cartilage of immature joints (before physis closure) suggest a unique self-regeneration potential, which diminishes with increasing skeletal maturation. Normal articular cartilage has an intermediate signal on both T1- and T2-weighted MR images. Inflamed immature cartilage in JIA patients may show an accentuated "spoke wheel" enhancement caused by hyperemia (see **Fig. 1**). This may prevent the formation of acute cartilage defects but contributes to growth disturbances. Cartilage defects ultimately occur with increasing progression of the disease and age of the patient (see **Fig. 3**). The pathologic classification of cartilage defects in mature bones is shown in **Table 3**. The size and extent of cartilage defects and the overall cartilage volume can be used to monitor anti-inflammatory treatment in advanced JIA.

Similarly, bone erosions are relatively rare in young patients with JIA, increasing in frequency with age. MR imaging shows a higher sensitivity for the detection of bone erosions compared with conventional radiographs and can be used to monitor their progression. Bone erosions are delineated as relatively low signal intensity areas on both T1- and T2-weighted images (**Figs. 4** and **5**). The MR imaging–detected erosions are clinically significant because one in four MR imaging erosions progress to radiographically visible and painful erosions within 1 year. MR imaging also detects osteophytes before conventional radiographs. Central osteophytes indicate cartilage damage. In addition, central osteophytes in the knee joints can push the menisci to the periphery of the joint, which may lead to meniscal abnormalities. Chronic inflammation of the knee joint may lead to meniscal atrophy with loss of the usual triangular shape, meniscal irregularity, or tears. Additional complications may include ligamentous injury, nerve dislocations, and osteochondral bodies in the joint.

Reactive marrow changes present as an edema-like process (T1 hypointense and T2 hyperintense) with variable extent and degree of contrast enhancement. Tenosynovitis most

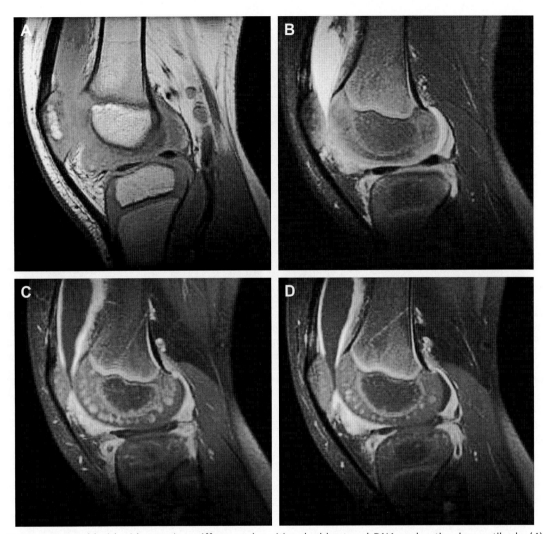

Fig. 1. A 3-year-old girl with morning stiffness and positive double strand DNA and antinuclear antibody. (*A*) Sagittal T1-weighted spin echo (SE), (*B*) fat-saturated (FS) T2-weighted fast spin echo (FSE), and (*C, D*) FS T1-weighted SE sequences after intravenous gadopentetate injection. Large rim-enhancing joint effusion with thickened synovial margins, compatible with synovitis. Some radially arrayed enhancement of the articular cartilage of the distal femur epiphysis following gadolinium administration represents prominent penetrating vessels.

commonly involves extensor tendons of the hand and ankle and is apparent as an area of swelling with T1 hypointensity and marked T2 hyperintensity and Gd enhancement. Signs of soft tissue inflammation may include myositis, fasciitis, and subcutaneous edema-like change. The extent of MR imaging signal edema-like change in muscle correlates with the activity of myositis. Acute and subacute myositis shows a markedly increased T2 signal and Gd uptake. Clinical improvement correlates with normalization of MR imaging muscle signal. In cases of chronic myositis, muscle atrophy and fatty replacement may be noted. Associated soft tissue masses may include inflamed bursae (subacromial-subdeltoid,

olecranon, iliopsoas, prepatellar); ganglia; and rheumatoid nodules (see **Fig. 4**).

Late sequelae of chronic JIA are growth disturbances with initial overgrowths of affected bones caused by hyperemia of the growth plates, followed by premature growth plate closure and growth arrest. Abnormalities in bone growth and development are relatively common, including shortening and abnormal shape of articular surfaces and flexion or valgus deformities. For example, in the knee joint, the femoral condyles may increase in size and the patella may show a typical "squaring" or angular remodeling. A scoliosis may develop because of asymmetric length of the lower extremities or compression

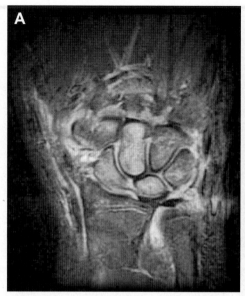
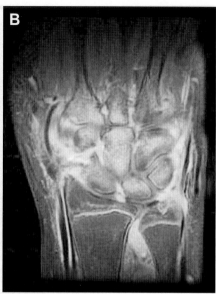

Fig. 2. A 10-year-old patient with JIA. (*A*) Coronal STIR sequences show a constellation of findings of marrow T2 hyperintensity in various carpal bones, fluid within the first carpometacarpal joint and the distal radioulnar joint. (*B*) FS T1-weighted SE sequences after intravenous gadopentetate injection demonstrate a diffuse enhancement of the joint spaces consistent with synovitis. There is also enhancement of the marrow, compatible with osteitis.

fractures related to steroid therapy. Temporomandibular joint involvement may lead to early growth arrest and micrognathia. The cervical spine may show vertebral fusion, especially at C2/3, with subluxations of more distal vertebrae. A spinal cord compression is a significant risk in adolescents and young adults. Steroid treatment may lead to compression fractures of vertebrae or weight-bearing bones and osteonecrosis, particularly affecting the hip joints.

To date, monitoring of pharmacotherapy of JIA is primarily done based on clinical findings, radiographs, and ultrasound. MR imaging is an emerging tool for monitoring drug treatment in patients with JIA, and is already helpful for evaluating complications of the disease. Prospective clinical studies are under way to determine whether clinical outcomes are improved by using MR imaging over standard radiographs to monitor disease progression in these patients.

There are several methods for determining treatment response. (1) A semiquantitative approach with definition of a grading score (eg, no enhancement, mild enhancement, severe enhancement, severe + erosions) is used in many institutions. It is easily feasible for clinical routine assessments, but is subjective and related to a high interobserver variability. (2) Assessments of dynamic time versus synovial signal enhancement curves provide a more objective means of synovial

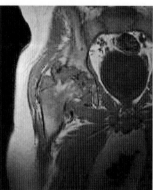
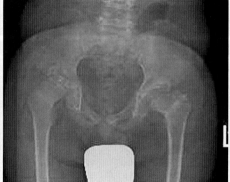
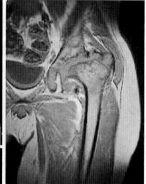

Fig. 3. A 7-year-old patient with JIA. The radiograph of the pelvis (*middle*) shows a bilateral femoral epiphysis flattening and destruction. Coronal T1-weighted MR images of both hips confirm an extensive destruction of the femoral epiphyses and bilateral effusion.

Table 3	
Classification of pathologic cartilage	
Grade	**Cartilage Pathology**
1	Cartilage softening/swelling
2	Cartilage fragmentation/fissuring <1.3 mm in area
3	Cartilage fragmentation/fissuring >1.3 mm in area
4	Full-thickness erosion to subchondral bone

From Outerbridge RE, Dunlop JA. The problem of chondromalacia patellae. Clin Orthop Relat Res 1975;110:177–96; with permission.

enhancement, but may vary with the rate of contrast agent injection, the heart rate of the patient, and the area and location of measurement. It is important to keep the injection mode and the location and area of analysis as constant as possible on follow-up studies to avoid a technique-related bias. (3) Quantifying the volume of enhancing synovium and synovial proliferation does not assess the vascularity of the synovium. In addition, synovial volumetry is time-consuming and requires data postprocessing, which makes it difficult to integrate into clinical routine assessments. With successful treatment, the extent and rate of synovial enhancement and the volume of synovial proliferation decrease. Active, hypervascularized pannus can transform into an inactive fibrous pannus, which is relatively low signal intensity on both T1- and T2-weighted MR images and shows minimal or no Gd enhancement.

Most children are initially treated with nonsteroidal anti-inflammatory drugs and intra-articular steroid injections. Intra-articular steroid injections may limit local disturbances of bone growth (initial accelerated bone growth followed by premature growth plate closure). Patients with systemic JIA often need intravenous steroid therapy to control the disease. In these patients, attention should be paid to possible related complications, such as osteonecrosis or stress fractures. Methotrexate is a powerful drug that helps suppress joint inflammation in patients with polyarthritis and systemic arthritis. These patients receive folic acid supplementation. Anemia may occur as a side effect of this therapy, however, and if severe may be apparent on MR images as bone marrow conversion to red marrow. Newer drugs have been developed recently, such as tumor necrosis factor-α blockers, which have provided significant improvement in patients with refractory disease to conventional therapies.[4,5] Patients receiving tumor necrosis factor inhibitors have an increased risk of developing neoplasms and in particular lymphoproliferative diseases, such as Hodgkin and non-Hodgkin lymphomas. Close attention should be

given to lymphadenopathy on MR imaging studies of tumor necrosis factor–treated patients. New biologic agents that target specific cytokine abnormalities are being increasingly investigated in pediatric rheumatic diseases, and several related clinical trials are currently under way.

In approximately 60% of patients, JIA burns out before adulthood. Persistent and long-term abnormalities may be found in these patients on imaging studies, however, such as persistent abnormal synovial enhancement (about 30%); joint deformities; cartilage or bone defects; bone growth abnormalities; limb asymmetries; functional impairments; and osteoporosis.

ENTHESIS-RELATED ARTHRITIS

Enthesis-related arthritis encompasses a diverse group of arthritides, such as ankylosing spondylitis, reactive arthritis, and undifferentiated spondyloarthropathy, and is associated with two of the following criteria: sacroiliac or spinal pain, HLA-B27 positivity, HLA-B27 family history, anterior uveitis, or arthritis onset in a boy aged 8 or more. An enthesitis is an inflammation of tendons or ligaments at their attachment site to bone. MR imaging features of enthesitis are swelling of the entheseal region, increased T2-signal of the usually uniform low signal intensity of tendons and ligaments, distention of adjacent bursae, peritendinous soft tissue swelling, and inflammation of bone adjacent to the insertion. Characteristic sites are the joints of the hands and feet, particularly the insertion of the Achilles tendon, and the sacroiliac joints. Isolated hip disease may also occur. Spinal involvement is usually not seen in children. It is a relatively late sequela of the disease and usually presents in adulthood. A possible associated extra-articular manifestation is aortic insufficiency.

Ankylosing spondylitis develops in boys and young men between the ages of 15 and 30 years. Girls are rarely affected. Ankylosing spondylitis is the least erosive of the inflammatory arthropathies

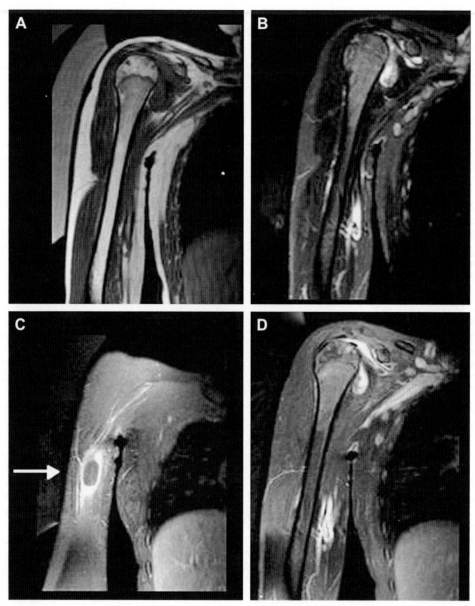

Fig. 4. A 15-year-old girl with advanced polyarticular JIA. (*A*) T1-weighted and (*B*) FS T2-weighted MR image show erosions of the humeral head, subchondral cysts, a joint effusion and axillary lymph nodes. (*C, D*) FS T1-weighted images after intravenous gadopentetate injection show a severe synovitis. Large inflamed bursa extending off biceps sheath (*arrow*).

and the most ossifying. The sacroiliac joints are most frequently involved, usually in an asymmetric fashion. STIR and fat saturated T2-weighted and post-Gd images show a hyperintense signal of the affected sacroiliac joint, often associated with a localized edema of the adjacent bone marrow of the sacrum and ilium (**Fig. 6**). Erosions are small and localized. Subchondral cysts and subluxations are rare. Joint ankylosis is a late sequela of the disease. Anti-inflammatory treatment of chronic sacroiliitis leads to fatty conversion of the juxta-articular bone marrow (**Fig. 7**). Other features of ankylosing spondylitis are enthesitis and asymmetric arthritis of peripheral joints. Inflammatory bowel disease (Crohn's, ulcerative colitis, and Whipple disease) affects the joints in a similar manner. The activity of the arthropathy parallels the activity of the bowel disease.

Reactive arthritis (formerly known as "Reiter syndome") is relatively common and may be secondary to an infection with enteric bacterial

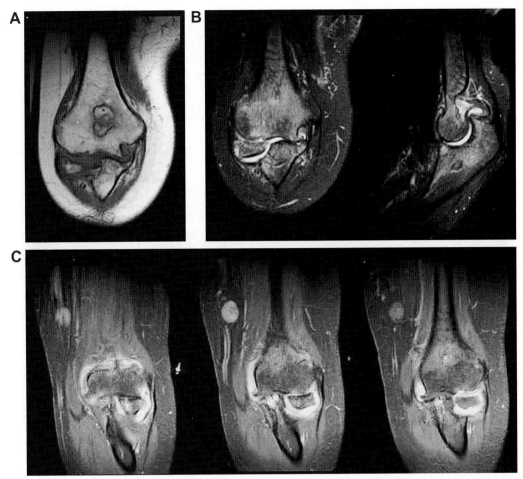

Fig. 5. A 17-year-old girl with end-stage polyarticular JIA. Coronal T1-weighted (*A*) and coronal and sagittal STIR images (*B*) of the left elbow show an intra-articular effusion with synovitis, bone-on-bone appearance, absence of cartilage, bone marrow edema, subchondral cyst formation, and osteophytosis caused by secondary degenerative osteoarthritis. (*C*) Contrast-enhanced FS T1-weighted MR images of the left elbow show marked abnormal enhancement and thickening of the synovium with debris bilaterally, consistent with an active synovitis.

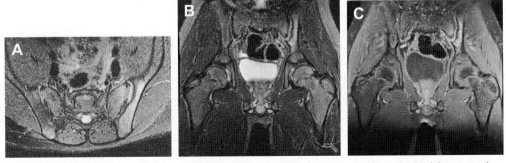

Fig. 6. A 10-year-old boy with moderate left sacroiliitis. Axial FS T2-weighted (*A*) and STIR (*B*) images show an effusion in the left sacroiliac joint with abnormal T2 hyperintensity in the adjacent left ilium and sacrum. (*C*) T1-weighted images after gadopentetate injection show a mild enhancement of the left sacroiliac joint and the adjacent bone marrow.

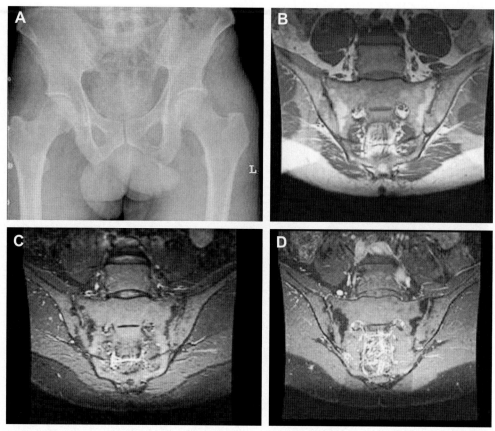

Fig. 7. A 23-year-old man with ankylosing spondylitis and chronic sacroiliitis on tumor necrosis factor-α therapy. Radiograph (*A*), T1-weighted SE (*B*), FS T2-weighted (*C*), and contrast-enhanced T1-weighted (*D*) MR images. Essentially symmetric erosions of the bilateral sacroiliac joints and partial bilateral fusion. No evidence of enhancement or fluid within the sacroiliac joints to correlate with active synovitis. Increased fatty changes in the bilateral sacroiliac joints are consistent with chronic sacroiliitis.

organisms, a viral infection, a vaccination, or *Chlamydia* infection. Reactive arthritis presents in sexually active teenagers with arthropathy and an associated urethritis and conjunctivitis. The reactive arthritis often affects a single joint of the lower extremity, most frequently the interphalangeal joint of the great toe. In addition, these patients may also show a bilateral, asymmetric sacroiliitis. An enthesitis is common around the calcaneus, with or without calcaneal erosions, and there can be a retrocalcaneal bursitis. Other common areas of enthesitis are the patella and insertion sites of the plantar fascia, with or without spur formation.

JUVENILE PSORIATIC ARTHRITIS

Juvenile psoriasis manifests before 16 years of age with a peak age of 6 to 11 years. Patients are usually rheumatoid factor negative. Typical symptoms, such as dactylitis and onychopathy, may present before occurrence of typical skin changes. A tenosynovitis of the fingers may produce a characteristic sausage digit and may be associated with an effusion of the involved joints. The tenosynovitis appears as T2-hyperintense signal around tendons on MR images and affects flexor tendons more often than extensor tendons. In addition, a diffuse T2-hyperintense soft tissue swelling is often seen, which is usually more extensive than that seen in JIA. A concomitant small joint synovitis is relatively rare. The arthritis is usually bilateral and asymmetric and may affect the small joints of the hands and feet, the knee joint, and the sacroiliac joints. In the hands, the arthritis may involve either several distal interphalangeal joints or all joints of one digit. The larger diarthrodial joints are occasionally involved. MR imaging of affected joints may show joint space narrowing or joint effusion, synovial enhancement, erosions, and ligamentous disruptions. Erosions at the joint periphery may produce "mickey mouse ears." Occasionally, the eroded articular ends may be separated by enhancing proliferative granulation tissue, which is highly suggestive of psoriatic arthritis. The typical "pencil-in-cup" deformity of interphalangeal joints is rare in children. Periostitis with occasionally extensive extra-articular periosteal new bone formation may be present. In approximately 5% to 10% of patients, an arthritis mutilans may develop.

DIFFERENTIAL DIAGNOSES IN PEDIATRIC ARTHRITIS
Collagen Vascular Disease

The collagen vascular diseases include dermatomyositis, scleroderma, systemic lupus erythematosus, polyarteritis nodosa, and mixed connective tissue disease. Articular symptoms are minor and there is little involvement of the joint itself.

Systemic lupus erythematosus is the most common of the collagen vascular diseases, with articular symptoms present in up to 90% of patients. MR imaging findings include soft tissue swelling, tenosynovitis, subluxations, and dislocations, with absence of erosions or joint space narrowing (**Fig. 8**). The periarticular, capsular, and ligamentous supporting structures are involved, resulting in easily reducible subluxations. Periarticular calcification and osteonecrosis may be seen. The most common deformity in the hand and wrist is ulnar deviation and volar subluxation of the metacarpophalageal joints, hyperextension of the proximal interphalageal joints and flexion of the distal interphalageal joints with ulnar drift of the

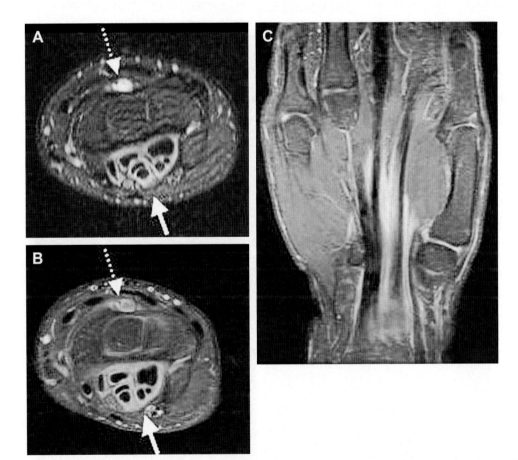

Fig. 8. A 17-year-old girl with systemic lupus erythematosus. Axial FS T2-weighted scans (*A*), axial (*B*) and coronal (*C*) fat-suppressed T1-weighted post-IV gadopentetate MR images through the wrist show T2 hyperintensity and enhancement of the tendon sheaths in the flexor compartment, consistent with a tenosynovitis of the flexor tendons, extending from the carpal tunnel and to the level of the mid metacarpals (*solid arrow*). Associated median nerve neuropathy is seen with enlargement and high signal intensity in the median nerve. The extensor tendons demonstrate normal signal characteristics. In the dorsal aspect of the wrist, there is a small ovoid mass measuring approximately 9 × 9 mm, deep to the flexor tendons at the level of the capitate (*dashed arrow*). This mass demonstrates a high signal on T2-weighted MR images and a mild rim enhancement, consistent with a ganglion.

radiocarpal joint. The joints are involved bilaterally and symmetrically with the most common involvement in the hand, wrist, hip, knee, and shoulder. Jaccoud arthropathy, which is seen in patients with prior history of rheumatic fever, can have an appearance similar to systemic lupus erythematosus.

Scleroderma is rare in children. There is a systemic form with involvement of internal organs and a localized form. The latter is confined to the skin and subcutaneous soft tissues and relatively more frequent in children. MR imaging findings include decreased soft tissue thickness of the finger tips (which correlates closely with the clinical appearance of Raynaud phenomenon); acro-osteolysis (which usually begins along the palmar aspect); and subcutaneous calcification (a late manifestation). Osseous erosions may be seen at the clavicles, distal radius, and ulna. Joint effusions are rare. Late in the disease, the hand joints may demonstrate uniform loss of cartilage and flexion deformities.

Juvenile dermatomyositis is an inflammatory myopathy in children and young adults. MR imaging is a sensitive tool to detect the distribution of the disease. Muscle involvement is usually nonuniform and the adductor muscles of the thigh are most commonly affected (**Fig. 9**). Areas of inflammation present as high signal intensity areas in T2-weighted and STIR images and may extend from affected muscles to the tendons (tenosynovitis) and adjacent fat (**Fig. 10**). In late stages of the disease sheet-like calcifications in the fascial planes and subcutaneous tissues appear hypointense on all pulse sequences, although some areas of calcification with increased proton content may appear paradoxically hyperintense on T2-weighted MR images. Of note, MR imaging

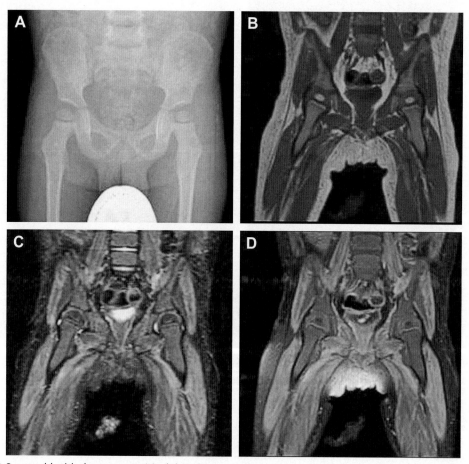

Fig. 9. A 2 year old with dermatomyositis. (*A*) Radiograph of the pelvis shows multiple areas of subtle linear and clumped soft tissue calcifications projecting over the perineal region, adductor muscular groups of the thighs, left sartorius, and lateral soft tissues of the lateral abdominal and pelvic walls. (*B*) T1-weighted SE images show a relatively low muscle signal. FS T2-weighted (*C*) and contrast-enhanced T1-weighted MR images (*D*) show a diffusely increased signal of all visualized muscles with marked contrast enhancement. These findings are consistent with myositis.

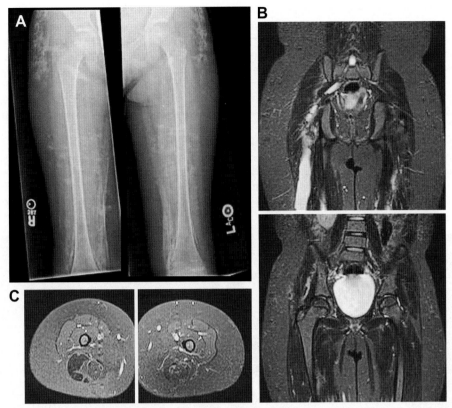

Fig. 10. X-rays of both thighs in an 8-year-old girl with dermatomyositis (*A*) shows diffuse fine soft tissue calcifications and vascular calcifications. Coronal FS-T2-weighted (*B*) and FS contrast enhanced T1-weighted (*C*) MR scans show several fluid collections in the bilateral thighs, adjacent to and intercalating between multiple muscles. The largest collection is in the posterior compartment of the right thigh, containing several septations. The bony structures are normal.

is not sensitive for the detection of these calcifications and may miss even large calcifications. Joints are usually spared.

Septic Arthritis

Septic arthritis is a common emergency in infants and children. The disease is usually caused by a hematogenous infection, most commonly by *Staphylococcus aureus*. Other possible pathogens include group B streptococci and gram-negative bacteria (eg, *Escherichia coli*) in neonates and *Pseudomonas*, pneumococci, and *Kingella kingae* (gram-negative organism) in young children (3 months to 3 years of age). A gonococcal arthritis may be found in neonates caused by a birth canal infection or in sexually active teenagers. Rarely, septic arthritis may develop because of a penetrating wound or cellulites. Septic arthritis is a medical emergency because it may lead to severe joint destruction and impairment or loss of the growth plate if not immediately and adequately treated. An early diagnosis is essential to successful treatment. The most commonly

affected joints are the knee, hip, and ankle joints. Clinically, fever, joint pain and swelling, an erythrocyte sedimentation rate of 40 or more mm/h, and a leukocytosis of greater than 12,000 cells/mm^3 can be found. Laboratory parameters are nonspecific and unreliable, however, being also elevated after trauma or with other infections, such as an otitis media. Blood cultures and evaluations of joint aspirates provide a more specific and more reliable diagnosis. A pyogenic joint effusion typically shows the presence of more than 40,000 leukocytes per field and more than 90% polymorphonuclear leukocytes. A Gram stain can provide a presumptive immediate diagnosis. False-negative results are possible, however, and the responsible organism cannot be identified in about 30% of cases. Prompt surgical drainage and antibiotic therapy are necessary to prevent complications.

The diagnosis of septic arthritis is based on clinical presentation and joint aspiration. MR imaging in patients with septic arthritis should be reserved for clinically equivocal cases, an inconclusive diagnosis based on a joint aspiration, therapy-refractory disease, or suspected complications. Of note, there is a high association of osteomyelitis and septic arthritis in infants younger than age 18 months. In these patients, blood vessels traverse the growth plate and can spread hematogenous infections from the metaphysis to the epiphysis and joint space or vice versa. In older patients, these vessels have regressed and the epiphyseal plate serves as a barrier for spread of pathogens.

MR imaging of septic joints shows an effusion and synovial thickening and contrast enhancement. The joint space turns into a self-contained abscess cavity. It has recently been suggested that the pyogenic abscess in a joint can be differentiated from reactive joint fluid based on diffusion-weighted MR imaging.[6,7] A pyogenic abscess shows an increased signal intensity on diffusion-weighted imaging, whereas a reactive effusion shows a low signal intensity on diffusion-weighted imaging. Other MR imaging findings in septic arthritis are a T2-hyperintense, T1-hypointense, and contrast-enhancing edema of the bone marrow and periarticular soft tissues. Abnormal diffuse marrow signal on T1-weighted images has a high association with concomitant osteomyelitis (**Fig. 11**).

It is important to distinguish pyogenic and tuberculous joint infections, because these require

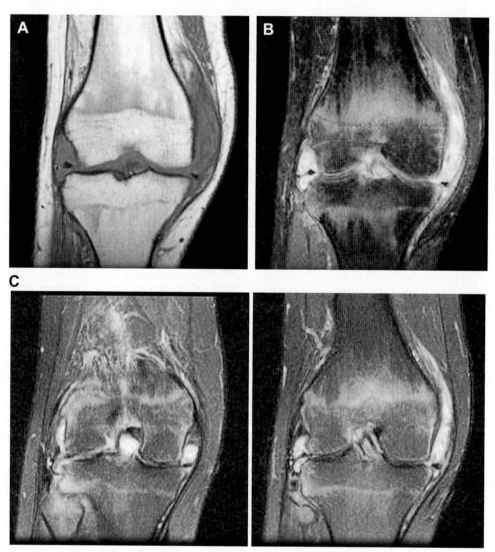

Fig. 11. An 18-year-old girl with tuberculous infection of the right knee joint. Coronal T1-weighted SE (*A*), FS T2-weighted FSE images (*B*), and FS contrast-enhanced T1-weighted SE images (*C*) show a diffuse inflammatory process involving the knee joint. There is synovial thickening and enhancement and generalized thinning of the cartilaginous surfaces and menisci. Nonenhancing debris is noted within the knee joint. Associated T2-hyperintensity and enhancement of the marrow of the distal femur and tibia could represent osteomyelitis or reactive inflammation.

different treatment regimens. Although MR imaging cannot replace serologic and joint fluid analyses, MR imaging may provide some hints for the correct diagnosis. The presence of bone erosions and absence of subchondral marrow signal intensity abnormality favor a diagnosis of tuberculous arthritis rather than pyogenic arthritis. In case of abscess formation, a thin and smooth abscess rim favors tuberculous arthritis, whereas a thick and irregularly enhancing rim is more indicative of a pyogenic arthritis.[8,9] Lyme disease, a *Borrelia burgdorferi* infection transmitted by a tick bite, can simulate a oligoarticular JIA or pyogenic arthritis. Clinical signs that lead to the correct diagnosis are history of a tick bite and a subsequent red macular skin lesion with centrifugal expansion; however, few patients or parents recall or notice these characteristic signs. Late associated neurologic abnormalities, such as headache, nausea, rigidity, and myalgias, are rare in children. Children most commonly present with an oligoarthritis of the knee joint within 2 weeks to 2 years after inoculation. The hip, ankle, elbow, and wrist are other potentially affected sites. There is a rapid test that provides the diagnosis within hours; however, this test is not widely available. The diagnosis by serum enzyme immunoassay and Western blot or polymerase chain reaction–based detection of *B burgdorferi* in synovial fluid can take several days. Recognizing typical imaging features may help to suggest the correct diagnosis and accelerate an early treatment of these patients. Inflammatory responses of the joint itself, such as extent and distribution of synovitis, joint effusion, and erosions, are not significantly different compared with pyogenic arthritides.[10] Ecklund and colleagues[10] identified three specific MR imaging features that are frequently seen in Lyme arthritis, but rare in pyogenic arthritis: (1) myositis, (2) lymphadenopathy, and (3) lack of subcutaneous edema.[10] A transient arthritis of the hip joint is a self-limited disease after a viral infection of the upper respiratory tract or urinary tract. It predominantly affects boys with an age of 3 to 10 years who present with joint pain, mild fever, and mildly elevated erythrocyte sedimentation rate or white blood count. The disease is often bilateral. If clinically suspected, an ultrasound is sufficient for evaluation of the affected joint. In equivocal cases, MR imaging may be performed to rule out other differential diagnoses. MR imaging shows a joint effusion and synovial enhancement. In addition, patients with transient arthritis frequently show involvement of the contralateral joint, whereas contralateral involvement is rare in patients with septic arthritis. Conversely, bone marrow signal alterations, erosions, and periarticular soft tissue edema are rare in transient arthritis, but frequently seen in septic arthritis. The treatment of transient arthritis is conservative with observation or nonsteroidal anti-inflammatory drug administration. A small proportion of affected patients develop a cyclic disease with recurrence after several months. Acute rheumatic fever presents with a polyarthritis, carditis, erythema, and subcutaneous nodules. The diagnosis can be confirmed by a streptococcal antibody test. The associated polyarthritis is relatively nonspecific on MR imaging studies, may present with an effusion and synovitis, is typically not associated with joint erosions, and may migrate to other joints. It may regress spontaneously or may be treated with nonsteroidal anti-inflammatory drugs.

Hemophilia

Hemophilia is characterized by an impaired blood coagulation caused by x-linked recessive deficiencies of clotting factor VIII or IX. Affected patients develop chronic hemarthrosis and intraosseous hemorrhage. The distribution is asymmetric and sporadic with involvement commonly in the knees, elbow, ankle, hip, and shoulder. Radiographic changes resemble those of JIA except that there is usually no inhibition of bone growth, periostitis, or osseous ankylosis (except in carpals and tarsals). Abnormalities include osteopenia, increased density in the soft tissues secondary to hemosiderin deposition, enlarged epiphyses and subchondral cysts, late joint space loss, and secondary osteoarthritic changes. Involvement of growth plates may produce deformity of joints, such as tibiotalar slant. MR images show bleeding and hemosiderin deposition within the joint and periarticular soft tissues. Acute hematomas have a similar signal as fluid, being isointense to muscle on T1-weighted sequences and hyperintense on T2-weighted sequences. Subsequently, the signal increases on T1-weighted sequences (progressing from the periphery to the center of the hematoma) and decreases on T2-weighted sequences. Old hematomas show signs of hemosiderin deposition, which appears of very low signal on both T1- and T2-weighted sequences. Additional findings within hemophilic joints on MR images are synovial thickening and enhancement; ligamentous tears; focal cartilage defects; diffuse cartilage thinning; subchondral cysts (especially in the area of cartilage defects); bone erosions; and joint space narrowing. Bleeding into soft tissues can cause the formation of pseudotumors, which are most commonly seen in the muscles of the thigh.

Neuroarthropathy

Neuropathic joints represent a severe arthropathy caused by autonomic nervous dysfunction, impaired proprioception, and recurrent microtrauma in patients with diabetes or other neuropathies, such as syringomyelia. Neuropathic arthropathy affects one or several joints with asymmetric involvement and presents with a combination of bone resorption and production. There are hypertrophic and atrophic forms of neuropathic joints. The hypertrophic form is usually seen in weight-bearing joints, such as the knee, hip, or ankle joints. Hallmarks of the hypertrophic form include increased bone production and severe degenerative changes. The atrophic form is often seen in the shoulder and elbow, or in a non–weight-bearing hip or knee. The imaging appearance of the atrophic joint occasionally simulates infection or an aggressive bone tumor.

One sees pseudosurgical bone erosions with absence of bone repair. MR imaging may show early signs of the disease at a time where joint architecture and function may still be preserved by dedicated treatment, such as rest, anti-inflammatory drugs, and orthoses. In the early stage of the disease, MR imaging shows extensive bone marrow edema of affected bones on T1-, fat-saturated T2-, and STIR sequences. Marked synovial enhancement and cartilage defects and bone resorption may also be seen. If not or inadequately treated, the disease rapidly progresses to an exaggerated osteoarthropathy with extensive cartilage and bone defects, joint disorganization, osseous debris, and soft tissue swelling.

Pseudoarthritis

Other differential diagnoses include epiphyseal dysplasias, which are typically not associated

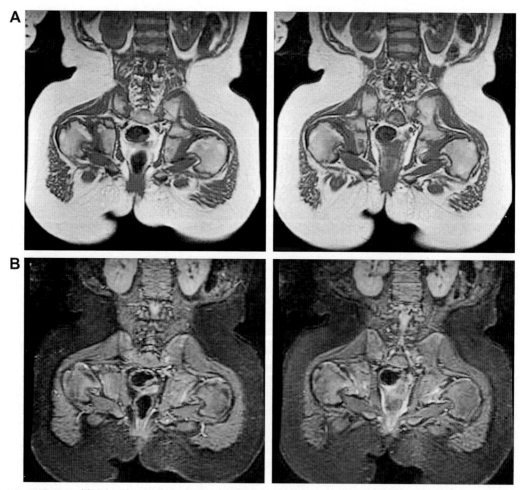

Fig. 12. A 13-year-old girl with spondyloepiphyseal dysplasia. Coronal T1-weighted SE (*A*) and FS T2-weighted FSE images (*B*) show a posterior, superior, and lateral hip subluxation, right greater than left, and moderate hip effusions with intra-articular debris. Without good clinical correlation, this could be confused with erosive arthropathy.

with fever, clinical signs of inflammation, or imaging features of synovitis. These pseudoarthritides include hereditary late spondyloepiphyseal dysplasia, an x-linked recessive or rarely autosomal-dominant skeletal dysplasia, which is characterized by a mild short trunk dwarfism and marked osteoarthritis of the hip and knee joints. Patients are normal at birth and slowly develop progressive spinal deformities with platyspondyly (flattened vertebrae) and intervertebral disk calcifications. The patients show marked deformities of both hip and knee joints (**Fig. 12**). The head of the femur remains cartilaginous until about age 5 years, the proximal femoral epiphysis is markedly flattened and irregular in shape, and a progressive coxa varus deformity develops. The iliac bones are short and the acetabular roof is flattened. Likewise, ossification of the epiphyseal centers of the distal femur and proximal tibia is markedly delayed, and the medial condyles of the distal femurs show a relative overgrowth and lead to a genu valgus deformity with increasing age. MR imaging shows these skeletal deformities. Unlike JIA or infectious arthritides, however, these patients usually do not show joint effusions, synovial thickening, or enhancement of bone marrow or periarticular soft tissue edema. One important practical aspect about this disease is the knowledge of associated spinal column defects and atlantoaxial instability that may lead to spinal cord injury with general anesthesia and forced neck retroflexion during intubation. The diagnosis can be confirmed by DNA analysis of a blood sample.

REFERENCES

1. Johnson K, Gardner-Medwin J. Childhood arthritis: classification and radiology. Clin Radiol 2002;57: 47–58.

2. Lawrence RC, Helmick CG, Arnett FC, et al. Estimates of the prevalence of arthritis and selected musculoskeletal disorders in the United States. Arthritis Rheum 1998;41(5):778–99.

3. Mason TG, Reed AM. Update in juvenile rheumatoid arthritis. Arthritis Rheum 2005;53(5):796–9.

4. Glys-Morin VM, Graham TB, Blebea JS, et al. Knee in early juvenile arthritis: MR imaging findings. Radiology 2001;220:696–706.

5. Petty RE, Southwood TR, Manners P, et al. International league of associations for rheumatology classification of juvenile idiopathic arthritis: second revision. J Rheumatol 2004;31:390–2.

6. Park JK, Kim BS, Choi G, et al. Distinction of reactive joint fluid from pyogenic abscess by diffusion-weighted imaging. J Magn Reson Imaging 2007; 25(4):859–61.

7. Greenstein AS, Marzo-Orthega H, Emery P, et al. MR imaging as a predictor of progressive joint destruction in neuropathic joint disease. Arthritis Rheum 2002;46(10):2814–5.

8. Hong SH, Kim SM, Ahn JM, et al. Tuberculous versus pyogenic arthritis: MR imaging evaluation. Radiology 2001;218:848–53.

9. Weissman BN, editor. Arthritis imaging. Radiol Clin North Am 2004;42.

10. Ecklund K, Vargas S, Zurakowski D, et al. MRI features of Lyme arthritis in children. AJR Am J Roentgenol 2005;184:1904–9.

MR Imaging of Primary Bone Tumors and Tumor-like Conditions in Children

Sandra L. Wootton-Gorges, MD[a,b,]*

KEYWORDS
- Bone tumor • MR imaging • Pediatrics
- Skeletal neoplasm • Children

Radiographs remain the primary imaging modality in characterizing primary bone tumors and tumor-like conditions of bone (**Table 1**). The appearance, location (**Boxes 1** and **2**), and patient age are all important features that allow the radiologist to offer a succinct differential diagnosis of the mass being evaluated. MR imaging also plays a valuable role in evaluating pediatric bone tumors because it is superior in assessing the extent of bony, intramedullary, joint, and soft tissue involvement by the neoplasm.[1,2]

It is preferable to perform the initial MR imaging for intraosseous tumor before biopsy to prevent distortion by postbiopsy changes.[2] In addition, MR imaging can help to determine the optimal site for biopsy. The examination must include imaging of the entire bone to evaluate for skip lesions, and to assess the longitudinal extent of the tumor because this helps with surgical planning.[2,3] Longitudinal imaging may either be in the sagittal or coronal plane. Highest specificity for tumor extent is defined on T1-weighted images,[3] where the tumor is typically low signal and distorts the normal marrow architecture. Highest tumor sensitivity is defined on short tau inversion recovery images (STIR) images, where the tumor is typically of high signal. Axial imaging with small field of view phased-array coil fast spin echo T2-weighted fat-saturated or STIR sequences through the tumor are most useful to determine the relationship of the tumor to the adjacent soft tissues, muscles, nerves, and vascular structures.[2,3] Gradient echo sequences can confirm blood flow within the blood vessels. Postgadolinium T1-weighted fat-saturated images can define areas of viable tumor and areas of tumor necrosis.[2] The growth plate and adjacent joint must be carefully analyzed for tumor involvement. Although most tumors have relatively nonspecific MR imaging signal characteristics (low signal on T1-weighed images and high signal on T2-weighted images) low signal on both T1- and T2-weighted images may suggest osteoblastic or fibrous matrix or chronic hemorrhage.[4] Most lesions containing fat, which is high signal on T1-weighted images and low signal on STIR images, are benign.[4] This hyperintensity on T1-weighted images must be distinguished from subacute hemorrhage.

Peritumoral edema may be seen with either benign or malignant tumors.[4] It may be intraosseous or extraosseous in location. Its signal characteristics are similar to the tumor, and so care must be taken to distinguish it from tumor. Intraosseous edema does not alter the normal architecture of the marrow space, and soft tissue edema does not demonstrate mass effect.[4] Marrow edema is intermediate between fat and muscle on T1-weighted sequences, and is high signal on T2 or STIR images, whereas most tumors are more heterogeneous. Edema also has a poorly defined margin in bone, and a feathery appearance, which

[a] Department of Radiology, University of California, Davis Medical Center, UC Davis Children's Hospital, 4860 Y Street, Suite 3100, Sacramento, CA 95817, USA
[b] Shriner's Hospital of Northern California, 2425 Stockton Boulevard, Sacramento, CA 95817, USA
* Department of Radiology, University of California, Davis Medical Center, UC Davis Children's Hospital, 4860 Y Street, Suite 3100, Sacramento, CA 95817.
E-mail address: sandra.gorges@ucdmc.ucdavis.edu

Magn Reson Imaging Clin N Am 17 (2009) 469–487
doi:10.1016/j.mric.2009.03.010

Table 1
Pediatric primary bone tumors and tumor-like lesions

Tumor Type	Benign	Malignant
Bone-forming tumors	Osteoid osteoma, Osteoblastoma	Osteosarcoma
Cartilage-forming tumors	Enchondroma, chondroblastoma, chondromyxoid fibroma, osteochondroma	Chondrosarcoma
Giant cell tumors	Giant cell tumor	—
Small round cell tumors	—	Ewing sarcoma, lymphoma
Vascular tumors	Hemangioma, Lymphangioma	Hemangiopericytoma
Fibro-osseous lesions	Nonossifying fibroma, fibrous dysplasia, osteofibrous dysplasia	Fibrosarcoma, malignant fibrous histiocytoma
Cystic lesions	Unicameral (simple) bone cyst, aneurysmal bone cyst	—
Others	Langerhans cell histiocytosis	—

follows muscle and fascial planes in soft tissue.[4] After gadolinium, edema enhances less than the tumor.

Periosteal reaction may be seen with a variety of benign and malignant bone tumors, and is seen well by MR imaging.[5] It is low signal on all pulse sequences and is located just outside the cortical surface. The periosteal reaction may be defined as lamellated (single or multilayer); solid; speculated; Codman triangle; or expanded shell.[5] It is important to remember that lamellated periosteal reaction may be seen with malignant tumors (especially Ewing sarcoma) and Codman triangle may be seen with benign lesions, such as osteo-myelitis or aneurismal bone cyst (ABC). Spiculated periosteal reaction is seen with aggressive tumors, with the orientation of the spicules resulting from the direction of tumor growth.

Flow voids correlate with pathologic vessels.[4] Hypervascular lesions, however, do not always demonstrate flow voids.

There are two different staging systems for bone tumors, and the reader is referred to the article by Yaw[6] for further discussion.

MALIGNANT TUMORS

About 6% of all childhood malignancies are malignant bone tumors, most commonly osteosarcoma and Ewing sarcoma.[7]

Osteosarcoma

Osteosarcoma (**Figs. 1** and **2**) is the most common primary malignant bone tumor in children.[8] Usually, the patient is an adolescent (second decade) with a painful mass. Serum alkaline phosphatase levels are elevated in about half of cases.[6] Boys are affected twice as often as girls. There is an increased risk of osteosarcoma in patients with retinoblastoma, Li-Fraumeni syndrome, and those with prior radiation therapy. Multifocal osteosarcoma may rarely be seen in children.

Osteosarcoma may be pathologically described as osteoblastic, chondroblastic, or fibroblastic based on the predominant tissue element within the tumor.[9] It may be further subtyped as giant cell-rich, telangiectatic, or small cell. Most children, however, have conventional, high-grade osteosarcoma.[6] Alterations in the tumor suppressor genes p53, RD, and the MDM2 oncogene are found in about half of patients with osteosarcoma.[10] In addition, heterozygosity for chromosomes 3q, 13q, and 18q may be found.

Pediatric osteosarcoma is usually metaphyseal and medullary in origin. The most common sites include (in order) the distal femur, proximal tibia, proximal humerus, pelvis, jaw, fibula, and ribs.[6] The tumor is characterized by production of bone. On plain radiographs, it may be a lytic, blastic, or mixed aggressive bony lesion, typically of large size, with indistinct margins, cortical destruction, aggressive periosteal reaction (Codman triangle or sunburst), and a soft tissue mass. Pathologic fracture is uncommon,[6] except in the rare telangiectatic osteosarcoma.[11]

About 20% of children with osteosarcoma have detectable metastases at presentation,[3] most frequently within the lung. High-resolution CT examination of the thorax is necessary in the initial evaluation of these patients.

Osteosarcoma is usually hypointense on T1-weighted images, and hyperintense on STIR imaging (see **Figs. 1** and **2**). The neoplastic bone is dark on all imaging sequences.[3] The longitudinal extent of the soft tissue mass usually matches that of the intramedullary tumor.[3] Marrow and soft

---

Box 1

Typical skeletal locations of pediatric primary bone tumors

Small tubular bones

Enchondroma

Osteoid osteoma

Long tubular bones

Most benign and malignant bone tumors and tumor-like lesions

Metastases

Ribs

Cartilaginous tumors

Ewing sarcoma

Fibrous dysplasia

Langerhans cell histiocytosis

Metastases

Spine: vertebral body

Giant cell tumor

Lymphoma

Langerhans cell histiocytosis

Hemangioma

Chordoma

Metastases

Spine: posterior elements

Osteoblastoma, osteoid osteoma

Aneurysmal bone cyst

Skull and facial bones

Fibrous dysplasia

Osteoma

Langerhans cell histiocytosis

Metastases

Pelvis

Osteochondroma

Fibrous dysplasia

Ewing sarcoma

Chondrosarcoma

Metastases

Box 2

Common location of pediatric primary bone tumors and tumor-like lesions

Epiphysis

Chondroblastoma

Metaphysis

Giant cell tumor

Aneurismal bone cyst

Unicameral bone cyst

Fibrous dysplasia

Osteochondroma

Enchondroma

Chondromyxoid fibroma

Nonossifying fibroma

Osteosarcoma

Malignant fibrous histiocytoma

Ewing sarcoma

Lymphoma

Metastases

Diaphysis

Osteoid osteoma

Ewing sarcoma

Lymphoma

Adamantinoma

Osteofibrous dysplasia

---

tissue edema, sometimes massive, may be seen.[10] Skip lesions may be present in up to 15% of patients. Fluid-fluid levels (FFL) are typical in the telangiectatic variety,[11] suggesting tumoral hemorrhage.

The tumor burden, measured by tumor size at diagnosis, correlates with response to chemotherapy and with survival,[8,12] but histologic response (indicated by percent necrosis) to preoperative chemotherapy is the strongest prognostic factor.[13–15] The soft tissue mass of an osteosarcoma tends to ossify with treatment, however, and the tumor size remains unchanged.[16] Further, the intramedullary tumor margins may become blurred by the yellow to red marrow conversion resulting from granulocyte-stimulating factor.[17] Not surprisingly, there is significant interobserver variability in the subjective assessment of tumor necrosis by MR imaging.[16] Functional imaging studies are useful quantitatively to assess tumor response to neoadjuvant therapy. Apparent diffusion coefficients increase with the development of tumoral necrosis.[18] Dynamic contrast-enhanced MR imaging measures tumor viability based on the accumulation of gadolinium within the tumor. The dynamic vector magnitude is a dynamic contrast-enhanced MR imaging measurement calculated from the contrast accumulation rate over time and maximal intensity of the tumor. Using a threshold dynamic vector magnitude of 1.8, those with a high dynamic

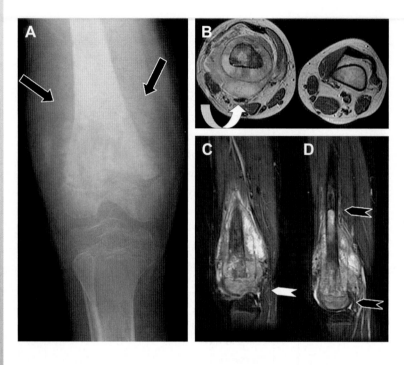

Fig. 1. Ten-year-old boy who has osteosarcoma of the distal femur. (A) The plain radiograph shows a destructive, permeative metaphyseal bone tumor with an associated soft tissue mass and proliferation of osteoid (*black arrows*). (B) Axial T2-weighted fat-saturated image shows the marrow replacement, cortical destruction, and soft tissue extent of the tumor The popliteal vessels are displaced posteriorly by the mass (*curved arrow*). (C, D) Sagittal fat-saturated postgadolinium images show enhancement of the tumor, and its superior extent to the distal diaphysis (no skip lesions were seen more proximally), and distal extent to involve the epiphysis (*black arrowheads*), and knee joint space (*white arrowhead*).

vector magnitude are poor responders (<90% necrosis), whereas those with low dynamic vector magnitude are good responders (>90% necrosis).[16] Kep is the measure of the exchange of gadolinium between the vascular space (plasma) and the interstitial space. A high Kep at diagnosis (suggesting that gadolinium, and so chemotherapy, can get into the tumor) tends to

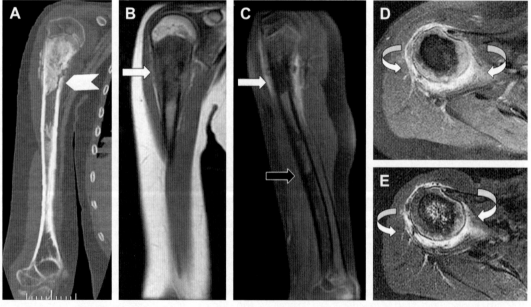

Fig. 2. Ten-year-old girl who has right proximal humeral osteosarcoma. (A) Coronal reformatted CT image shows the aggressive, metaphyseal osteoid-producing bone tumor with a pathologic fracture (*arrowhead*). (B) Coronal T1-weighted image demonstrates the tumor to be low signal intensity, including the relatively small soft tissue mass (*arrow*). (C) Sagittal STIR image again shows the soft tissue extension (*white arrow*) and medullary extension to the mid-diaphysis (*black arrow*). The epiphysis in this case was spared. Axial T2-weighted fat-saturated (D) and T1-weighted fat-saturated postgadolinium (E) images define the soft tissue extent of the tumor (*curved arrows*).

correlate with a favorable outcome,[13] as does a low Kep at week 9 of neoadjuvant therapy.[3,16]

Ewing Sarcoma

Ewing sarcoma (**Fig. 3**) is the second most common malignant bone tumor in children, and is predominantly seen in the second decade of life.[19] This highly malignant small blue round-cell tumor shows varying degrees of neuroectodermal differentiation. In greater than 85% of cases a balanced t(11:22) (q24:12) translocation is found.[20] This fuses the EWS gene with the FLI-1 gene, which is thought to then function as an abnormal transcription factor.[7] Ewing sarcoma is

more common in the white population. Males and females are equally affected. Patients usually present with local pain and swelling, and may also have constitutional symptoms. A palpable mass is usually present, and there may be overlying erythema.[6] An elevated white blood cell count and erythrocyte sedimentation rate may be seen.

The most common site of involvement by Ewing sarcoma is the pelvis, followed by the metadiaphysis of the long bones (femur > tibia > humerus > rib).[19] At plain film analysis, one sees a permeative, poorly marginated, mixed sclerotic and lytic bony diametaphyseal mass with significant cortical destruction and a surrounding (often extensive) noncalcified soft tissue mass.[1,19] Diaphyseal

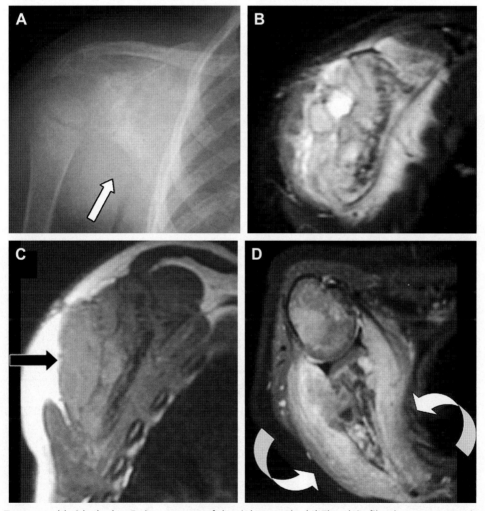

Fig. 3. Two-year-old girl who has Ewing sarcoma of the right scapula. (*A*) The plain film shows a permeative. lytic, destructive lesion of the scapula, with a very thin incomplete rim of immature periosteal reaction (*arrow*). A large soft tissue mass is seen surrounding the scapula. Oblique-sagittal T2-weighted fat-saturated (*B*), T1-weighted (*C*), and axial postgadolinium fat-saturated T1-weighted (*D*) images of the scapula show the inhomogeneous soft tissue mass (*black arrow, curved white arrows*) surrounding the tumor-infiltrated scapula. Feathery soft tissue edema is noted on the T2-weighted image.

tumors are typically central; those in the metaphysis are eccentrically located.[21] Epiphyseal extension is rare.[19] Aggressive periosteal reaction may be spiculated or onion peel in character.

MR imaging shows the mass to be heterogeneous and T1 isointense to mildly hypointense and T2 hyperintense; with a variable enhancement pattern.[19,22] Skip lesions are present in about 14%.[19] Joint involvement may be seen, but MR imaging may overestimate this because of inflammation of the synovium. Transverse T2-weighted images best display the interface between tumor and adjacent soft tissues and the relationship with neurovascular structures.

With radiotherapy or chemotherapy, the soft tissue mass decreases in size, and the intramedullary tumor undergoes myxoid degeneration. In addition, dynamic contrast-enhanced MR imaging may be used to differentiate tumor and necrosis.[3] Apparent diffusion coefficient also increases in areas of necrosis.[18]

In addition to assessment of the primary tumor site, imaging is performed to evaluate for metastatic disease, which occurs most commonly in the lungs, followed by bone and bone marrow.[2] CT is the preferred modality to evaluate for lung metastases.

Chondrosarcoma

Chondrosarcoma (**Fig. 4**) is an uncommon tumor in the pediatric population.[9] This tumor generally arises in large bones, including the pelvis and shoulder girdle, and the metaphysis of long bones, ribs, and spine. It may be primary or secondary. It is an osteolytic tumor that is expansile, destructive, and often large at presentation. Matrix calcification, if present, may be amorphous or chondroid in nature. At MR imaging, chondrosarcoma is often heterogeneous with overall low signal intensity on T1-weighted sequences, and overall low to intermediate signal intensity on T2-weighted images. The heterogeneity results from areas of calcification, intratumoral hemorrhage, and cystic change.[23] Bright signal on T2 images may correlate with hyaline cartilage islands.[24] Soft tissue extension may be seen, but marrow edema is

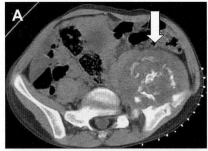

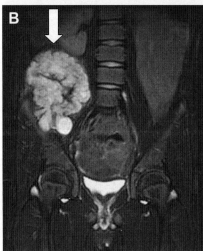

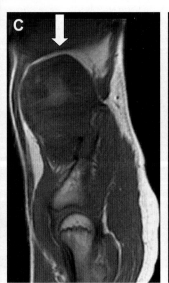

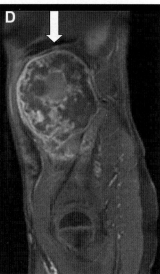

Fig. 4. Nineteen-year-old man who has left iliac wing primary chondrosarcoma. Axial CT (*A*), coronal T2-weighted fat-saturated (*B*), sagittal T1-weighted (*C*), and postgadolinium sagittal fat-saturated (*D*) images show the chondrosarcoma arising from the inner aspect of the iliac wing. There is a large soft tissue mass (*white arrows*) with chondroid calcifications, which is heterogeneous, but overall T2 hyperintense and T1 hypointense. Postenhancement, patchy central and peripheral tumor enhancement is seen.

underwhelming.[23] These tumors enhance following gadolinium administration, but the enhancement may also be heterogeneous.

Lymphoma

About 5% of children with lymphoma present with primary bone disease (**Fig. 5**), and most of these are high-grade, diffuse, large B-cell lymphomas.[9] The spine and diaphysis of long bones are the most common location for primary bone lymphoma in children. The imaging appearance is most commonly lytic and destructive, with associated layered periosteal reaction, but occasionally the bone lymphoma may be nearly undetectable on plain radiography.[25] Cortical breakthrough and sequestra are better seen by CT.

MR imaging shows low T1 signal intensity and high T2 signal of the involved bone marrow. Peritumoral edema may also be seen[25] as high signal on T2-weighted or STIR images. The tumor typically enhances after gadolinium. Surrounding soft tissue mass may be seen. One rather unique feature of small round cell tumors, such as lymphoma or Ewing sarcoma, may be a soft tissue mass without significant cortical destruction resulting from tumor cells growing through small cortical vascular channels.[25]

Malignant Fibrous Histiocytoma

Most cases of pediatric malignant fibrous histiocytoma (**Fig. 6**) occur in adolescence, but these are still very unusual tumors in the pediatric population. They are most commonly seen centrally within the metaphysis of a long bone. The tumor is lytic, and ranges from geographic to permeative. When geographic, they may mimic a nonaggressive tumor. Diaphyseal malignant fibrous histiocytoma tends to appear much more aggressive and permeative.[26] Unlike many other bone neoplasms, however, periosteal reaction is uncommonly seen in malignant fibrous histiocytoma.[26] The MR imaging features of this tumor are not specific, with T1 signal similar to muscle, and T2 hyperintensity, but MR imaging is again very useful in defining the extent and anatomic relationships of this neoplasm.

BENIGN TUMORS AND TUMOR-LIKE LESIONS
Cystic Lesions

Unicameral or simple bone cyst

Most simple bone cysts (**Fig. 7**) occur in the long tubular bones, especially the proximal humerus, proximal femur, and proximal tibia, and are seen in children between 9 and 15 years of age.[27]

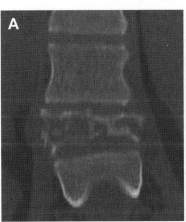
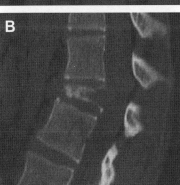
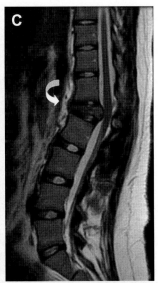
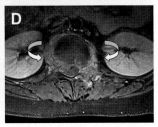

Fig. 5. Fifteen-year-old girl who has primary bony lymphoma of the L1 vertebra. Coronal (*A*) and sagittal (*B*) reformatted CT images show a collapsed L1 vertebra with a permeative, lytic destructive underlying lesion. A small adjacent noncalcified soft tissue mass is seen. Sagittal T2-weighted (*C*) and postgadolinium axial fat-saturated T1-weighted (*D*) images better define the soft tissue mass (*arrows*) and retropulsion of the posterior aspect of the vertebral body. Overall, the vertebral body marrow is T1 hypointense and T2 isointense, with predominantly enhancement seen within the soft tissue mass (*arrows*).

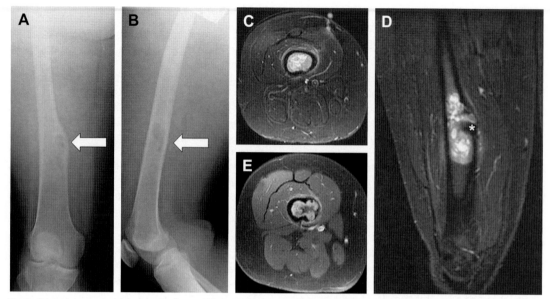

Fig. 6. Seventeen-year-old girl who has malignant fibrous histiocytoma of the diaphysis of the right femur. (*A, B*) Plain films demonstrate an eccentric sclerotic-rimmed geographic lytic lesion (*arrows*) with vague cortical destruction. Axial and coronal STIR (*C, D*) and axial postgadolinium (*E*) images better define the intramedullary extent of the mass. There is a small amount of T2 hyperintense and enhancing edema or inflammation surrounding the femur. The hypointense focus seen on the coronal image (*) is a postbiopsy artifact.

Patients usually present with pain caused by pathologic fracture. The lesion arises centrally in the metaphysis, but may extend into the diaphysis, and is a well-defined lytic expansile lesion that may show internal trabeculation, especially after prior fracture. A fallen fragment may be seen in the dependent part of the cyst after fracture through the cyst.[9]

At MR imaging the fluid-filled cyst is high signal on T2-weighted images,[9] and intermediate signal on T1-weighted images.[27] Simple bone cysts do not demonstrate FFLs.[27] Hemosiderin deposition may also be observed.[4] Fatty change may be seen within the cyst, especially in the calcaneus.[4]

Aneurysmal bone cyst

The name "aneurysmal bone cyst" is a misnomer. ABC are not true cysts, nor are they true aneurysms.[28] ABC consists of large vascular spaces, filled with blood and hemosiderin, and lined with giant cells.[27] ABC may be primary (**Fig. 8**), or may arise secondarily (**Fig. 9**) in a pre-existing benign or malignant bone lesion (eg, giant cell tumor (GCT), osteoblastoma, chondroblastoma, fibrous dysplasia, hemangioma, or nonossifying fibroma).[4,29] Patients usually present with pain or pathologic fracture during the second decade of life. They are most commonly found in the metaphyseal region of long bones (femur, tibia, and humerus); the pelvis; and the posterior elements

of vertebra.[4,27] They may be seen in any bone, however, and anywhere within the bone. Plain radiographs show a radiolucent, expansile mass without matrix production, but often with septations.[27]

ABC are low signal on T1-weighted images, and high signal on T2-weighted images,[27] with low signal fibrous tissue lining the spaces.[30] ABC are usually septated, and after gadolinium administration enhancement of the septations and "cyst" walls may be seen.[30,31] Surrounding soft tissue edema may be present. Although solid components may be present within ABC, the presence of solid tissue should alert the radiologist to consider a secondary ABC, or an alternative diagnosis (eg, osteosarcoma).[30]

FFL were first described in ABC, and result from separation of blood and serum in the cavernous spaces.[4] FFL may also result from hemorrhage with breakdown of blood products, however, or from tumor necrosis with sedimentation of cells and tissue fluid, and are not specific for the diagnosis of ABC;[1,4] they may be seen in both benign and malignant tumors (eg, osteoblastomas, osteoid osteomas, GCT, chondroblastomas, and osteosarcomas). As a general rule, however, lesions that are composed of greater than two thirds FFL are generally benign, whereas those that are less than one third FFL are often malignant.[4]

The MR imaging appearance of FFL varies based on the composition of the superior and

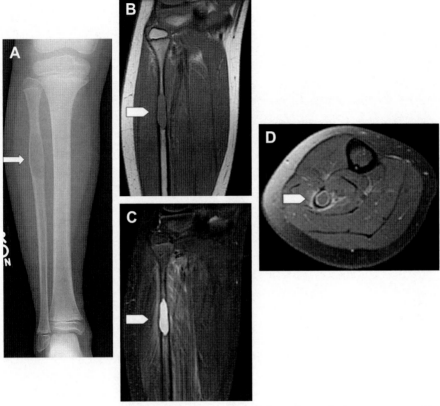

Fig. 7. Nine-year-old boy who has calf pain after trauma. (A) Plain radiograph shows a geographic, expansile, fibular proximal diaphyseal bone lesion without definite pathologic fracture (*arrowhead*). Coronal T1-weighted (B), coronal STIR (C), and axial postgadolinium fat-saturated (D) images show a T1 intermediate intensity and T2 hyperintense simple bone cyst (*arrowhead*). There is, however, surrounding edema and a small amount of enhancement in the adjacent soft tissues, likely posttraumatic. No fracture is seen.

inferior fluid, and the pulse sequences used.[4] On T1-weighted sequences high signal in the superior layer suggests methemoglobin and low signal serum. On T2-weighted sequences high signal in the superior layer suggests extracellular methemoglobin or serous fluid. The lower layer is usually isointense to slightly hyperintense to muscle on all sequences resulting from layering cellular debris or blood.

GIANT CELL TUMOR

GCT are very rare in children under 15 years of age,[9,32] and are seen more commonly in girls. Radiographically, these tumors are solitary, well-defined, eccentric lytic lesions usually located about the knee. They lack matrix calcification and have a nonsclerotic margin. Cortical thinning is common, but periosteal reaction is unusual. GCT are located in the metaphysis and do not cross the open physis,[32] but may extend to the subchondral bone if the physis is closed. At MR imaging, GCT

frequently demonstrates peripheral low signal on T1-weighted images and generalized hypointensity on T2-weighted images.[4,32] This T2-hypointensity may result from the tumor cellularity, or from recurrent hemorrhage within the lesion. In either case, it is a useful feature in characterizing this tumor. The solid portions of GCT enhance diffusely after gadolinium administration, whereas cystic components demonstrate a delicate septal and peripheral enhancement pattern.[32] Secondary ABC components are seen in about 14% of GCT (see **Fig. 9**).

CARTILAGINOUS LESIONS
Osteochondroma

Solitary osteochondroma (**Fig. 10**) is the most common benign tumor of bone in children,[33] and occurs more commonly in boys. Some question if this lesion is a tumor, or a developmental abnormality of physeal growth. Multiple hereditary exostoses (diaphyseal aclasis) is an autosomal-dominant disease characterized by multiple

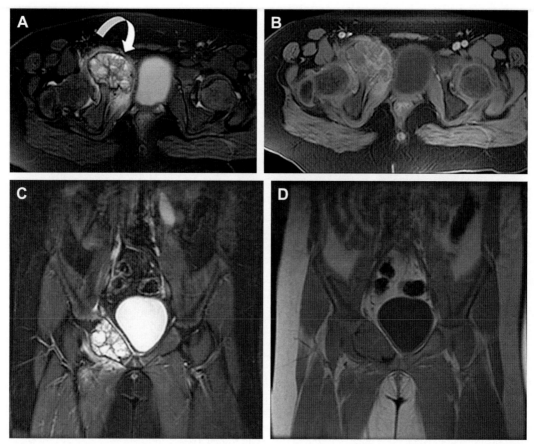

Fig. 8. Eight-year-old boy who has aneurysmal bone cyst of the right pubic bone. Axial T2-weighted fat-saturated (*A*), postgadolinium T1-weighted fat-saturated (*B*), coronal STIR (*C*), and coronal T1-weighted (*D*) images show the expansile, septated mass with multiple fluid-fluid levels (*curved arrow*). The "cystic" spaces are T1 isointense and T2 hyperintense. Enhancement is predominately along the septa. A small amount of surrounding soft tissue edema and inflammation is noted.

osteochondromas. Osteochondromas may also be found in the radiation field of children who have undergone radiation therapy.[9] Osteochondromas may grow during childhood, but should cease to grow when skeletal maturity is reached. Although often asymptomatic, symptoms may result from osseous deformity, adjacent vascular injury or neurologic compromise, fracture, or bursa formation. In about 1% of solitary and 5% to 25% of patients with multiple hereditary exostoses, malignant transformation to (often low grade) chondrosarcoma may occur.[4,30]

Osteochondromas develop in bone formed by enchondral ossification. In the long bones, these exostotic sessile or pedunculated lesions arise on the surface of the metaphysis and grow away from the nearest epiphysis. They are most commonly found about the knee or at the proximal humerus. The key imaging feature of osteochondroma is its continuity with the medullary cavity of the parent bone.[4] A cartilage cap, which is intermediate signal on T1-weighted images and high signal on T2-weighted or STIR images, may be seen. An overlying thin rim of low signal, representing the perichondrium, may be present.[4] In children, the cap may be thicker than in an adult. A cap greater than 3 cm in thickness in children or 2 cm in adults, however, should raise concern for malignant degeneration.[4,29,33] MR imaging, specifically axial T2-weighted or STIR images, is the best modality to measure the cartilage cap.[4,30] Other features worrisome for malignant change include increase in cap size after skeletal maturity, irregularity of the cap, multiple foci of calcification, soft tissue mass, irregular interface between the cartilage and the bone, or bony destruction.

Enchondroma

Enchondromas (**Fig. 11**) are the second most common benign tumor of bone in childhood,[9]

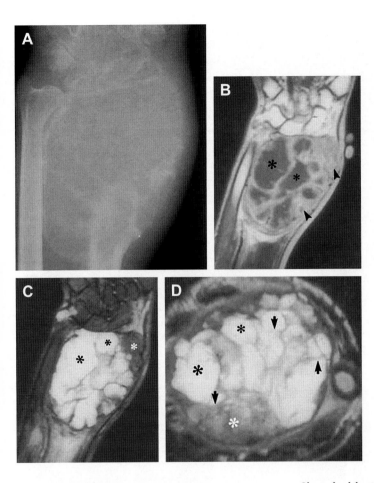

Fig. 9. Giant cell tumor of the distal radius with a large secondary ABC component in a 17-year-old girl. (*A*) Radiograph shows marked expansion caused by a multiloculated lytic lesion of the distal radius extending to sub-chondral bone. (*B*) Coronal contrast-enhanced T1-weighted image reveals diffuse enhancement of solid portions of the giant cell tumor (*arrowheads*) and peripheral enhancement about the ABC regions (*). Coronal (*C*) and axial (*D*) T2-weighted images reveal markedly increased signal intensity in the ABC areas (*black ***), with fluid levels (*arrows in D*) and low signal intensity in the small solid regions (*white ***). (*From* Murphey MD, Nomikos GC, Flemming DJ, et al. Imaging of giant cell tumor and giant cell reparative granuloma of bone: radiologic-pathologic correlation. Radiographics 2001;21:1283–309; with permission.)

and are characterized by formation of abundant mature hyaline cartilage. They are most commonly seen during the second decade, and are most frequently found in the small tubular bones of the hands and feet, but can arise in any bone. Ollier disease, or enchondromatosis, is a nonhereditary disease that results from abnormal production of growth plate cartilage leading to the development of multiple enchondromas. Maffucci syndrome consists of multiple enchondromas and hemangiomas.

Enchondromas are central, well-defined, expansile masses with endosteal scalloping. Chondroid calcifications may be seen. MR imaging usually shows a lobulated T1 hypointense and T2 hyperintense lesion.[33] Small foci of low signal may represent calcification. A chemical shift artifact may be noted. Contrast-enhanced images may show a "ring and arc" pattern, corresponding to fibrovascular tissue at the periphery of the avascular lobules of hyaline cartilage.[30]

Malignant transformation of enchondroma to (usually) chondrosarcoma may occur in up to 30% of patients who have Ollier disease or Maffucci syndrome.[9]

Chondroblastoma

Chondroblastoma (**Fig. 12**) is an uncommon benign primary cartilage tumor of the second and third decades of life.[34] This geographic epiphyseal or apophyseal medullary tumor is most commonly found in the femur, humerus, and tibia. It may extend into the adjacent metaphysis in about half of cases, or into the adjacent joint. MR imaging shows a lobulated, heterogeneous predominantly low T1 and variable (predominantly low) T2 signal lesion.[35] Matrix calcification is very low signal on both T1- and T2-weighted sequences, whereas islands of cartilage are T1 hypointense and T2 hyperintense. Other factors that may affect the T2 signal include tumor cellularity and the presence of an associated ABC. A characteristic peripheral thin (<1 mm) hypointense rim (which may be incomplete) corresponds to marginal sclerosis seen with this tumor.[35] Associated marrow edema, best seen on STIR images, is common and may be extensive,[33,35] and soft tissue edema may also be present. After gadolinium administration, lobular enhancement is seen in about 60% of cases.[34] The presence of septal enhancement should suggest an associated ABC.

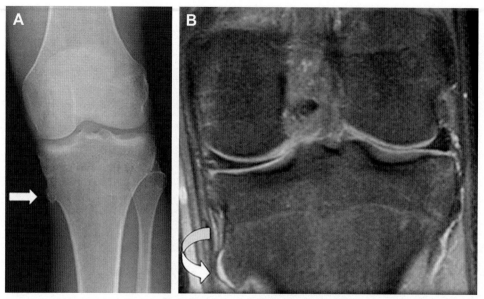

Fig. 10. Osteochondroma of a 16-year-old boy being evaluated after knee trauma. (*A*) Plain radiograph shows a small medial proximal tibial bony exostosis (*arrow*). (*B*) Coronal proton density fat-saturated image shows continuity of the medullary marrow, and the bright cartilage cap (*arrow*).

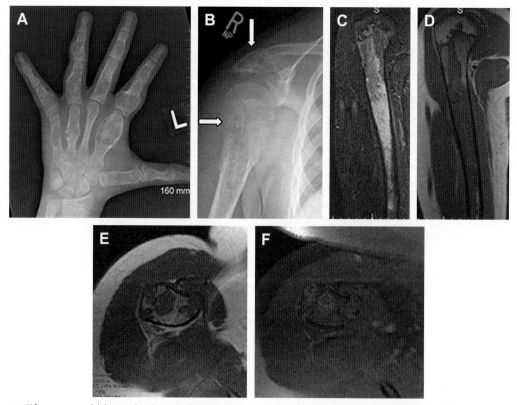

Fig. 11. Fifteen-year-old boy who has enchondromatosis. (*A*) Frontal radiograph of the hand shows extensive multiple expansile lytic enchondromas. (*B*) Multiple enchondromas are also seen at the right proximal humerus and right scapula (*arrows*). Sagittal T1-weighted (*C*) and STIR (*D*) images define the extent of the humeral enchondroma, which is predominantly low signal on T1 images and high signal on STIR. Axial pregadolinium (*E*) and postgadolinium (*F*) images demonstrate cartilage nodules with rim enhancement.

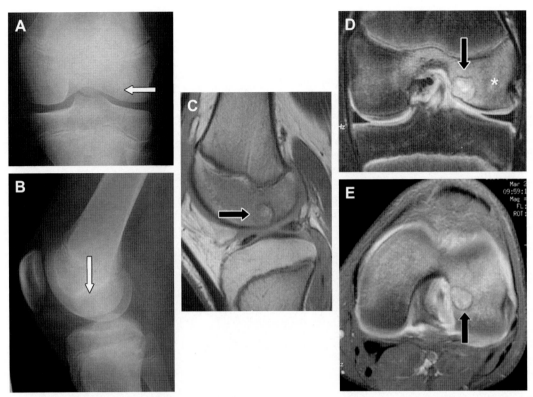

Fig. 12. Chondroblastoma. Frontal (*A*) and lateral (*B*) radiographs demonstrate a well-defined lytic round epiphyseal lesion at the distal lateral femur (*arrow*). Sagittal T1 (*C*), coronal T2 fat-saturated (*D*), and axial postgadolinium fat-saturated (*E*) MR images show the chondroblastoma (*arrow*) with a rim of hypointensity on all pulse sequences. Adjacent marrow edema and inflammation (*) is noted.

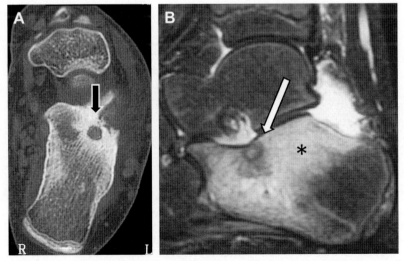

Fig. 13. Twelve-year-old boy who has calcaneal osteoid osteoma. (*A*) Noncontrast CT shows a well-defined hypodense nidus (*arrow*) with surrounding bony sclerosis at the anterolateral calcaneus. (*B*) Sagittal T2-weighted fat-saturated image shows an intermediate-intensity nidus (*arrow*) with marked adjacent marrow edema (*). An ankle joint effusion is also noted. (*Courtesy of* John Hunter, MD, Sacramento, CA.)

OSSEOUS LESIONS
Osteoid Osteoma

Osteoid osteoma (**Fig. 13**) is a benign tumor most common in the second decade of life, and more common in boys. This hypervascular tumor composed of primitive woven bone and osteoid is painful, with the pain typically described as worse at night and relieved by aspirin.[9,36] It is found most commonly in the shafts of tubular bones, with the femur and tibia being most common. It may also be seen in the posterior elements of the vertebra.

Radiographically, this tumor is characterized by intense osteosclerotic thickening of the cortex in which a paracortical radiolucent nidus (<1.5–2 cm) may be seen. At MR imaging, the cortical thickening is very hypointense on all pulse sequences.[33] The nidus varies in signal intensity from isointense to muscle on T1-weighted images and high signal on T2-weighted images, to low signal on all pulse sequences depending on the amount of matrix production and osteoid,[29,30] and enhances with gadolinium. Edema, often very prominent, in the marrow or soft tissues is high signal on STIR or T2-weighted sequences.[33]

Osteoblastoma

Osteoblastoma (**Fig. 14**) differs from osteoid osteoma in that the nidus is greater than 1.5 to 2 cm in diameter. These tumors also show greater

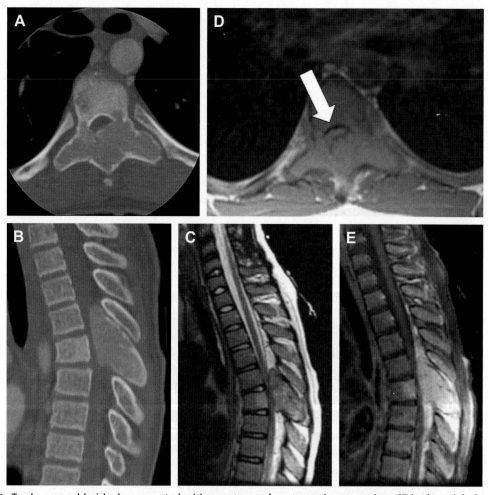

Fig. 14. Twelve-year-old girl who presented with symptoms of acute cord compression. CT in the axial plane (*A*) and sagittal reformatted images (*B*) show an expansile mass with hazy osteoid involving predominantly the posterior elements of the T6 vertebral body. There is associated narrowing of the spinal canal, and a focal thoracic kyphosis at the level of the tumor. Sagittal T2-weighted image (*C*), axial T1-weighted image (*D*), and sagittal postgadolinium fat-saturated image (*E*) demonstrate the expansile posterior element T6 osteoblastoma, which is slightly T1 hyperintense, T2 heterogeneous, and which enhances after gadolinium. There is probably a mixture of marrow edema and tumor extension into the back of the vertebral body. Cord compression (*arrow*) is noted.

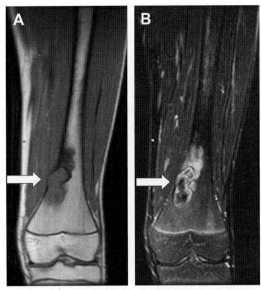

Fig. 15. Nonossifying fibroma. Coronal T1-weighted (*A*) and T2-weighted fat-saturated (*B*) images of this teenage boy (who has neurofibromatosis) show a T1 hypointense to isointense cortically based lobular mass (*arrow*), which is heterogeneous on T2-weighted images.

histologic variability.[30] The MR imaging appearance is variable depending on the amount of matrix and osteoid development. As with osteoid osteoma, there is often prominent surrounding edema. In the spinal posterior elements osteoblastoma may present as an osteolytic expansile tumor with shell-like periosteal reaction. MR imaging can define epidural or paraneural tumor extent, but may overestimate the size of the lesion because there may be intense inflammatory

response and enhancement that may extend over several vertebral levels.[29,30] A secondary ABC may be associated with osteoblastoma, and may result in a cystic appearance with FFL.

FIBRO-OSSEOUS LESIONS
Nonossifying Fibroma and Fibrous Cortical Defect

Nonossifying fibromas (**Fig. 15**) and fibrous cortical defects are common in children and adolescents, and are usually a painless, incidental finding. They regress over time, and are not seen after 25 years of age.[29] There is an association between multiple nonossifying fibromas and neurofibromatosis. Nonossifying fibromas and fibrous cortical defects are eccentric, well-defined, and cortically based lesions with marginal sclerosis.[36] Fibrous cortical defects measure less than 2 cm in size, whereas nonossifying fibromas are larger. At MR imaging, they are low signal intensity on T1-weighted images. T2 signal varies based on the degree of hypercellular fibrous tissue, with high signal intensity seen during the development of these lesions, and low signal intensity as the lesions heal.[4,33] After gadolinium administration, a thin, hyperintense rim is seen.[29]

Fibrous Dysplasia

Fibrous dysplasia (**Fig. 16**) is a nonhereditary developmental abnormality of bone[9] composed of cellular fibrous tissue and irregular bone trabeculae. Most cases are monostotic and asymptomatic, but about one fifth of cases are polyostotic. In McCune-Albright syndrome, one sees polyostotic fibrous dysplasia with precocious puberty

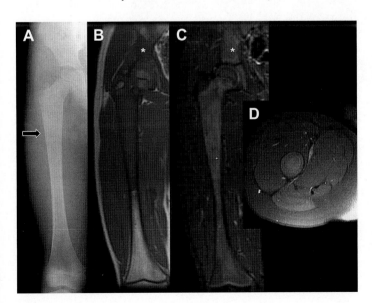

Fig. 16. Five-year-old boy who has polyostotic fibrous dysplasia. (*A*) Frontal radiograph demonstrates the classical ground-glass opacity and mild bony expansion of the proximal femoral metaphysis and diaphysis (*arrow*). Near the femoral neck, the lesion is more lytic appearing. Coronal T1-weighted (*B*), STIR (*C*), and axial postgadolinium (*D*) images show this marrow-based lesion is T1 hypointense, predominantly T2 hyperintense, and shows homogeneous enhancement. Note the multifocal lesions also involving the iliac wing (*). This patient went on to develop a shepherd crook deformity about 4 years later.

and endocrine dysfunction. Lesions of fibrous dysplasia become quiescent at puberty.[37]

Fibrous dysplasia may develop in any bone. Radiographically, fibrous dysplasia is a well-defined, often sclerotic-rimmed, expansile ground-glass lesion that may have endosteal scalloping.[37] If the lesion contains a significant amount of cartilage, popcorn-like or more confluent calcification may be seen.

MR imaging is better at defining the extent of fibrous dysplasia. It is a sharply defined intramedullary lesion with no evidence of cortical destruction that is T1 hypointense to isointense and T2 hyperintense but inhomogeneous. This inhomogeneity results from areas of calcification, cysts, fatty areas, or septations. The lesions are typically surrounded by a rim of hypointense signal on all pulse sequences, corresponding to the sclerotic rim seen by plain radiography.[37] Enhancement varies from rim to patchy to homogeneous.

The main complications of fibrous dysplasia are deformity or pathologic fracture. Malignant sarcomatous degeneration is quite rare.

Osteofibrous Dysplasia

Osteofibrous dysplasia (**Fig. 17**) is seen in young children who present with painless anterior bowing of the tibia (or rarely fibula), which may be associated with a mass.[29] This lesion arises in the anterior cortex of the diaphysis and slowly spreads longitudinally. It is cortically based, loculated, and expansile with sclerotic margins. Periosteal reaction is absent unless pathologic fracture has occurred. The MR imaging appearance includes T1 hyperintensity compared with muscle, and high signal on T2-weighted images.[38] Surrounding soft tissues seem normal.

VASCULAR LESIONS

Most vascular lesions rarely present as primary bone tumors in the pediatric population.[9]

Hemangioma

Less than 5% of hemangiomas are detected in children and adolescents.[39] Hemangiomas are most frequently seen in the spine or skull,[30] and are discovered incidentally. They are composed of capillaries and vascular spaces lying between the bony trabeculae. The MR imaging appearance of a hemangioma depends on the proportions of lipomatous tissue and vascular elements.[30] Fatty elements are high signal intensity on T1-weighted sequences, intermediate to high signal on T2-weighted sequences, and low signal on STIR or fat-suppressed sequences.[39] Vascular elements are low signal on T1-weighted images, and high signal on T2 or STIR imaging. Contrast enhancement after gadolinium may be moderate to marked.

OTHER
Histiocytosis

Langerhans cell histiocytosis results from an abnormal proliferation of antigen- presenting

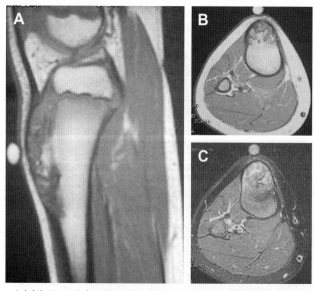

Fig. 17. Sagittal (*A*) and axial (*B*) T1-weighted, and axial T2-weighted (*C*) MR images show an anterior cortical metadiaphyseal tibial mass that is heterogeneous but overall T1 hypointense and T2 hyperintense in this 5-year-old child with osteofibrous dysplasia. The mass is marked anteriorly by a vitamin E capsule.

histiocytes, or Langerhans cells.[40,41] The etiology is unknown. Patients may be asymptomatic, or may develop bone pain.[9] Early in the course of the disease, there is an inflammatory infiltrate within the lesion, followed by a granulomatous phase, and lastly a fibrous phase.[40] Solitary bony lesions occur more commonly than multifocal disease.[9] The lesions may arise in any bone, but the skull (**Fig. 18**), jaw, ribs, vertebral bodies, and proximal long bones are most often affected. Extraskeletal involvement may include the liver, spleen, lymph nodes, and lungs.[41]

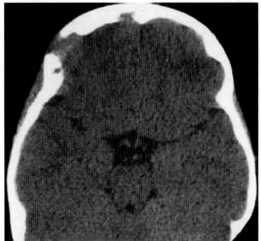

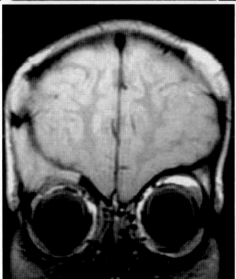

Fig. 18. Langerhans cell histiocytosis. Unenhanced axial CT showing beveled edge appearance of the lytic right frontal lesion, and the associated high density soft-tissue component in this child with histiocytosis. Coronal proton density MR image shows bilateral frontal high signal bony and soft tissue masses. (*From* Willatt JMG, Quaghebeur G. Calvarial masses of infants and children: a radiological approach. Clin Radiol 2004;59:474–86; with permission.)

Bony Langerhans cell histiocytosis may vary on plain film from well-defined ovoid osteolytic lesions without surrounding sclerosis, to large lytic lesions, to poorly defined permeative lesions.[9] MR imaging best demonstrates the bone marrow involvement, soft tissue mass, and inflammation.[40,42] The lesions are focal, variable on T1-weighted images, and hyperintense on T2 and STIR images.[40,42,43] Early in the course of the disease, the lesions markedly enhance after gadolinium administration.[40] A bony sequestration may be seen. Lesions outside the skull may show surrounding marrow soft tissue edema,[40,43] best seen on STIR images. Cortical breech and soft tissue masses may also be seen. Vertebral plana may be present with vertebral involvement. An important differential feature is noninvolvement of the adjacent disks with this disease.[40]

Whole-body coronal MR imaging including STIR and T1 sequences is better than skeletal survey or bone scintigraphy in delineation of extent of disease.[41,44] Some have also found postgadolinium whole-body coronal MR imaging helpful.

MR imaging also is able to demonstrate healing within the lesion,[41,44] seen as decrease in T2 signal, size, and contrast enhancement. A visible endosteal rim of decreased signal intensity on STIR imaging suggests early healing with marginal sclerosis.[42] Marrow and soft tissue edema also resolve with healing.[40]

SUMMARY

This article has reviewed the MR imaging features of both benign and malignant tumors and tumor-like conditions of the pediatric skeleton with focus on their MR imaging features. Although the plain radiographic features remain the primary tool for the initial analysis of a pediatric bony neoplasm, MR imaging plays an important role. MR imaging offers superior assessment of the extent of bony, intramedullary, joint, and soft tissue involvement by the tumor. Certain anatomic MR imaging features, discussed previously, can also help to define the neoplasm. Recent advances in functional imaging (dynamic contrast-enhanced MR imaging, apparent diffusion coefficient, and so forth) allow improved analysis of tumor response to therapy.

REFERENCES

1. Vade A, Eissenstadt R, Schaff HB. MRI of aggressive bone lesions of childhood. Magn Reson Imaging 1992;10:89–96.
2. Meyer JS, Nadel HR, Marina N, et al. Imaging guidelines for children with Ewing sarcoma and

osteosarcoma: a report from the Children's Oncology Group Bone Tumor Committee. Pediatr Blood Cancer 2008;51:163–70.

3. Hoffer FA. Primary skeletal neoplasms: osteosarcoma and Ewing sarcoma. Top Magn Reson Imaging 2002;13:231–40.

4. Alyas F, James SL, Davies AM, et al. The role of MR imaging in the diagnostic characterization of appendicular bone tumours and tumour-like conditions. Eur Radiol 2007;17:2675–86.

5. Wenaden AET, Szyszkoa TA, Saifuddina A. Imaging of periosteal reactions associated with focal lesions of bone. Clin Radiol 2005;60:439–56.

6. Yaw KM. Pediatric bone tumors. Semin Surg Oncol 1999;16:173–83.

7. Caudill JSC, Arndt CAS. Diagnosis and management of bone malignancy in adolescence. Adolesc Med 2007;18:62–78.

8. Longhi A, Errani C, De Paolis M, et al. Primary bone osteosarcoma in the pediatric age: state of the art. Cancer Treat Rev 2006;32:423–36.

9. Vlychou M, Athanasou N. Radiological and pathological diagnosis of paediatric bone tumours and tumour-like lesions. Pathology 2008;40(2):196–216.

10. Weiss A, Khoury JD, Hoffer FA, et al. Telangiectatic osteosarcoma: the St. Jude Children's Research Hospital's experience. Cancer 2007;109:1627–37.

11. Arndt AS, Crist WM. Common musculoskeletal tumors of childhood and adolescence. N Engl J Med 1999;341:342–52.

12. Kaste SC, Liu T, Billups CA, et al. Tumor size as predictor of outcome in pediatric nonmetastatic osteosarcoma of the extremity. Pediatr Blood Cancer 2004;43:723–8.

13. Reddick WE, Wang S, Xiong X, et al. Dynamic magnetic resonance imaging of regional contrast access as an additional prognostic factor in pediatric osteosarcoma. Cancer 2001;91:2230–7.

14. Bacci G, Ferrari S, Bertoni F, et al. Histologic response of high-grade nonmetastatic osteosarcoma of the extremity to chemotherapy. Clin Orthop Relat Res 2001;386:186–96.

15. Provisor AJ, Ettinger LJ, Nachman JB, et al. Treatment of nonmetastatic osteosarcoma of the extremity with preoperative and postoperative chemotherapy: a report from the Children's Cancer Group. J Clin Oncol 1997;15:76–84.

16. McCarville MB. New frontiers in pediatric oncologic imaging. Cancer Imaging 2008;8:87–92.

17. Fletcher BD, Wall JE, Hanna SL. Effect of hematopoietic growth factors on MR images of bone marrow in children undergoing chemotherapy. Radiology 1993;189:745–51.

18. Hayashida Y, Yakushiji T, Awai K, et al. Monitoring therapeutic responses of primary bone tumors by diffusion-weighted image: initial results. Eur Radiol 2006;16:2637–43.

19. Peersman B, Vanhoenakcker FM, Heyman S, et al. Ewing's sarcoma: imaging features. JBR-BTR 2007;90:368–76.

20. Szuhai K, Ijszenga M, Tanke HJ, et al. Molecular cytogenetic characterization of four previously established and two newly established Ewing sarcoma cell lines. Cancer Genet Cytogenet 2006;166:173–9.

21. Laor T, Jaramillo D, Oestreich AE. Musculoskeletal system. In: Kirks DR, Griscom NT, editors. Practical pediatric imaging: diagnostic radiology of infants and children. 3rd edition. Philadelphia: Lippincott-Raven; 1998. p. 328–510.

22. Mar WA, Taljanovic MS, Bagatell R, et al. Update on imaging and treatment of Ewing sarcoma family tumors: what the radiologist needs to know. J Comput Assist Tomogr 2008;32:108–18.

23. Collins M, Koyama T, Swee RG, et al. Clear cell chondrosarcoma: radiographic, computed tomographic and magnetic resonance findings in 34 patients with pathologic correlation. Skeletal Radiol 2003;32:687–94.

24. Kaim AH, Hugli R, Bonel HM, et al. Chondroblastoma and clear cell chondrosarcoma: radiological and MRI characteristics with histopathological correlation. Skeletal Radiol 2002;31:88–95.

25. Krishnan A, Shirkhoda A, Tehrznzadeh J, et al. Primary bone lymphoma: radiographic-MR imaging correlation. Radiographics 2003;23:1371–87.

26. Murphey MD, Gross TM, Rosenthal HG. Musculoskeletal malignant fibrous histiocytoma: radiologic-pathologic correlation. Radiographics 1994;14:807–26.

27. Sullivan RJ, Meyer JS, Dormans JP, et al. Diagnosing aneurysmal and unicameral bone cysts with magnetic resonance imaging. Clin Orthop Relat Res 1999;(366):186–90.

28. Bollini G, Jouve JL, Cottalorda J, et al. Aneurysmal bone cyst in children: analysis of twenty-seven patients. J Pediatr Orthop B 1998;7:274–85.

29. Azouz EM. Magnetic resonance imaging of benign bone lesions: cysts and tumors. Top Magn Reson Imaging 2002;13:219–29.

30. Woertler K. Benign bone tumors and tumor-like lesions: value of cross-sectional imaging. Eur Radiol 2003;13:1820–35.

31. Mahnken AH, Nolte-Ernsting CCA, Wildberger JE, et al. Aneurysmal bone cyst: value of MR imaging and conventional radiography. Eur Radiol 2003;13:1118–24.

32. Murphey MD, Nomikos GC, Flemming DJ, et al. Imaging of giant cell tumor and giant cell reparative granuloma of bone: radiologic-pathologic correlation. Radiographics 2001;21:1283–309.

33. Stacy GS, Heck RK, Peabody TD, et al. Neoplastic and tumorlike lesions detected on MR imaging of the knee in patients with suspected internal derangement: part 1, intraosseous entities. Am J Roentgenol 2002;178:589–94.

34. Jee WH, Park YK, McCauley TR, et al. Chondroblastoma: MR characteristics with pathologic correlation. J Comput Assist Tomogr 1999;23:721–6.

35. Oxtoby JW, Davies AM. MRI characteristics of chondroblastoma. Clin Radiol 1996;51:22–6.

36. Yildiz C, Erler K, Altesalp AS, et al. Benign bone tumors in children. Curr Opin Pediatr 2003;15:58–67.

37. Shah ZK, Peh WCG, Koh WL, et al. Magnetic resonance imaging appearances of fibrous dysplasia. Br J Radiol 2005;78:1104–15.

38. Dominguez R, Saucedo J, Fenstermacher M. MRI findings in osteofibrous dysplasia. Magn Reson Imaging 1989;7:567–70.

39. Ma LD. Magnetic resonance imaging of musculoskeletal tumours: skeletal and soft tissue masses. Curr Probl Diagn Radiol 1999;28:33–62.

40. DeSchepper AMA, Ramon F, Van Marck E. MR imaging of eosinophilic granuloma: report of 11 cases. Skeletal Radiol 1993;22:163–6.

41. Goo HW, Yang DH, Ra YS, et al. Whole-body MRI of langerhans cell histiocytosis: comparison with radiography and bone scintigraphy. Pediatr Radiol 2006;36:1019–31.

42. Davies AM, Pikoulas C, Griffith J. MRI of eosinophilic granuloma. Eur J Radiol 1994;18:205–9.

43. Beltran J, Aparisi F, Bonmati LM, et al. Eosinophilic granuloma: MRI manifestations. Skeletal Radiol 1993;22:157–61.

44. Steinborn M, Wortler K, Nathrath M, et al. [Whole-body MRI in children with langerhans cell histiocytosis for the evaluation of the skeletal system]. Rofo 2008;180:646–53 [in German].

MR Imaging of Soft Tissue Masses in Children

Rebecca Stein-Wexler, MD

KEYWORDS

- MR imaging • Soft tissue mass • Soft tissue tumor
- Pediatric

In approaching a child who has a soft tissue mass, clinical history and physical examination (including lesion location) play a critical role in diagnosis, and patient age also can narrow the differential. The typical presenting complaint is a palpable mass; larger masses are more likely to present with pain. Reactive processes and benign neoplasms are the most common lesions, whereas malignant tumors are rare. Radiography and CT offer limited assistance, being most useful for characterization of calcification or ossification, as in myositis ossificans. Ultrasonography can be helpful in the evaluation of small, superficial masses and in determining the cystic nature of some lesions. In general, however, MR imaging provides the most information, determining lesion extent and, in some cases, specific diagnoses.

MR imaging sometimes provides definitive diagnosis of common benign lesions. The most common benign lesions are hemangioma/lymphangioma, lipoma, periarticular cyst, inflammatory masses, fat necrosis, neurofibroma, and giant cell tumor of the tendon sheath.[1] Coincidentally, this list correlates well with those lesions for which definitive diagnosis at MR imaging is possible: hemangioma, lymphangioma, and other vascular tumors; lipoma; periarticular cysts; hematoma; giant cell tumor of the tendon sheath; benign neural tumors; and fat necrosis.

Many benign and malignant soft tissue masses have common imaging characteristics.[2–5] Many lesions are iso- or hypointense to muscle on T1-weighted (T1-W) imaging and hyperintense on T2-weighted (T2-W) imaging. Although some investigators have found MR imaging capable of determining the benignity of specific lesions

(discussed previously), accuracy often is uncertain, necessitating biopsy. When MR imaging appearance is nondiagnostic, benign origin may be more likely if a patient is less than 20 years old, the mass measures less than 10 cm, its position is subcutaneous or fascial, and it appears well circumscribed, homogeneous on T2-W imaging, and with no surrounding edema.[6] Enhancement characteristics may facilitate diagnosis of malignant lesions, which may show less rapid enhancement and more rapid washout.[7] MR imaging also defines the cystic nature of some lesions, provided T1 and T2 characteristics are evaluated carefully and contrast is administered in equivocal cases.[8] Only 1% to 6% of soft tissue masses are malignant.[1] Of the malignant tumors in the 0- to 5-year age group, fibrosarcoma is most common, followed by rhabdomyosarcoma. In the older age group, 6 to 15 years old, malignant fibrous histiocytoma is most common, followed by synovial sarcoma and rhabdomyosarcoma.[9]

Even when MR imaging fails to differentiate between benignity and malignancy or provide a tissue diagnosis of a malignant tumor, it does provide essential information, delineating the extent of the lesion, extension beyond facial planes, and involvement of adjacent structures, such as the neurovascular bundle, joints, and bone. It also is useful in assessing response to therapy, although differentiation of residual or recurrent tumor from postoperative edema, hemorrhage, or inflammation often is difficult.[10] If high T2-W signal is present without mass effect, differential considerations include seroma, hematoma, postradiation change, packing material, fat necrosis, or hygromas.[1] Mass effect increases

Department of Radiology, University of California, Davis, 4860 Y Street, Suite 3100, Sacramento, CA 95817, USA
E-mail address: rebecca.steinwexler@ucdmc.ucdavis.edu

Magn Reson Imaging Clin N Am 17 (2009) 489–507
doi:10.1016/j.mric.2009.03.009

concern for tumor recurrence,[1] as does gadolineum enhancement.[10]

MR IMAGING TECHNIQUE

The goal of MR imaging is to evaluate the entire lesion with as small and tight a coil as possible and to image with as small a field of view possible, within the limitation of obtaining adequate signal to noise. T1 and fat-suppressed T2 sequences in at least two orthogonal planes provide essential information. Coronal T1 sequences reveal contour changes and signal alterations due to the presence of fat or hemorrhage, although the lesion itself usually is poorly defined, often iso- or slightly hypointense to muscle. At T2-W sequences, the lesion and adjacent edema are hyperintense; thus, there is excellent contrast with adjacent tissues, delineating lesion extent, along with peritumoral edema. This allows determination of encasement of the neurovascular bundle, extension to bone, and the presence of tumor within nearby joints. Gadolinium rarely helps narrow the differential diagnosis, but it can provide important information regarding the cystic or solid nature of the lesion, and it also can help locate viable tissue for biopsy. Gradient-recalled echo imaging may help assess the presence of high flow, which assists in differentiation of vascular lesions; it also helps define adjacent vasculature. Occasionally, magnetic resonance angiography or magnetic resonance venography provides similar assistance and may simplify preoperative planning.

BENIGN PROCESSES: SOFT TISSUE MASSES
Fibrous Lesions

Many kinds of fibrous tumors occur in children, and all except for fibrosarcoma are benign. In general, these tumors are more common in boys.[11] Infantile myofibromatosis and desmoid tumor are the most common,[12] with the former usually diagnosed during the first year of life and the latter during the second decade. Fibromatosis colli and fibrous hamartoma of infancy are also discussed, but a thorough discussion of the less common fibrous lesions is beyond the scope of this article.

Fibromatosis Colli

Fibromatosis colli presents as fusiform or eccentric expansion of the sternocleidomastoid muscle. Found in approximately 0.4% of infants,[13] it usually presents at age 2 or 3 weeks with a firm anterior neck mass, often on the right, rarely bilateral, and sometimes followed by development of torticollis.[14] The mass typically increases in size over the course of several weeks and in 90% of cases resolves spontaneously during the next 4 to 8 months.[13] Cause is uncertain. There often is a history of birth trauma,[15] but pathologic evaluation demonstrates myoblasts, fibroblasts, and myofibroblasts in various stages of differentiation,[16] arguing for a developmental origin. The younger the baby, the more immature the cells appear.[16]

Ultrasound usually is diagnostic, demonstrating well-defined, unilateral, fusiform expansion of the sternocleidomastoid muscle. At MR imaging, the mass is isointense to muscle on T1-W images and hyperintense on T2-W images, with subtle patchy and linear areas of decreased signal intensity.[14] An atypical imaging appearance—such as irregular margins, extension of the mass beyond the sternocleidomastoid muscle, lymphadenopathy, or encasement of vascular structures—suggests an alternative diagnosis, such as lymphoma, rhabdomyosarcoma, neuroblastoma, or an inflammatory process.[15]

Infantile Myofibromatosis

Infantile myofibromatosis manifests itself in infancy, usually in the neonatal period, with presentation after 2 years of age unusual.[17] It consists of nodules composed of spindle cells, having features of smooth muscle and fibroblasts at histologic evaluation. Although unifocal disease can occur, the typical appearance is that of multiple soft tissue nodules confined to the subcutaneous tissues or involving the skeleton, intestinal tract, heart, and lungs. Subcutaneous masses typically involve the head, neck, and trunk. Pulmonary involvement may result in interstitial fibrosis and pleural and pulmonary nodules.[18] If visceral involvement is present, the disease is lethal in 75%, but otherwise recovery is the rule, and spontaneous regression occurs in 30%.[19] Boys tend to have solitary lesions, whereas multicentric lesions are more common in girls.[17]

The lesions are round and may be well or ill defined. They usually are isointense to muscle on T1-W imaging and hyperintense on T2-W sequences, but signal intensity is variable (**Fig. 1**).[17] The center may appear mildly hyperintense on T1. Enhancement often is intense and may demonstrate a target appearance, with a nonenhancing center.[20]

Desmoid Tumor

Also known as infantile fibromatosis and aggressive fibromatosis, this nonmetastasizing and technically benign but locally infiltrative tumor consists of intertwining fibroblasts and myofibroblasts.[21] It is most common within muscle tissue of the

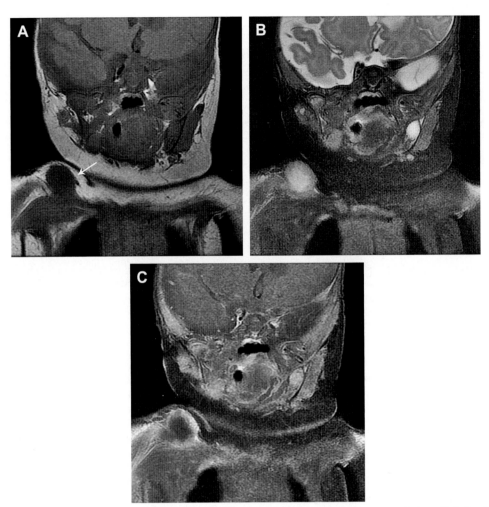

Fig. 1. Infantile myofibromatosis. (*A*) T1-W, coronal, MR image demonstrates a rounded, well-defined right shoulder mass (*arrow*), slightly hypointense on T1. The center is hyperintense on T2-W imaging (*B*), and there is marginal enhancement, resulting in a target appearance on T1 fat-suppressed, gadolinium-enhanced imaging (*C*).

extremities, followed in frequency by the head/neck and trunk. It typically appears in the third decade, but up to 30% of cases occur before age 20 (mean age 13 years).[12] Its behavior is more aggressive in children than in adults. A history of antecedent major trauma to the area may be present in as many as 30% of patients, and 1% to 2% of patients who have this lesion have a history of Gardner's syndrome.[22]

The MR imaging appearance of desmoid tumor is variable, dependent in part on the amount of collagen that is present. Although it may appear encapsulated, microscopic infiltration is the rule. The mass is typically iso- to slightly hyperintense to muscle at T1-W imaging and of intermediate[23] or variably increased[20,24,25] signal intensity on T2-W imaging, secondary to variable cellularity,

collagen, and myxoid material (**Fig. 2**). Linear and curvilinear strands of decreased signal on T1-W and T2-W sequences may represent collagen[23] and if extensive should suggest the diagnosis.[1] Enhancement is often—but not always—intense.[24,26] The tumor's relatively aggressive appearance at MR imaging can lead to the supposition that it is malignant.[2] Because desmoid tumor tends to infiltrate and invade nearby structures, assessment of critical adjacent structures, such as joints and the neurovascular bundle, is essential.

Treatment consists of broad resection, as the tumor margins almost invariably extend beyond what is apparent at imaging or surgical palpation. Even with wide margins, the recurrence rate is approximately 60% in children.[27] Radiation and

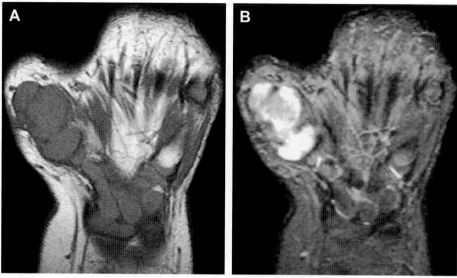

Fig. 2. Desmoid tumor. Coronal, T1-W (*A*) and fast spin-echo, T2-W, fat-suppressed images (*B*) of the hand in a 4-year-old girl demonstrate a lobulated mass that developed after resection of a duplicated thumb. (*Courtesy of* Shriners Hospital for Children Northern California, Sacramento, CA.)

medical therapy often are required,[21,28,29] but occasionally residual tumors involute without therapy.

Fibrous Hamartoma of Infancy

Fibrous hamartoma of infancy, a painless, benign, freely movable, subcutaneous tumor, is most common in boys less than 2 years old. It is composed of immature round to spindle cells, distributed in an orderly fashion within a mucoid matrix admixed with mature fat. Most common in the shoulder girdle, it can occur elsewhere (although not in the hands and feet).[20] The tumor demonstrates intermediate signal intensity strands of fibrous tissue, interspersed with fat.[20,30] It usually is approximately 2.5 to 5 cm, but can be as large as 15 cm.[11,31] Treatment is excision.

Popliteal Cysts

Popliteal cysts are encountered in approximately 6% of pediatric knee MR studies, at an average age of approximately 8 years; they are more common in boys.[32] Although their appearance is similar to those in adults, cause differs. Popliteal cysts in adults almost always are accompanied by joint pathology, but in children the joint usually is normal, although there may be osteochondritis dissicans or synovial pathology.[32] They may result from irritation of a weak portion of the posterior joint capsule. This occurs when seated children dangle their legs; the presence of acute and

chronic inflammation, along with bursal thickening, supports this theory.[33]

Synovium protrudes between the medial head of the gastrocnemius tendon and that of the semitendinosus, but the cyst may extend medial, lateral, deep, or superficial to the adjacent muscles.[33] Most popliteal cysts are unilocular,[34] but septations occur.[32] They typically have decreased signal on T1 and increased signal on T2, unless complicated by hemorrhage or infection (**Fig. 3**). Because the connection to the joint in children is usually inapparent, differential considerations include—in addition to meniscal cyst—ganglion cyst, synovial sarcoma, and popliteal vein varix. To be certain the cystic lesion is a popliteal cyst, a "tail" must track to the joint space.[1] Most pediatric popliteal cysts resolve spontaneously.

Lipoblastic Tumors

Lipoblastoma and lipoblastomatosis are benign neoplasms composed of immature adipocytes that are most common in the extremities. They usually occur during the first 3 years of life and are more common in boys than in girls.[35] Composed of a spectrum of different types of fat cells, including immature mesenchymal cells and mature fat cells, they also contain variable amounts of myxoid stroma. On MR imaging, the tumors usually are bright on T2-W sequences and variable on T1-W sequences (**Fig. 4**), depending on the maturity of the fat cells, as lipoblasts have slightly lower signal than do mature lipocytes

A

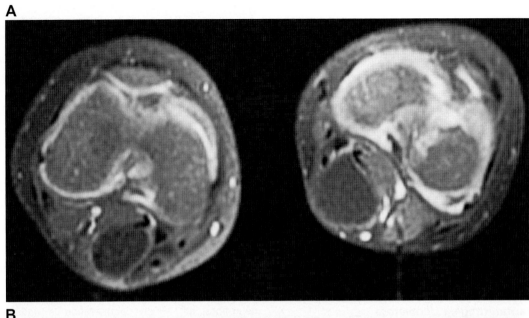

B

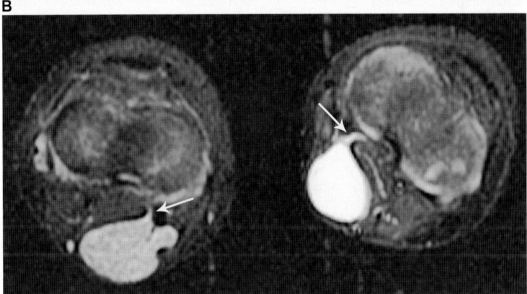

Fig. 3. Popliteal cysts. (*A*) Axial, fat-suppressed, gadolinium-enhanced, T1-W image in a 3-year-old girl demonstrates bilateral cystic structures posterior to the knee. (*B*) Axial short-tau inversion recovery image shows that the lesion on the right is hemorrhagic, whereas that on the left is a simple cyst. Both have tails (*arrows*) between the medial head of the gastrocnemius tendon and that of the semitendinosus, directed to the joint capsule. Both resolved spontaneously with no recurrence.

on T1.[36] The amount of myxoid material also affects signal characteristics. Enhancement is limited when the lesions are composed predominantly of fat.[35] These tumors are less homogeneous than the typical lipoma,[36] which is in any case unusual in childhood.

Lipoblastoma is encapsulated and appears as a well-defined mass; recurrence is uncommon after resection. Lipoblastomatosis, alternatively,

is unencapsulated and infiltrative; it may recur locally if resection is incomplete, and recurrences rarely differentiate into a mature lipoma.[37,38] Metastases have not been reported. Liposarcoma is extremely rare in children,[39] especially under age 5,[37] when lipoblastoma/lipoblastomatosis is most common. Of the liposarcomas, myxoid is the type that tends to occur in children and cannot be differentiated from lipoblastomatosis at MR

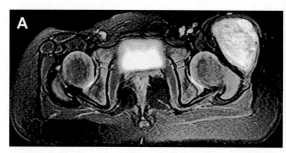

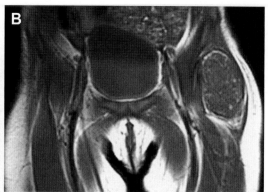

Fig. 4. Lipoblastoma. (*A*) On axial T2-W image the mass is hyperintense, with only a few hypointense foci. (*B*) Coronal T1-W image shows a heterogeneous ovoid well defined septated hypointense mass with a few hyperintense foci.

imaging[37] or histologic examination. Tumor karyotype, however, allows differentiation.[35,40]

Macrodystrophia Lipomatosa

Macrodystrophia lipomatosa involves overgrowth of all mesenchymal elements, resulting in gross enlargement of one or several digits, usually the second and third toes of the lower extremity. Adipose tissue proliferates the most, embedded within a mesh of fibrous tissue. There also is bony overgrowth. At T1-W MR imaging, hyperintense signal of fat mingles with linear fibrous hypointense bands, and on T2-W imaging most of the tissue follows the signal of fat, demonstrating intermediate signal intensity (**Fig. 5**).[41] The fatty tissue is less well defined than the typical lipoma.[42]

Nerve Sheath Tumors

Neurofibromas are common in patients who have neurofibromatosis type I and result from proliferation of the connective tissue of nerve sheaths. The extracellular matrix of plexiform neurofibromas is more extensive, growing along the course of a major nerve and following its small branches to involve adjacent structures. They can be differentiated into superficial, displacing, and invasive growth patterns.[43] They typically demonstrate a beaded, undulating appearance, isointense to muscle on T1-W MR imaging and hyperintense on T2-W sequences, enhancing vigorously (**Fig. 6**). In cross section, neurofibromas demonstrate a "target" appearance on T2-W sequences, resulting from a central zone of tightly packed hypointense dense collagen surrounded by hyperintense myxomatous matrix.[44]

Absence of the target sign results from cystic, hemorrhagic, or necrotic degeneration and also raises concern for degeneration into a malignant

peripheral nerve sheath tumor. This occurs in approximately 10% of patients who have neurofibromatosis I, usually in a pre-existing plexiform neurofibroma.[45] Such degeneration is unusual before age 10. It presents as a rapidly enlarging and sometimes painful subcutaneous or deep soft tissue mass in the extremity or trunk. Patients who have neurofibromatosis I are at 10 to 10,000 times increased risk for this type of tumor.[46] Absence or presence of the target sign is not entirely reliable, but, if it is present in the largest area of the tumor, malignant degeneration is unlikely.[44] Inhomogeneity due to hemorrhage or necrosis, along with patchy contrast enhancement, infiltrative margins, and bone destruction also may indicate malignant degeneration, but

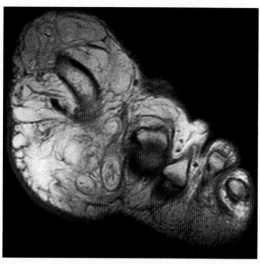

Fig. 5. Macrodystrophia lipomatosa. An axial T1-W image through the metatarsals demonstrates hyperintense adipose tissue mingled with linear fibrous hypointense bands. Nerve sheath tumors.

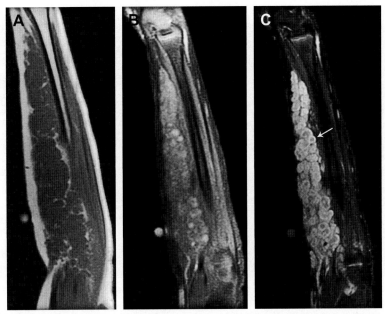

Fig. 6. Plexiform neurofibroma. (*A*) Sagittal T1-W image of the lower arm demonstrates a lobulated mass isointense to muscle. (*B*) Gadolineum-enhanced, fat-suppressed, T1-W image shows intense enhancement. The inversion recovery image (*C*) demonstrates the target appearance (*arrow*) typical of this entity.

this too is not entirely reliable.[45] Surgical excision of a malignant peripheral nerve sheath tumor is necessary, but this is undesirable in a benign tumor, as neuronal tissue also is excised.

BENIGN PROCESSES: REACTIVE
Soft Tissue Infection

Patients who have a soft tissue infection usually present with fever, pain, and elevated white blood cell count, triggering the correct diagnosis. Occasionally, the clinical presentation may be misleading, or there may be concern for the presence of abscess formation or osteomyelitis, leading to performance of MR imaging. When cellulitis progresses to abscess formation, solitary or multiple lesions develop, with extensive adjacent soft tissue inflammation and skin thickening.[47] The central portion of an abscess is iso- to hypointense on T1-W images and hyperintense on T2-W images (**Fig. 7**);[48] marginal enhancement, especially if irregular, may raise concern for the presence of a necrotic tumor. The penumbra sign (an area of relative T1-W hyperintensity positioned between the intermediate or low signal abscess and the adjacent soft tissue edema) may be present, however, in soft tissue infection but not tumor.[49]

Hematoma

Unrecognized trauma is common in children, which can make clinical diagnosis of a hematoma difficult, especially when the overlying skin is not discolored. Many investigators have evaluated the characteristics and timing of soft tissue hemorrhage, and a thorough discussion of this is beyond the scope of this article.[50–52] In brief, MR imaging appearance depends on changes in the structure of the hemoglobin molecule. At less than 48 hours, hematomas usually are decreased to isointense on T1-W images and hypointense on T2-W images. Up to 2 weeks they are bright on T1-W and dark on T2-W imaging. Subacute hematomas (2 weeks to several months) are hyperintense at T1-W and T2-W imaging due to extracellular methemoglobin. With conversion to hemosiderin, a rim develops that is hypointense on T1-W and T2-W imaging.

The differentiation between subacute hematoma and hemorrhagic sarcoma can be challenging; fortunately, the latter is rare among children. Both demonstrate central decreased to intermediate T1-W signal and heterogeneous increased signal intensity on T2-W sequences.[53] The wall of both entities can be thick and demonstrate enhancement, but the wall of a tumor tends to be thicker and more irregular;[54] delineation of an enhancing nodule after gadolinium administration suggests the presence of neoplasm.[5] The presence of ecchymosis in the overlying skin favors hematoma, as a tumor capsule may prevent extravasation of blood components.[54] At minimum, follow-up clinical examination or MR imaging is needed. If it still is not possible to establish that the lesion is not a hemorrhagic tumor, open biopsy is required, as

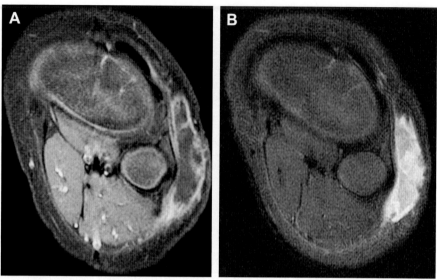

Fig. 7. Abscess. (*A*) Axial, T1-W, gadolinium-enhanced, fat-suppressed image through the lower leg of a 3-year-old girl demonstrates a septated hypointense rim-enhancing mass, with some surrounding enhancement also. On axial inversion recovery sequence (*B*), the central portion is slightly less intense than the rim.

fine-needle aspiration does not provide satisfactory sampling.[53]

Myositis Ossificans Traumatica

Myositis ossificans traumatica is a benign, self-limiting, non-neoplastic proliferative mesenchymal response to soft tissue injury, resulting in formation of mature bone in the periphery of the soft tissue lesion by 6 to 8 weeks.[55] History of antecedent trauma, however, often is absent in children, and presenting complaints of pain and swelling may suggest the presence of infection or soft tissue neoplasm. Most common during the second and third decades, it is extremely rare before age 10.[55] It usually occurs in the large muscles of the anterior thigh or, less often, the upper arm. As the lesion matures, it shrinks, and 30% of cases resolve entirely.[55]

The imaging appearance evolves with maturation. Initially, the lesion consists of fibroblasts, myoblasts, and myxoid stroma,[5] and the MR imaging characteristics are similar to those of many soft tissue tumors.[10,56,57] Surrounding edema, however, often is more intense than is usually seen with primary neoplasms.[5] Fluid-fluid levels may occur, and rim enhancement sometimes suggests early abscess formation or tumor necrosis. A hypointense bony rim gradually develops and is reported to be diagnostic.[57] Mature myositis ossificans, which develops by 6 to 8 weeks, demonstrates signal characteristics of bone, with a well-defined, hypointense rim and

trabeculae, dense fibrosis, and central adipose tissue (**Fig. 8**).

Early myositis ossificans appears malignant at pathology, and MR imaging often is nonspecific and misleading until the chronic phase, but correlative CT may be diagnostic. CT demonstrates a well-defined geometric hypodense mass with peripheral calcification in the earlier phases;[55] when mature, dense calcification can be seen.

BENIGN PROCESSES: VASCULAR ANOMALIES
Vascular Anomalies

A general classification scheme for vascular anomalies groups these lesions based on their flow characteristics.[58] Lesions with arterial components are defined as high flow, and those without arterial components are defined as low flow. High-flow lesions include the common hemangioma (which is the only true vascular neoplasm of this group) along with arteriovenous malformations and arteriovenous fistulas. Unlike the latter two entities, hemangiomas have a mass-like appearance. Low-flow lesions include the relatively common venous malformation and lymphatic malformations. Enhancement characteristics help differentiate these lesions. Anomalies that combine characteristics of several lesions defy classification. Lesions also are characterized by their rate of endothelial turnover. Hemangiomas have a high rate of initial endothelial proliferation, followed by plateau and then involution, whereas vascular malformations have a normal rate of endothelial turnover.[58]

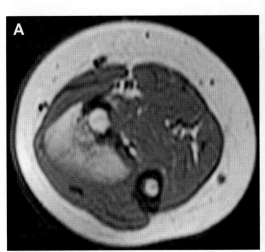
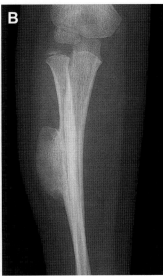

Fig. 8. Mature myositis ossificans. (*A*) Axial T1-W image reveals a central hyperintense matrix similar to that of adjacent marrow, along with a thin, hypointense rim of cortical bone. Radiograph (*B*) demonstrates the typical appearance. (*Courtesy of* Leslie Grissom, Wilmington, DE.)

Imaging is important to define high flow, tissue characteristics, lesion location, and involvement of adjacent structures, such as the neurovascular bundle and nearby joints. Ultrasound can characterize high flow, but its contribution is otherwise limited for large or deep lesions. Gadolinium is helpful to characterize the lesion and to identify slow flow vessels. Gradient-recalled echo sequences define hyperintense high flowing blood along with the presence of phleboliths and hemosiderin.[59] Dynamic contrast-enhanced MR imaging may be used to diagnose venous malformations with high specificity.[60]

High Flow Lesions

Hemangiomas

Occurring in 12% of infants, hemangiomas are the most common vascular tumor of childhood and are especially common in girls.[61] Composed of proliferating endothelial cells, which form a syncytial mass with or without vascular lumens,[62] they usually develop during the first 3 months of life. Influenced by vascular endothelial growth factor and fibroblast growth factor,[62] they proliferate until age 8 to 10 months, when they plateau and begin to involute. By age 5, 50% are gone[63] and most have regressed by 10 to 12 years.[63,64] Most are readily diagnosed by the crimson appearance of overlying skin at physical examination, but occasionally deep or extensive neoplasms require imaging characterization. Visceral lesions may be present in children who have multiple cutaneous hemangiomas.[63]

The MR imaging appearance varies with lesion phase. During proliferation and plateau, hemagiomas appear isointense to muscle on T1 and hyperintense on T2. On T2-W imaging, the typical appearance is of a focal, well-marginated, lobulated mass, although margins may be indistinct at T1-W imaging (**Fig. 9**). Enhancement is homogeneous and diffuse. Enlarged, high-flow vessels, within and around the mass, demonstrate increased signal on gradient-recalled echo and signal voids on spin-echo sequences.[59] Enlarged veins also are seen. Central low-signal-intensity dots are common, probably representing fibrofatty septa viewed in cross section, or perhaps thrombosed vascular channels.[65] Phleboliths and calcifications are not encountered. With involution, vascularity and enhancement decrease, and with progressive fibrofatty replacement, only a few scattered hyperintense vessels remain. Treatment is required for those with unusually rapid growth, visceral location, critical ulceration, or accompanying congestive heart failure.

Differential considerations include neonatal soft tissue sarcomas, such as rhabdomyosarcoma and infantile fibrosarcoma. Sarcomas tend to demonstrate more poorly defined margins, however, and a more heterogeneous appearance before and during contrast administration. The triad of lobulation, septation, and central low-signal-intensity dots are more common in hemangiomas.[65] T2 signal and enhancement also are generally more

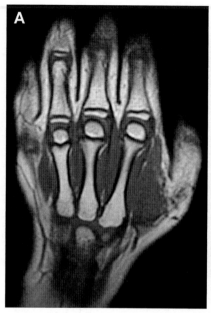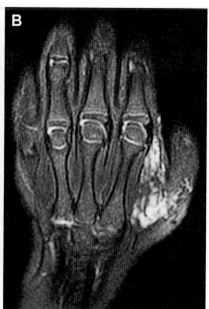

Fig. 9. Hemangioma. (*A*) Coronal, T1-W, image of the right hand shows contour alteration due to an isointense mass at the thenar eminence. (*B*) At fat-suppressed T2-W imaging, this mass appears focal, well marginated, and lobulated.

intense in hemangiomas than in soft tissue sarcomas.[65] Indeterminate masses require biopsy. Unusual hemangiomas include noninvoluting and intramuscular subtypes, which are encountered in older children and adults. Their imaging appearance is similar to that of infantile hemangiomas.[59]

Kaposiform hemangioendothelioma is associated with Kasabach-Merritt syndrome, wherein platelet trapping results in severe coagulopathy.[66] These tumors often are located in the liver or spleen but occasionally in the extremities.[66]

Arteriovenous malformations

These rare vascular malformations result from abnormal vessel development, which bypasses the capillary bed. Demonstrating a normal rate of endothelial turnover, they are composed of a focal or diffuse network of interconnecting arteries and veins, with a central nidus of tortuous, dysplastic vessels. Although present at birth, they usually manifest later on. Growth rate is commensurate with that of the child, although they may suddenly enlarge due to trauma or puberty. Patients present with pain, ischemia, embolism, hemorrhage, or, for large lesions, cardiac failure. Overlying skin may be warm and red, with a palpable thrill or pulsatile mass. Extremity overgrowth is common.

MR imaging identifies high flow as signal voids on spin-echo imaging or as increased signal with gradient-recalled echo.[67] Feeding and draining vessels without a focal soft tissue mass are seen, along with enlarged central vascular channels. Surrounding tissue may demonstrate edema and enhancement, but there is no associated mass. An arteriovenous malformation confined to a muscle sheath may resemble a vascular tumor.[59] The skin may appear thickened, and bony involvement results in lytic changes with cortical thinning. Treatment is transarterial hyperselective embolization.[61]

Arteriovenous fistulas

Arteriovenous fistulas usually occur as iatrogenic or posttraumatic lesions in older patients, but this single direct communication between an artery and a vein can occur as a congenital lesion, usually in the head and neck.

Low Flow Lesions

Venous malformations

Venous malformations are the most common vascular anomaly and consist of an easily compressed soft tissue mass that enlarges when dependent or with Valsalva's maneuver. Like arteriovenous malformations, these typically are present at birth, but they usually are recognized later as a blue mass or patch.[68] They grow proportionally with the child and usually become symptomatic after infancy. Absence of mural smooth muscle cells allows them to grow with the patient. These lesions may be localized or extensive, confined to the skin or infiltrating musculature, joints, and bone. They may present with pain or cause deformity or decreased range of motion.

An important diagnostic characteristic is the presence of phleboliths, which appear as round signal voids on T1-W and T2-W sequences. The venous malformation appears as a multilocular, lobulated, septated mass, iso- or hypointense to muscle on T1-W imaging and hyperintense on T2 (Fig. 10). Fluid-fluid levels are rare.[59,64] Low flow is seen on gradient-recalled echo sequences, and the dilated vascular channels enhance diffusely, which allows differentiation from lymphatic malformations and cystic lesions. Anomalies of the venous drainage system may be present. When venous malformations involve an extremity, undergrowth is more common than overgrowth. Involvement of the neuromuscular bundle must be evaluated. Extension into a joint may mandate excision, as recurrent hemorrhage may cause hemosiderin arthropathy. Pathologic fractures may occur when the lesion involves bone.

Lymphatic malformations

Lymphatic malformations are composed of masses of endothelial-lined, chyle-filled spaces that may be microcystic, macrocystic, or combined. They develop from sequestered lymphatic sacs due to congenital obstruction of lymphatic drainage.[69] Usually presenting in early childhood, these lesions are most common in the head and neck, axilla, and trunk. Involvement of the extremity may result in soft tissue and skeletal overgrowth along with swelling.

Cyst size determines the MR imaging appearance. Microcystic lesions may appear solid, hypointense on T1, and markedly hyperintense on T2. Enhancement is absent or diffuse, further complicating differentiation from a solid mass. However, the macrocystic form usually is readily identified as clearly defined cysts that are hypointense on T1 and hyperintense on T2 (unless there has been hemorrhage or infection) (Fig. 11). Fluid-fluid levels result from hemorrhage or infection. Vascular flow voids do not occur. Septae often enhance, yielding the characteristic "rings and arcs," but—unlike with venous malformations—the cysts do not enhance unless there has been treatment. In the extremities, there is considerable overlap in the appearance of venous and lymphatic malformations, and enhancement characteristics are essential for differentiation.[59] Dilated or anomalous veins may accompany this lesion.[70] Treatment usually is percutaneous sclerotherapy or resection.

Combined Malformations

Lesions often demonstrate crossover characteristics, and venous versus lymphatic malformations may be especially difficult to differentiate. Identification of high flow versus low flow is more important than definite tissue identification, as flow characteristics usually dictate treatment.[62]

Syndromes Associated with Vascular Anomalies

Klippel-Trenaunay syndrome consists of a port wine nevus, extensive capillary-lymphaticovenous malformation involving an entire extremity

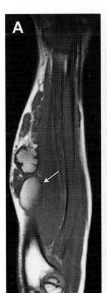
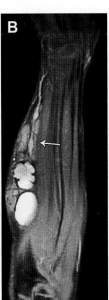
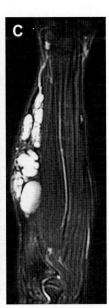

Fig. 10. Venous malformation. (A) Coronal T1-W image of the upper arm in an 11-year-old boy whose mass has grown with him demonstrates a multilobulated mass composed of a few hyperintense posthemorrhagic areas (arrow) and multiple tubular isointense areas. With administration of gadolinium (B), the tubular areas enhance (arrow). The full extent of this mass is evident at (C) coronal, fat-saturated, T2-W imaging.

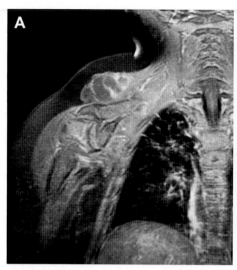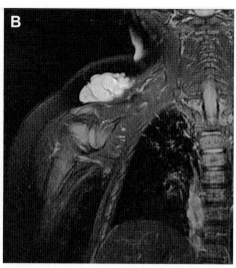

Fig. 11. Lymphatic malformation. (*A*) Coronal, T1-W, gadolinium-enhanced, fat-suppressed image of the right shoulder shows enhancing rings and arcs interposed between multiple nonenhancing cysts. (*B*) These cysts are uniformly hyperintense on coronal T2-W fat suppressed imaging.

(Fig. 12), and extremity overgrowth along with increased fat and muscle atrophy.[66] Anomalous veins have deformed or absent valves, and there is fibromuscular dysplasia.[61] MR imaging is useful to define the extent of this low flow lesion and to identify whether or not the deep venous system is anomalous. The gastrointestinal tract is involved in 20% of patients.[66] Bony enchondromas accompanied with soft tissue venous malformations constitute Maffucci's syndrome. Blue rubber bleb nevus syndrome is characterized by cutaneous vascular lesions and venous malformations of the gastrointestinal tract.[66]

MALIGNANT SOFT TISSUE TUMORS
Congenital or Infantile Fibrosarcoma

Fibrosarcomas constitute 11% of soft tissue sarcomas in children.[71] The incidence of this tumor peaks in the age group less than age 5 years old and then again in the 10- to 15-year age range. This discussion is limited to fibrosarcomas in the younger age group, as those in older children behave like those in adults.

Congenital/infantile fibrosarcoma is most common in neonates and infants less than 1 year old and most often is encountered in the extremities. It consists of anaplastic immature spindle-shaped cells arrayed in a herringbone pattern.[72] Behavior is more favorable than in adults,[20,71] for although these large tumors are bulky and disfiguring, they rarely metastasize.[18] Metastatic disease is more common when the tumors arise in the trunk than in the extremities;[72] when in the extremities, they tend to be distal.[71] Usually treated with

conservative resection,[18,46] they also may respond to adjuvant chemotherapy and have been noted to shrink after cessation of chemotherapy as well.[20] Local recurrence, however, is common.[72]

This tumor is isointense to muscle on T1-W sequences and inhomogeneously hyperintense on T2-W sequences; enhancement is heteroegeneous,[20] which may be due to hemorrhage and necrosis.[46] Margins usually are poorly defined.[72] Scattered areas of decreased signal intensity on all sequences may result from fibrous foci. Differential diagnosis includes desmoid tumor, myofibromatosis, rhabdomyosarcoma, and hemangiopericytoma.[72]

Rhabdomyosarcoma

Derived from primitive mesenchymal cells that have differentiated into rhabdomyoma cells, this tumor accounts for 10% to 15% of solid tumors in the extremities[73] and 4% to 5% of childhood cancers;[74,75] it constitutes more than half of pediatric soft tissue sarcomas.[71,76] It is most common in the head and neck, genitourinary tract, and retroperitoneum, but 18% of cases occur in the extremities.[71] Although this tumor sometimes arises in striated muscle, it can develop anywhere that its mesenchymal anlage occurs.[71] The relatively aggressive alveolar subtype is most common in the extremities.

Prognosis is based on tumor size (less than 5-cm maximum diameter fares better), local invasiveness, nodal spread, and distant metastases. Tumors in the extremities have a worse prognosis,

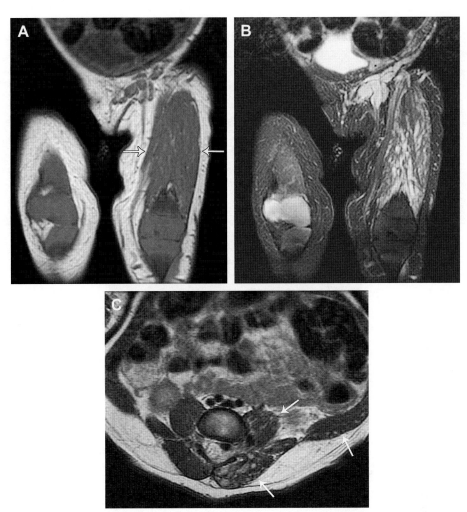

Fig. 12. Klippel-Trenaunay-Weber syndrome. (*A*) Coronal T1-W image of the left thigh in a newborn demonstrates an isointense lymphaticovenous malformation insinuated within atrophic musculature (*arrows*). (*B*) On T2-W, fat-suppressed, coronal imaging, the mass clearly extends to the inguinal area, and on (*C*), an axial T2-W image through the lower lumbar spine, hyperintense cystic infiltration of the left erector spinae and other musculature can be seen (*arrows*), along with enlargement of spinal veins.

metastasizing to lymph nodes in the first year in 74% of cases, but prognosis is better if the proximal, instead of distal, extremity is involved.[75] Complete excision is essential to a good prognosis,[75] as the survival rate for nonresectable alveolar rhabdomyosarcoma is only 50%.[74] The presence of metastases to lung, marrow, and bone confers a mere 20% 5-year survival.[74]

MR imaging provides detailed tissue characterization and can suggest the site of origin and local extent and nodal spread. After surgical resection, it is useful for evaluation of recurrence. The tumor appears isointense to muscle on T1-W and of intermediate to high signal intensity on T2-W imaging (**Fig. 13**). Enhancement usually is intense.[73] There may be signal voids due to vessels having high velocity flow.

Synovial Sarcoma

This malignant, high-grade tumor is not derived from the synovial membrane but from primitive mesenchymal cells, differentiated into spindle cells and sometimes epithelial cells. Although classically located near a joint, it can occur anywhere. Nearly half of cases occur in children and adolescents,[77] and it is the most common nonrhabdomyosarcoma soft tissue sarcoma to occur in this age group; however, it constitutes only 5% of all pediatric soft tissue sarcomas.[71] The typical presentation is a painless mass that has been present for weeks to years, although it can present with pain in the absence of a mass, acute arthritis, or joint contracture.[77] Completely resected disease has an excellent outcome, but

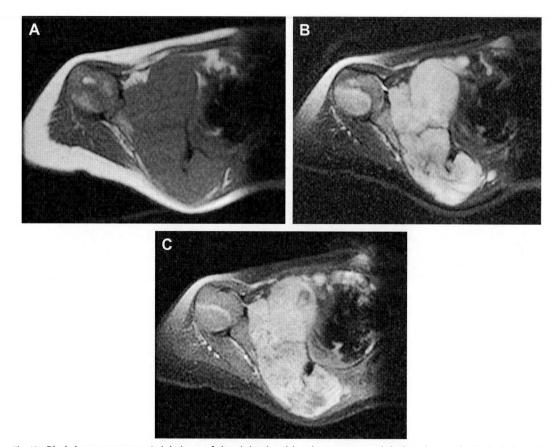

Fig. 13. Rhabdomyosarcoma. Axial views of the right shoulder demonstrate a lobulated mass that is isointense to muscle on T1-W (*A*), of intermediate to high intensity on T2, fast spin-echo, fat suppressed imaging (*B*), and that enhances intensely though heterogeneously (*C*). (*Courtesy of* Leslie Grissom, Wilmington, DE.)

the presence of metastases (usually to the lung) confers a dismal prognosis. Prognosis is best if the tumor is less than 5 cm or if it develops in a younger child around the hand, foot, or knee.[71]

More common in the lower extremities than in the upper and especially common around the knee,[71] synovial sarcoma usually occurs in the deep compartment, often within 7 cm of a joint.[78] It typically is large at diagnosis (mean diameter almost 9 cm), and margins usually are rounded or lobulated and well defined, with the suggestion of a capsule.[78] Although it appears to displace rather than invade adjacent structures, at surgery there usually is microscopic invasion beyond the pseudocapsule.[79] On T1-W imaging, it appears isointense to muscle, and on T2-W imaging, it appears heterogeneous but hyperintense (**Fig. 14**).[78,80] Hemorrhage may be present,[78] and fluid-fluid levels are seen in approximately 20% of cases. This tumor may appear purely cystic and has been mistaken for a Baker's cyst, hematoma, or ganglion cyst;[1,77] it is the most common

malignant tumor to be mistaken as benign.[2] Spotty mineralization occurs in approximately one fourth of tumors.[81] Complete resection is important, and re-resection is often required. Local radiation therapy may help if surgical margins are small.[79]

Other Nonrhabdomyosarcomatous Soft Tissue Sarcomas

Most other nonrhabdomyosarcomatous soft tissue sarcomas are rare during childhood but when present tend to occur in the second decade of life. Fibrosarcomas are rare (excluding congenital/infantile fibrosarcoma). Malignant fibrous hystiocytomas show some predilection for the upper arm as does epithelioid sarcoma.[82] Clear cell sarcoma is even less common and has a poor prognosis.[82]

Granulocytic sarcoma (**Fig. 15**) consists of primitive precursors of granulocytic white blood cells and occurs in approximately 5% of cases of acute myelogenous leukemia. It may precede onset of

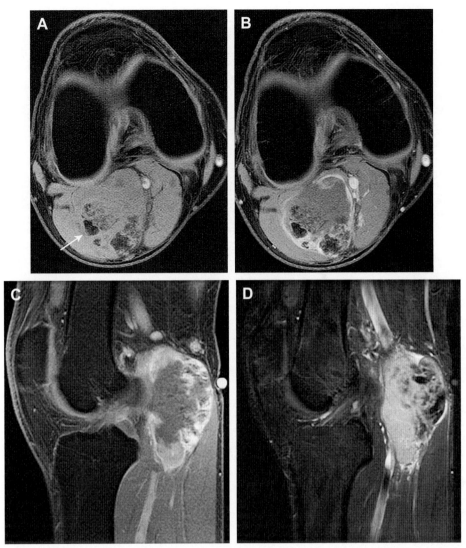

Fig. 14. Synovial sarcoma. (*A*) A heterogeneous mass in the popliteal fossa of a 17-year-old girl appears isointense on axial, T1-W, fast spoiled gradient-recalled echo sequence and demonstrates intense marginal enhancement on T1-W, fast spoiled gradient-recalled echo gadolineum-enhanced, axial (*B*) and coronal (*C*) sequences. Hypointense areas represent calcification (*arrow* in *A*), evident on radiographs. (*D*) The well-circumscribed mass appears hyperintense on sagittal inversion recovery sequences, which also demonstrate areas of hypointense calcification.

leukemia by as much as 8 years.[83] The tumor arises in the bone marrow and traverses haversian canals to extend to and then beyond the periosteum and thus often is encountered near bone. By far most common in the head and neck, it occasionally occurs in the extremities. Like many soft tissue tumors, it is isointense to muscle on T1 but also isointense to muscle on T2. Enhancement usually is uniform.[84]

Hemangiopericytoma

This usually painless, firm, rubbery subcutaneous mass consists of mesenchymal cells derived from pericytes and constitutes 3% of pediatric soft tissue sarcomas.[71] Approximately one third of tumors are located in the extremities,[46] with other common locations including retroperitoneum, head, and neck.[71] When this tumor occurs in children over 1 year old, metastatic disease (to lungs and bone) or unresectable disease is common, but its behavior is more benign in infants, in whom it sometimes demonstrates spontaneous regression or maturation into a hemangioma.[85] Spontaneous hemorrhage may be life threatening, and ulceration may result from extremely rapid growth.[46] In infants, treatment consists of wide local excision, with chemotherapy

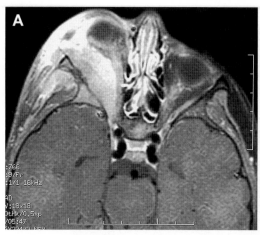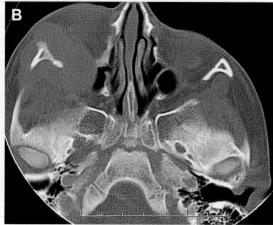

Fig. 15. Granulocytic sarcoma. (*A*) Axial, T1-W, gadolinium-enhanced MR imaging of the orbits demonstrates a large, enhancing, soft tissue mass centered on the bone of the lateral wall of the right orbit. Axial CT scan (*B*) demonstrates intact cortex and trabeculae, typical of this entity.

reserved for incomplete resection. MR imaging appearance is nonspecific but provides information about tumor extent.

SUMMARY

Soft tissue lesions in children usually are benign. Although tissue diagnosis often rests in the hands of a pathologist, MR imaging is able to suggest a specific benign diagnosis in approximately 30% to 45% of cases.[1] Malignant lesions share common features, however, and it is unusual for MR imaging to establish a specific malignant diagnosis. Also, there is significant overlap between the appearance of benign and malignant tumors. Although MR imaging often is nonconclusive, and biopsy is usually required, MR imaging provides essential information about lesion extent, which proves essential in planning biopsy and surgery.

REFERENCES

1. Bissett GS 3rd. MR imaging of soft-tissue masses in children. Magn Reson Imaging Clin N Am 1996;4(4): 697–719.
2. Berquist TH, Ehman RL, King BF, et al. Value of MR imaging in differentiating benign from malignant soft-tissue masses: study of 95 lesions. AJR Am J Roentgenol 1990;155(6):1251–5.
3. Kransdorf MJ, Murphey MD. Radiologic evaluation of soft-tissue masses: a current perspective. AJR Am J Roentgenol 2000;175(3):575–87.
4. Soler R, Castro JM, Rodriguez E. Value of MR findings in predicting the nature of the soft tissue lesions: benign, malignant or undetermined lesion? Comput Med Imaging Graph 1996;20(3):163–9.
5. Jelinek J, Kransdorf MJ. MR imaging of soft-tissue masses. Mass-like lesions that simulate neoplasms. Magn Reson Imaging Clin N Am 1995;3(4):727–41.
6. Moulton JS, Blebea JS, Dunco DM, et al. MR imaging of soft-tissue masses: diagnostic efficacy and value of distinguishing between benign and malignant lesions. AJR Am J Roentgenol 1995; 164(5):1191–9.
7. Mutlu H, Silit E, Pekkafali Z, et al. Soft-tissue masses: use of a scoring system in differentiation of benign and malignant lesions. Clin Imaging 2006;30(1): 37–42.
8. Ma LD, McCarthy EF, Bluemke DA, et al. Differentiation of benign from malignant musculoskeletal lesions using MR imaging: pitfalls in MR evaluation of lesions with a cystic appearance. AJR Am J Roentgenol 1998;170(5):1251–8.
9. Kransdorf MJ. Malignant soft-tissue tumors in a large referral population: distribution of diagnoses by age, sex, and location. AJR Am J Roentgenol 1995; 164(1):129–34.
10. Siegel MJ. Magnetic resonance imaging of musculoskeletal soft tissue masses. Radiol Clin North Am 2001;39(4):701–20.
11. Enzinger FM. Fibrous hamartoma of infancy. Cancer 1965;18:241–8.
12. Coffin CM, Dehner LP. Fibroblastic-myofibroblastic tumors in children and adolescents: a clinicopathologic study of 108 examples in 103 patients. Pediatr Pathol 1991;11(4):569–88.
13. Parikh SN, Crawford AH, Choudhury S. Magnetic resonance imaging in the evaluation of infantile torticollis. Orthopedics 2004;27(5):509–15.
14. Snitzer EL, Fultz PJ, Asselin B. Magnetic resonance imaging appearance of fibromatosis colli. Magn Reson Imaging 1997;15(7):869–71.

15. Ablin DS, Jain K, Howell L, et al. Ultrasound and MR imaging of fibromatosis colli (sternomastoid tumor of infancy). Pediatr Radiol 1998;28(4):230–3.

16. Tang S, Liu Z, Quan X, et al. Sternocleidomastoid pseudotumor of infants and congenital muscular torticollis: fine-structure research. J Pediatr Orthop 1998;18(2):214–8.

17. Laor T. MR imaging of soft tissue tumors and tumor-like lesions. Pediatr Radiol 2004;34(1):24–37.

18. Patrick LE, O'Shea P, Simoneaux SF, et al. Fibromatoses of childhood: the spectrum of radiographic findings. AJR Am J Roentgenol 1996;166(1):163–9.

19. Robbin MR, Murphey MD, Temple HT, et al. Imaging of musculoskeletal fibromatosis. Radiographics 2001;21(3):585–600.

20. Eich GF, Hoeffel JC, Tschappeler H, et al. Fibrous tumours in children: imaging features of a heterogeneous group of disorders. Pediatr Radiol 1998;28(7):500–9.

21. McCarville MB, Hoffer FA, Adelman CS, et al. MRI and biologic behavior of desmoid tumors in children. AJR Am J Roentgenol 2007;189(3):633–40.

22. Faulkner LB, Hajdu SI, Kher U, et al. Pediatric desmoid tumor: retrospective analysis of 63 cases. J Clin Oncol 1995;13(11):2813–8.

23. Kransdorf MJ, Jelinek JS, Moser RP Jr, et al. Magnetic resonance appearance of fibromatosis. A report of 14 cases and review of the literature. Skeletal Radiol 1990;19(7):495–9.

24. Ahn JM, Yoon HK, Suh YL, et al. Infantile fibromatosis in childhood: findings on MR imaging and pathologic correlation. Clin Radiol 2000;55(1):19–24.

25. Quinn SF, Erickson SJ, Dee PM, et al. MR imaging in fibromatosis: results in 26 patients with pathologic correlation. AJR Am J Roentgenol 1991;156(3):539–42.

26. Lee JC, Thomas JM, Phillips S, et al. Aggressive fibromatosis: MRI features with pathologic correlation. AJR Am J Roentgenol 2006;186(1):247–54.

27. Kingston CA, Owens CM, Jeanes A, et al. Imaging of desmoid fibromatosis in pediatric patients. AJR Am J Roentgenol 2002;178(1):191–9.

28. Abbas AE, Deschamps C, Cassivi SD, et al. Chest-wall desmoid tumors: results of surgical intervention. Ann Thorac Surg 2004;78(4):1219–23 [discussion: 1219–23].

29. Lackner H, Urban C, Benesch M, et al. Multimodal treatment of children with unresectable or recurrent desmoid tumors: an 11-year longitudinal observational study. J Pediatr Hematol Oncol 2004;26(8):518–22.

30. Loyer EM, Shabb NS, Mahon TG, et al. Fibrous hamartoma of infancy: MR-pathologic correlation. J Comput Assist Tomogr 1992;16(2):311–3.

31. Paller AS, Gonzalez-Crussi F, Sherman JO. Fibrous hamartoma of infancy. Eight additional cases and a review of the literature. Arch Dermatol 1989; 125(1):88–91.

32. De Maeseneer M, Debaere C, Desprechins B, et al. Popliteal cysts in children: prevalence, appearance and associated findings at MR imaging. Pediatr Radiol 1999;29(8):605–9.

33. Lang IM, Hughes DG, Williamson JB, et al. MRI appearance of popliteal cysts in childhood. Pediatr Radiol 1997;27(2):130–2.

34. Torreggiani WC, Al-Ismail K, Munk PL, et al. The imaging spectrum of Baker's (Popliteal) cysts. Clin Radiol 2002;57(8):681–91.

35. Moholkar S, Sebire NJ, Roebuck DJ. Radiological-pathological correlation in lipoblastoma and lipoblastomatosis. Pediatr Radiol 2006;36(8):851–6.

36. Reiseter T, Nordshus T, Borthne A, et al. Lipoblastoma: MRI appearances of a rare paediatric soft tissue tumour. Pediatr Radiol 1999;29(7):542–5.

37. Collins MH, Chatten J. Lipoblastoma/lipoblastomatosis: a clinicopathologic study of 25 tumors. Am J Surg Pathol 1997;21(10):1131–7.

38. Duhaime AC, Chatten J, Schut L, et al. Cervical lipoblastomatosis with intraspinal extension and transformation to mature fat in a child. Childs Nerv Syst 1987;3(5):304–6.

39. Jung SM, Chang PY, Luo CC, et al. Lipoblastoma/lipoblastomatosis: a clinicopathologic study of 16 cases in Taiwan. Pediatr Surg Int 2005;21(10):809–12.

40. Miller GG, Yanchar NL, Magee JF, et al. Lipoblastoma and liposarcoma in children: an analysis of 9 cases and a review of the literature. Can J Surg 1998;41(6):455–8.

41. Soler R, Rodriguez E, Bargiela A, et al. MR findings of macrodystrophia lipomatosa. Clin Imaging 1997; 21(2):135–7.

42. Wang YC, Jeng CM, Marcantonio DR, et al. Macrodystrophia lipomatosa. MR imaging in three patients. Clin Imaging 1997;21(5):323–7.

43. Mautner VF, Hartmann M, Kluwe L, et al. MRI growth patterns of plexiform neurofibromas in patients with neurofibromatosis type 1. Neuroradiology 2006; 48(3):160–5.

44. Bhargava R, Parham DM, Lasater OE, et al. MR imaging differentiation of benign and malignant peripheral nerve sheath tumors: use of the target sign. Pediatr Radiol 1997;27(2):124–9.

45. Mautner VF, Friedrich RE, von Deimling A, et al. Malignant peripheral nerve sheath tumours in neurofibromatosis type 1: MRI supports the diagnosis of malignant plexiform neurofibroma. Neuroradiology 2003;45(9):618–25.

46. McCarville MB, Kaste SC, Pappo AS. Soft-tissue malignancies in infancy. AJR Am J Roentgenol 1999;173(4):973–7.

47. Christian S, Kraas J, Conway WF. Musculoskeletal infections. Semin Roentgenol 2007;42(2):92–101.

48. Gylys-Morin VM. MR imaging of pediatric musculoskeletal inflammatory and infectious disorders. Magn Reson Imaging Clin N Am 1998;6(3):537–59.

49. McGuinness B, Wilson N, Doyle AJ. The "penumbra sign" on T1-weighted MRI for differentiating musculoskeletal infection from tumour. Skeletal Radiol 2007;36(5):417–21.

50. Rubin JI, Gomori JM, Grossman RI, et al. High-field MR imaging of extracranial hematomas. AJR Am J Roentgenol 1987;148(4):813–7.

51. Swensen SJ, Keller PL, Berquist TH, et al. Magnetic resonance imaging of hemorrhage. AJR Am J Roentgenol 1985;145(5):921–7.

52. Unger EC, Glazer HS, Lee JK, et al. MRI of extracranial hematomas: preliminary observations. AJR Am J Roentgenol 1986;146(2):403–7.

53. Imaizumi S, Morita T, Ogose A, et al. Soft tissue sarcoma mimicking chronic hematoma: value of magnetic resonance imaging in differential diagnosis. J Orthop Sci 2002;7(1):33–7.

54. Ward WG Sr, Rougraff B, Quinn R, et al. Tumors masquerading as hematomas. Clin Orthop Relat Res 2007;465:232–40.

55. Gindele A, Schwamborn D, Tsironis K, et al. Myositis ossificans traumatica in young children: report of three cases and review of the literature. Pediatr Radiol 2000;30(7):451–9.

56. Crundwell N, O'Donnell P, Saifuddin A. Non-neoplastic conditions presenting as soft-tissue tumours. Clin Radiol 2007;62(1):18–27.

57. Kransdorf MJ, Meis JM, Jelinek JS. Myositis ossificans: MR appearance with radiologic-pathologic correlation. AJR Am J Roentgenol 1991;157(6):1243–8.

58. Mulliken JB, Glowacki J. Hemangiomas and vascular malformations in infants and children: a classification based on endothelial characteristics. Plast Reconstr Surg 1982;69(3):412–22.

59. Konez O, Burrows PE. Magnetic resonance of vascular anomalies. Magn Reson Imaging Clin N Am 2002;10(2):363–88, vii.

60. van Rijswijk CS, van der Linden E, van der Woude HJ, et al. Value of dynamic contrast-enhanced MR imaging in diagnosing and classifying peripheral vascular malformations. AJR Am J Roentgenol 2002;178(5):1181–7.

61. Enjolras O. Classification and management of the various superficial vascular anomalies: hemangiomas and vascular malformations. J Dermatol 1997;24(11):701–10.

62. Donnelly LF, Adams DM, Bisset GS 3rd. Vascular malformations and hemangiomas: a practical approach in a multidisciplinary clinic. AJR Am J Roentgenol 2000;174(3):597–608.

63. Fishman SJ, Mulliken JB. Hemangiomas and vascular malformations of infancy and childhood. Pediatr Clin North Am 1993;40(6):1177–200.

64. Burrows PE, Laor T, Paltiel H, et al. Diagnostic imaging in the evaluation of vascular birthmarks. Dermatol Clin 1998;16(3):455–88.

65. Teo EL, Strouse PJ, Hernandez RJ. MR imaging differentiation of soft-tissue hemangiomas from malignant soft-tissue masses. AJR Am J Roentgenol 2000;174(6):1623–8.

66. Elsayes KM, Menias CO, Dillman JR, et al. Vascular malformation and hemangiomatosis syndromes: spectrum of imaging manifestations. AJR Am J Roentgenol 2008;190(5):1291–9.

67. Meyer JS, Hoffer FA, Barnes PD, et al. Biological classification of soft-tissue vascular anomalies: MR correlation. AJR Am J Roentgenol 1991;157(3):559–64.

68. Enjolras O, Ciabrini D, Mazoyer E, et al. Extensive pure venous malformations in the upper or lower limb: a review of 27 cases. J Am Acad Dermatol 1997;36(2 Pt 1):219–25.

69. Siegel MJ, Glazer HS, St Amour TE, et al. Lymphangiomas in children: MR imaging. Radiology 1989;170(2):467–70.

70. Laor T, Burrows PE. Congenital anomalies and vascular birthmarks of the lower extremities. Magn Reson Imaging Clin N Am 1998;6(3):497–519.

71. Miser JS, Pizzo PA. Soft tissue sarcomas in childhood. Pediatr Clin North Am 1985;32(3):779–800.

72. Lee MJ, Cairns RA, Munk PL, et al. Congenital-infantile fibrosarcoma: magnetic resonance imaging findings. Can Assoc Radiol J 1996;47(2):121–5.

73. Kim EE, Valenzuela RF, Kumar AJ, et al. Imaging and clinical spectrum of rhabdomyosarcoma in children. Clin Imaging 2000;24(5):257–62.

74. McCarville MB, Spunt SL, Pappo AS. Rhabdomyosarcoma in pediatric patients: the good, the bad, and the unusual. AJR Am J Roentgenol 2001;176(6):1563–9.

75. Tabrizi P, Letts M. Childhood rhabdomyosarcoma of the trunk and extremities. Am J Orthop 1999;28(8):440–6.

76. Arndt CA, Crist WM. Common musculoskeletal tumors of childhood and adolescence. N Engl J Med 1999;341(5):342–52.

77. McCarville MB, Spunt SL, Skapek SX, et al. Synovial sarcoma in pediatric patients. AJR Am J Roentgenol 2002;179(3):797–801.

78. Jones BC, Sundaram M, Kransdorf MJ. Synovial sarcoma: MR imaging findings in 34 patients. AJR Am J Roentgenol 1993;161(4):827–30.

79. Andrassy RJ, Okcu MF, Despa S, et al. Synovial sarcoma in children: surgical lessons from a single institution and review of the literature. J Am Coll Surg 2001;192(3):305–13.

80. Morton MJ, Berquist TH, McLeod RA, et al. MR imaging of synovial sarcoma. AJR Am J Roentgenol 1991;156(2):337–40.

81. Frassica FJ, Khanna JA, McCarthy EF. The role of MR imaging in soft tissue tumor evaluation: perspective of the orthopedic oncologist and musculoskeletal pathologist. Magn Reson Imaging Clin N Am 2000;8(4):915–27.

82. McGrory JE, Pritchard DJ, Arndt CA, et al. Nonrhab-domyosarcoma soft tissue sarcomas in children. The Mayo Clinic experience. Clin Orthop Relat Res 2000;374:247–58.

83. Pui MH, Fletcher BD, Langston JW. Granulocytic sarcoma in childhood leukemia: imaging features. Radiology 1994;190(3):698–702.

84. Stein-Wexler R, Wootton-Gorges SL, West DC. Orbital granulocytic sarcoma: an unusual presentation of acute myelocytic leukemia. Pediatr Radiol 2003;33(2):136–9.

85. Rodriguez-Galindo C, Ramsey K, Jenkins JJ, et al. Hemangiopericytoma in children and infants. Cancer 2000;88(1):198–204.

The Hip: MR Imaging of Uniquely Pediatric Disorders

Jerry R. Dwek, MD

KEYWORDS
- Hip • Perthes • Pediatric • Impingement
- Slipped epiphysis • MR Imaging

The hip joint is a deceptively complex ball and socket, which is the result of coordinated growth of four different bones: the femur, ilium, ischium, and pubis, centered around two main physeal cartilages, that of the triradiate cartilage and that of the proximal femur. Complex and coordinated growth at all these bony structures and physes culminates in the adult with a fully formed articulation, which must bear the entire weight of an individual for the rest of the individual's lifetime.

The hip joint endures great stresses throughout life and normal morphology is critical to its normal function. Errors in its development during childhood, whether congenital or acquired, commonly result in a shape that is ill suited to normal motion and prolonged weight bearing and places severe limitations on movement, ultimately ending in early osteoarthritis and joint replacement.

Throughout its development, pathologic processes are well imaged by MR imaging before, during, and after ossification. In infancy, MR imaging depicts well the cartilaginous model of the pelvis and is very useful for the preoperative and postoperative care of patients with developmental dysplasia of the hip (DDH), proximal focal femoral deficiency (PFFD), and some osteochondrodysplasias. Later in childhood, when the limping child is a major diagnostic dilemma, MR imaging is extremely helpful in the identification of such varied disease processes as osteomyelitis, septic arthritis, traumatic injuries, and especially Legg-Calvé-Perthes (LCP) disease where MR imaging is useful not only at the initial stage of diagnosis but in assessing disease progression and planning therapy. In adolescence, MR imaging is an exciting complement to conventional radiography in the early diagnosis of slip of the capital femoral epiphysis. Finally, as femoral acetabular impingement syndromes become more emphasized, MR imaging has a unique advantage as an imaging tool because it is able to image both the ossified and nonossified structures, such as the labrum, in a single examination and without exposure to ionizing radiation. Furthermore, with proper sequences an arthrogram-like effect can be produced that allows analysis of the central overarching question of femoral head coverage.

GENERALITIES

T1 sequences are excellent in portraying the ossified elements with good anatomic detail. T2 fat-saturated sequences are excellent at locating and characterizing pathologic processes by dint of the bright signal, which usually accompanies disease. They also have the ability to produce arthrogram-like image of the hip joint. Because commonly the involved hip has a joint effusion, the labrum can be visualized and at times labral tears identified. Cartilage-sensitive sequences are excellent at depicting the cartilaginous model of the pelvis. Because many of the cartilage sequences are obtained as a three-dimensional volume, multiplanar reconstructions with little loss in image detail are facilitated. These three-dimensional volume acquisitions have great value in allowing the retrospective analysis of various angles and relationships about the hips and pelvis with one acquisition.

Department of Radiology, Rady Children's Hospital and Health Center-San Diego, 3020 Children's Way, San Diego, CA 92123, USA
E-mail address: jdwek@yahoo.com

Magn Reson Imaging Clin N Am 17 (2009) 509–520
doi:10.1016/j.mric.2009.03.003

INFANCY

During infancy the main and most common clinical concern is DDH. Although the initial diagnosis of DDH is by ultrasound and conventional radiography, MR imaging has its place in preoperative planning and postoperative care.

The value of MR imaging in preoperative planning centers on its ability to portray the cartilaginous anlage of the pelvis and analyze the relationship of the femoral head to the acetabulum and labrum. Cartilage sequences that are primarily intermediate flip angle, fat-saturated, gradient sequences (SPGR) can be obtained as a volume and depending on how they are prescribed can be reformatted into any plane desired, in some cases isotropically, allowing multiplanar reconstructions critical for correct therapeutic intervention. With a flip angle of 34 to 45 degrees and fat saturation, epiphyseal cartilage is bright, ossified bone is dark, and the labrum is dark. The femoral head should ordinarily sit within the friendly confines of the acetabulum with a down-tilted labrum completing coverage laterally. In DDH the head is variably laterally displaced with posterior and superior displacement (**Fig. 1**). Possible blocks to reduction can be visualized especially in cases where closed reduction has been unsuccessful. These include a flipped labrum (**Fig. 2**); prominent pulvinar and a redundant ligamentum teres; capsule or iliopsoas tendon; or transverse acetabular ligament, which may become interposed into the joint (**Fig. 3**).

In the immediate postoperative period, MR imaging is useful in evaluation of proper reduction of the dislocated femoral head and in the assessment of its vascular health. To achieve a successful reduction with the femoral head normally seated within the acetabulum varying amounts of abduction, at time quite marked, at the hip is necessary. At times, excessive abduction can interrupt the

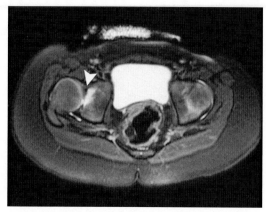

Fig. 2. Axial T2-weighted MR image. The femoral head is laterally displaced. Labrum (*arrowhead*) is flipped into joint and blocks successful reduction.

blood supply to the femoral head. The degree of abduction that causes this ischemia is variable so that the safe zone, in which reduction is maintained and the femoral head remains perfused, cannot be established clinically.[1] The blood supply to the cartilaginous femoral head is primarily from femoral circumflex vessels, which enter the femoral epiphysis and ramify within it in vascular canals. The vascular canals that are visible by MR imaging do not anastomose and contain an artery, vein, and a capillary plexus. Nutrients must diffuse from the vascular canals and perivascular tissues into the cartilaginous epiphysis.[2–4] In the immediate postoperative period, MR imaging with intravenous contrast enhancement is capable of identifying ischemia to the femoral head.[5] If interruption of the blood supply has occurred, that portion of the head that is ischemic does not enhance and it remains dark on T1 fat-saturated sequences. Because the vascular canals do not anastomose, the boundary between enhancing and nonenhancing femoral head is usually sharp

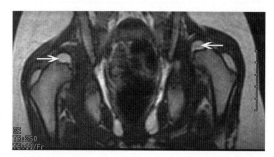

Fig. 1. Coronal T1-weighted MR image. A 7-year-old ballerina with difficulty in abduction. Both hips are chronically dislocated. Both femoral heads are superiorly displaced (*arrows*).

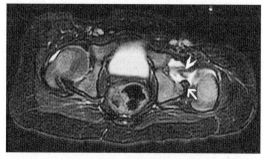

Fig. 3. Axial T2-weighted MR image. The femoral head is laterally displaced. Redundant posterior capsule and labrum (*arrow*) blocks successful reduction. Note thickened ligamentum teres (*arrowhead*).

and geographic. The anterolateral portion of the head is most commonly at risk. If identified early enough such ischemia is reversible before the femoral head is damaged.

A normally located femoral head has the head placed within the cup of the acetabulum. Frequently, in difficult reductions a slightly posterior axis of the femoral head relative to the acetabulum is present and although is not optimal, is acceptable. Care must be taken in these tenuous situations that adequate reduction is maintained. Prominent pulvinar is visualized as fibrofatty material in the joint, which does not allow normal seating of the femoral head within the joint. Some pulvinar is within the range of normal and although the head may be slightly laterally displaced, as long as the femoral head is encompassed by the confines of the acetabulum and pointing at the triradiate cartilage, the pulvinar usually atrophies and allows the hip to seat normally. Here, follow-up MR imaging is also of use.

Long after the initial treatment for DDH, morphologic changes in the hip whether it is from the original pathology or postoperative ischemia may be present and in these cases MR imaging is invaluable in the assessment of pain and planning therapy.

DYSPLASIA

The femoral head normally ossifies between 4 and 6 months of age. After ossification, conventional radiography well delineates the relationship of the already ossified elements of the hip and pelvis. In some skeletal dysplasias, however, ossification may be severely delayed and in those patients, many of whom are no longer infants, MR imaging is helpful in evaluating for appropriate coverage and size of the femoral heads relative to the acetabulum. Type II collagenapathies are typified by a delay in femoral head ossification, and MR imaging is helpful with this patient population as it is in other disorders in which either femoral head ossification delay is present, such as multiple epiphyseal dysplasia, pseudoachondroplasia, or Morquio's disease. In general, cartilage is very abundant in these syndromes, and especially with type 2 collagenopathies has bright signal on T2 fat-saturated sequences, whereas cartilage sensitive sequences are underwhelming (**Fig. 4**).

PFFD stands out as one congenitally dysplastic syndrome in which MR imaging is especially helpful. In PFFD, the femoral head is variably small or absent and the femur is short. The prognosis and treatment options depend on appropriate staging of the abnormalities. The most common grading system is the Aitken classification, which assigns types A to D to the abnormality depending on the presence or absence of the femoral head and the acetabulum and osseous integrity of the remainder of the femoral shaft. In patients with type A PFFD, the femur is short. The femoral head and acetabulum are present. There is frequently a pseudoarthrosis at the femoral neck. In type D the femur is very short and head and acetabulum are absent.

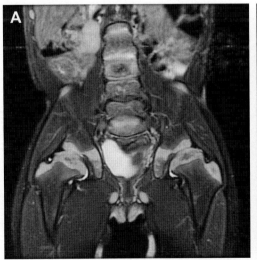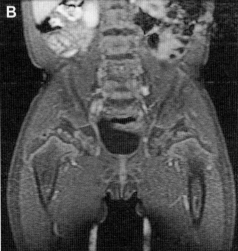

Fig. 4. (*A*) Coronal T2-weighted fat-saturated MR image. (*B*) Coronal three-dimensional SPGR fat-saturated image. A 4-year-old girl with spondyloepiphyseal congenital. Both acetabula are shallow and dysplastic with the left femoral head showing less coverage. Note the hyperintensity of the epiphyseal cartilage signal compared with low signal from the abundant epiphyseal cartilage on the cartilage-sensitive three-dimensional SPGR image.

Acetabular deformity is correlated with the presence or absence of the femoral head. Although the presence of a femoral head can be somewhat inferred from the relative development of the acetabulum, it is inexact. Careful MR imaging with appropriate fields of view can usually identify correctly the size and position of the femoral head if present. If the femoral head is present it may be quite small and not be immediately apparent so that thin-section coronal and axial imaging are of greatest use. An ossified femoral head has normal fatty T1 marrow signal (**Fig. 5**). Nonossified elements being formed of cartilage portray cartilage signal. In addition to the position of the femoral head its relationship and any continuity to the remainder of the femur should also be assessed. Because patients with PFFD frequently do not have cruciate ligaments at the knee or a fibula (fibular hemimelia), MR imaging can also be useful in assessing existing ligamentous support at the knee.

CHILDHOOD

The typical presentation of a child with LCP is the limping child who refers pain to the medial aspect of the distal thigh or knee. Physical examination usually reveals pain at the hip and limitation of range of motion.

The differential diagnosis of the limping child includes infectious causes, such as osteomyelitis, septic arthritis, and myositis; sterile inflammatory etiologies including toxic synovitis and juvenile rheumatoid arthritis; various traumatic etiologies; and LCP. If symptoms and signs point to an infectious etiology centered at the hip, sonographic confirmation of a hip effusion followed by aspiration is usually the preferred clinical pathway because early therapy of a septic arthritis is important in decreasing damage to the articular surface. Relief of some of the pressure in the joint may also help in maintaining perfusion of the femoral head.

MR imaging examination should include imaging of the whole pelvis because the differential diagnosis is broad. Osteomyelitis is identified by bright signal on T2 fat-saturated sequences in the bony pelvis, commonly in the acetabulum, which is a metaphyseal equivalent centered on the triradiate cartilage, or at the femoral metaphysis. Low T1 signal and postcontrast enhancement is usually present. A septic joint usually shows a large effusion with some measure of synovitis, although in early cases the synovial inflammation may be underwhelming. Both osteomyelitis and septic arthritis frequently occur together and care must be taken when an obvious effusion is present to examine diligently the periarticular bony structures for subtle edema or enhancement indicative of osteomyelitis (**Fig. 6**).

Toxic or transient synovitis is a common condition in this age group. Signs and symptoms are similar to that with infectious causes, although usually not quite as severe. On MR imaging a joint effusion is apparent with mild synovial enhancement. There should be no osseous edema, and if present mitigates in favor of an infectious cause.

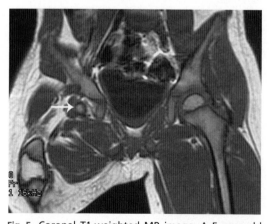

Fig. 5. Coronal T1-weighted MR image. A 5 year old with proximal focal femoral deficiency. The femoral head (*arrow*) is laterally displaced and is very small. The acetabulum, although also small, is fairly well formed.

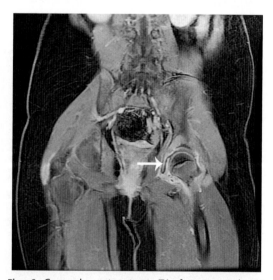

Fig. 6. Coronal postcontrast T1 fat-saturated MR image. A 9-year-old girl septic hip and osteomyelitis. Left hip joint shows enhancing effusion with marked synovitis. Enhancement is also present in the acetabulum (*arrow*). Cultures were positive for *Staphylococcus aureus* from joint fluid and acetabulum.

Juvenile inflammatory arthritis has a similar appearance to septic arthritis and differentiation cannot be made on MR imaging alone. The presence of an abnormal effusion on the contralateral hip or sacroiliac joint effusion and enhancement mitigates in favor of a sterile synovial inflammatory process.

Although synovial enhancement is nonspecific, MR imaging can be helpful in confirming and assessing disease activity and severity. Postcontrast imaging shows synovial enhancement and pannus formation well. Because synovial tissue lacks tight junctions or a basement membrane, contrast begins to diffuse into the joint quickly postinjection so that care should be exercised to ensure that scanning begins immediately after injection. If multiple joints are to be imaged the order of scan acquisition should be considered. If bilateral extremities are scanned it is usually helpful to image both extremities in a larger coil sacrificing field of view to acquire the images as soon as possible after injection. Quantitative imaging can also be helpful in providing a clear objective indicator of disease severity.

LEGG-CALVÉ-PERTHES DISEASE

LCP disease initially may be seen simply as a small-to-moderate size joint effusion. Differentiation from infectious processes should be somewhat aided by the lack of infectious markers, although some C-reactive protein elevation is common. The patient frequently complains of knee pain usually along the medial aspect of the distal thigh. Close examination reveals pain and limitation of motion at the hip joint.

Initial MR imaging in all these situations should include postintravenous gadoteridol contrast dynamic imaging of the head to assess for proper femoral head perfusion. Acquisition is usually obtained in the coronal plane to allow easy comparison between involved and noninvolved sides. Because the critical upstroke of enhancement occurs quickly, within the first 2 minutes, early and prompt acquisition is essential immediately after contrast enhancement to avoid confusion because the enhancement of the early vascular phase decreases after about 2 to 5 minutes postinjection.[6] After the early vascular phase, the disparity between normal and abnormal sides is less clear. Dynamic subtraction imaging has also been successful.[6] Most recently, new fast gradient sequences have become available, which have better signal to noise than standard SPGR dynamic sequences with less imaging time. Image acquisition time is 1 minute or less but it remains to be seen whether these are as sensitive to perfusion changes dynamically.

It is important to note that lack of perfusion on MR imaging in the acute situation does not necessarily mean that necrosis has occurred or will occur. Various interventions may interrupt the ischemic pathway. Most obviously, prompt operative intervention in cases of sepsis with arthrotomy may help relieve the intra-articular pressure. Even in cases where the effusion is sterile and symptomatology is consistent with LCP, lack of perfusion does not mean that standard LCP ensues. At the authors' institution, where dynamic imaging is commonly used, they have observed cases where perfusion is absent but there are no long-term sequelae (**Fig. 7**).

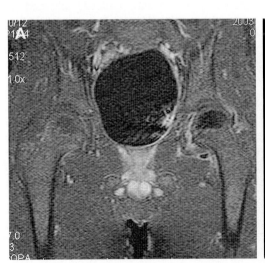 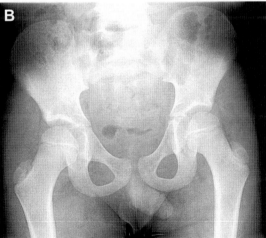

Fig. 7. (*A*) Coronal SPGR fat-saturated dynamic postcontrast image. A 5-year-old boy with left hip pain. Severely diminished enhancement is present at the left femoral head. Left hip effusion is present. (*B*) Follow-up conventional radiograph 5 months later shows no abnormalities.

Diffusion-weighted imaging may be of use. Recent investigations show that early restricted diffusion is present. This soon shifts to increased diffusion, which remains increased through the period of experimental reperfusion. Diffusion-weighted imaging may be a better indicator of cell damage and necrosis than postcontrast gadolinium imaging.[7,8]

After LCP diagnosis, MR imaging scanning is an excellent complement to plain film imaging. MR imaging has been shown to be more accurate in evaluating the extent of epiphyseal necrosis and can be used to stage the hip and identify when the revascularization period begins.

Imaging of LCP should include images in all three planes. The coronal plane is best for comparative analysis of one hip with the other, whereas the sagittal plane is most accurate in estimating the volume of necrotic bone.[9] Axial planes are more useful in examination of the surrounding structures rather than the femoral head itself. Three-dimensional volume acquisitions are also helpful. Early imaging may show a subchondral fracture line ordinarily seen as linear low intensity on T1 in the subchondral zone. Bright fluid intensity T2 signal may be seen within the linear fracture line. The subchondral fracture line correlates well within the extent of epiphyseal necrosis,[10] although MR imaging provides a more accurate assessment (**Fig. 8**).[11] Necrotic bone is usually but not always dark on all imaging sequences.

An assessment of femoral head coverage should be made. A well-seated hip should have majority bony coverage. The labrum completes coverage laterally and should have an obliquely inferior course. If the femoral head is lateralized, there is likely to be significant synovial inflammation medially. The acetabular cartilage also is slightly thickened. Frequently, an effusion is present. Even if small, the labrum and its position are apparent. With larger effusions and smaller fields of view, labral tears can be diagnosed as bright signal within or traversing the labral tissue. Some caution is necessary because there is some controversy in the literature over whether normal variants of labral clefting can occur anterosuperiorly.[12,13] In addition, on certain imaging planes the attachment of the transverse acetabular ligament can simulate a labral tear.

The reparative interface is subdivided into an outer curvilinear focus of decreased signal intensity and an inner layer, which is bright on T2 at the margin of the necrotic, signal void bone (**Fig. 9**). The outer layer corresponds to thickened trabecular bone and fibrous repair tissue, whereas the inner layer represents the inner edge of the granulation tissue.[11] Dynamic postcontrast images accurately indicate the viable bone, which should enhance brightly postcontrast. Early enhancement of the lateral pillar (the lateral one third of the femoral head) is consistent with a better prognosis. More accurately, inasmuch as enhancement indicates viability, enhancement of the lateral pillar indicates that no more loss of height of the pillar should occur. It can then be staged according to the Herring classification, which grades LCP according to the relative height of the lateral pillar, with whatever loss of height is present at that time. Transphyseal neovascularity is associated with a longer and less satisfactory course with physeal bridging[14] and growth abnormality. Metaphyseal signal abnormality, which is representative of cartilaginous metaphyseal ingrowth, also indicates a higher risk of growth abnormalities caused by physeal bridges. Loose intra-articular bodies are unusual but can occur particularly in the medial joint space where more room is available.

It is interesting to note that not all gadolinium contrast products are created equal. Bashir and colleagues[15–17] showed that intra-articular ionic negatively charged gadopentetate pools in areas of proteoglycan loss in the articular cartilage. Proteoglycans or glycosaminoglycans are long-chain negatively charged molecules that form a major component on articular cartilage. Focal loss of these large negatively charged molecules theoretically allows puddling of negatively charged ionic gadopentetate contrast in areas bereft of proteoglycan. Menezes and colleagues[18] have added to this body of evidence with the fact that nonionic gadolinium is seen to enhance more evenly neutrally charged fat marrow. It is helpful to use nonionic gadoteridol when working with dynamic imaging for the analysis of perfusion of the normally fatty femoral head epiphysis.[18]

ADOLESCENCE

There are two main focuses of imaging of the hip in the adolescent: slipped capital femoral epiphysis (SCFE) and recently femoral acetabular impingement (FAI). The latter is a newcomer but seems to be a major cause of early degenerative disease. Interestingly, SCFE and FAI may be linked.

With the knowledge that hip pain in the adolescent can occur from multiple etiologies about the hip including osteomyelitis, septic joints, and especially traumatic causes some of which include subtle stress injuries at the apophyses, a complete MR imaging examination in the adolescent with hip pain should include fluid-sensitive imaging of the

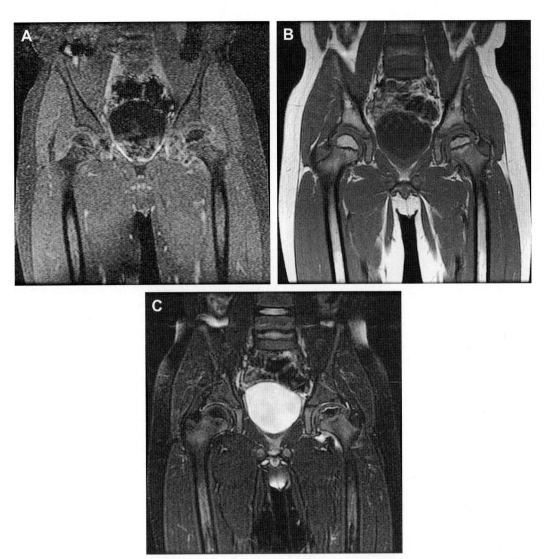

Fig. 8. A 6-year-old boy with LCP. (*A*) Coronal SPGR fat-saturated dynamic postcontrast image. Complete diminished left femoral head enhancement. (*B*) Coronal T1-weighted MR image. Low-intensity linear subchondral fracture line is seen deep to most of the femoral head articular surface consistent with epiphyseal necrosis and LCP. Note that T1 fat marrow is still maintained, although there is already slight volume loss. (*C*) Coronal T2-weighted fat-saturated MR image. Subchondral fracture line shows bright fluid intensity signal. Note only minimal bright T2 signal in remainder of epiphysis.

entire pelvis. Axial T2 fat-saturated sequences are well suited for the examination of the pelvic bones outside the femoral head neck junction. For close investigation of the femoral head and metaphysis, coronal and sagittal fluid-sensitive imaging are superior to straight axial imaging because some of the physis is in plane on axial imaging leading to suboptimal definition and conspicuity of the physis. Reconstructed sagittal and axial oblique images can be very helpful because the sagittal and axial oblique planes allow a confident analysis of morphologic alterations about the hip joint.

SLIPPED CAPITAL FEMORAL EPIPHYSIS

Slipped capital femoral epiphysis is simply a Salter I fracture through the proximal femoral physis. The process is complex, however, in that there are recognized chronic and acute factors. Probably all SCFE should be considered a chronic morphologic abnormality with acute factors. Although some hormonal factors are probably contributory, the major change in this condition is a morphologic change in the relationship of the femoral head to the femoral neck centered at the physeal level

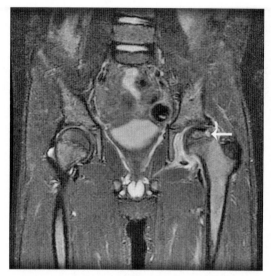

Fig. 9. Coronal T2-weighted fat-saturated MR image. A 5-year-old boy with LCP. The repair zone interface is identified as bright signal along the lateral margin of the ossified epiphysis (*arrow*). This is the lateral pillar. Slight loss of height is present. There was no progression on follow-up conventional radiographs.

possibly caused by obesity. The femoral head becomes relatively retroverted at the physeal level placing the head and physis at a significant mechanical disadvantage when subjected to either normal or supernormal stressors, such as might be present in an obese individual.[19,20] Accurate MR imaging diagnosis relies on identification of these two factors: recognition of a morphologic change at the head neck junction and abnormal signal intensity centered on the physis indicating mounting stress and edema at the physeal level.

On coronal images a line drawn along the lateral aspect of the femoral neck should intersect a portion, usually about one sixth of the lateral aspect of the femoral epiphysis. At the Rady Children's Hospital and Health Center-San Diego, staff make frequent use of three-dimensional volume acquisition to reconstruct sagittal oblique images along the axis of the femoral neck to identify any retroversion at the epiphysis-metaphyseal junction. The femoral head should sit squarely atop the femoral metaphysis without any posterior displacement. Bright signal on fluid-sensitive images at the physis is indicative of a chronic slip condition frequently with a recent acute component. Abnormal bright T2 signal is usually but not invariable seen on both sides of the physis in unambiguous cases (**Fig. 10**). More subtle abnormalities include edema on the metaphyseal side alone usually at the extreme medial aspect of the physis. Because the subphyseal zone of the metaphysis normally has some signal elevation caused by residual hematogenous marrow, coronal sequences that provide easy comparison with the contralateral hip are of the greatest use. It must be kept in mind, however, that because SCFE is a bilateral process with retroversion usually present, bilateral abnormalities are common. Patients with SCFE are at risk for osteonecrosis of the femoral head, and chondrolysis.

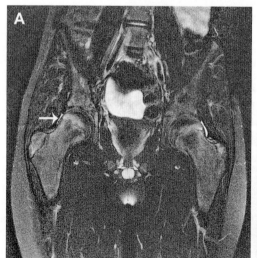

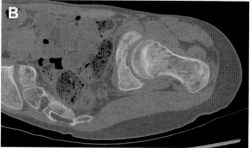

Fig. 10. (*A*) Coronal T2-weighted fat-saturated MR image of a 12-year-old boy with right hip pain. Edema is seen bilaterally on both sides of the proximal femoral physis greater on the epiphyseal side. Note slight medial slip on right (*arrow*). (*B*) Reconstructed CT axial oblique image. Image reconstructed along the plane of the femoral neck shows slight retroversion at the level of the proximal femoral physis.

With femoral head screws in place, MR imaging is of limited usefulness, although at times some diagnostic information can be obtained. Frequently, in complicated cases of SCFE as the head collapses the screw tip protrudes into the articular surface of the femoral head and it is removed to avoid further joint damage; then, MR imaging is of greater use.

As was seen in LCP disease, MR imaging is useful to evaluate for the vascular integrity of the head with the use of postcontrast T1 fat-saturated sequences. A lack of enhancement is consistent with nonviability. A subchondral fracture line may occur with impending collapse of the head. The articular space can be examined for degradation of the articular cartilage consistent with chondrolysis. Edema in the subchondral zones is usually present with joint space narrowing.

FEMORAL ACETABULAR IMPINGEMENT

Recently, Ganz and colleagues[21] brought attention to the contribution of the geometry of femoral neck and acetabulum to long-term degenerative disease. Normally, the femoral neck has a definite narrowing or waist, which allows the femur to abduct fully without impingement on the lateral aspect of the acetabulum. In patients with FAI the femoral neck is not tubulated normally. Instead of having an identifiable constriction, a so-called "pistol grip" deformity is seen in which tubulation is lacking. A small bump or protuberance is frequently identified at the anterior femoral neck.

There is some discussion of the relationship of SCFE to femoral waist deficiency and FAI. Slight slips where there is slight posterior and medial displacement of the femoral head could result in the pistol grip deformity and certainly FAI is a problem for patients[22] with SCFE, although it is unlikely that SCFE is the only contributing factor.

Axial oblique images prescribed along the axis of the femoral neck, or again reconstruction of the three-dimensional volume acquisition into the axial oblique plane, allows measurement of the alpha angle. First the center of the femoral head is identified using the contour of the head to fit a circle to outline and define the position of the center of the head. Two lines are extended from the center point of the head, one down the axis of the femoral neck and the second to the intersection point between the head and the neck where the convexity of the femoral head becomes the concavity of the femoral neck. Angles under 55 degrees are abnormal or if the head-neck line measures greater than the radius of the circle defining the femoral head then a femoral waist deficiency is present.[23,24]

Synovial herniation pits or fibroosseous defects in the femoral neck, formerly thought to be a normal variant, are highly correlated with FAI.[25] They can be recognized as a lucent lesion with a thin sclerotic rim at the femoral neck on conventional radiography. On MR imaging the lesion is seen as a small excavation in the anterior aspect of the femoral neck filled with moderately hyperintense signal (**Fig. 11**). Fragmentation of the

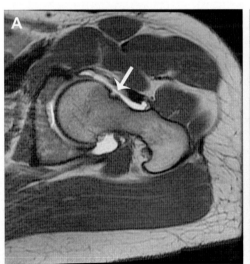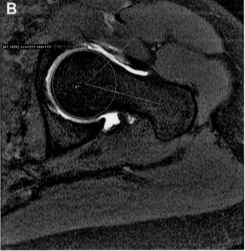

Fig. 11. (*A*) Axial oblique T1-weighted MR arthrogram. A synovial herniation pit (*arrow*) is seen at the anterior femoral neck. (*B*) Axial T1-weighted fat-saturated MR arthrogram. The alpha angle is over 55 degrees consistent with femoral waist deficiency and cam impingement. Note lack of offset of femoral neck (compare with posterior femoral neck).

superolateral aspect of the acetabulum and labral tears may be present, although it needs to be recognized that osseous and degenerative abnormalities may not become apparent until adulthood and this entity is an active area of current investigation and research. Labral tears are frequently in continuity with chondral defects on the articulating surface of the roof of the acetabulum. MR arthrography is necessary in most cases accurately to diagnose labral pathology (**Fig. 12**).

In addition to femoral waist deficiencies, overcoverage of the femoral head and neck may be caused by acetabular retroversion. In normal individuals the acetabulum has its lateral opening directed slightly anteriorly. In the abnormal case, the anterolateral edge of the acetabulum extends further laterally than the posterolateral edge so that the acetabular opening is directed posteriorly. By conventional radiography this is visualized as the acetabular crossover sign, which is a reliable indicator of acetabular retroversion on a well-aligned AP pelvis film. The crossover sign is present when the anterior lip of the acetabulum crosses over the posterior lip on a standard frontal view of the pelvis.[26] The ischial spines may also be prominent (**Fig. 13**).[27] This causes variable limitation on the ability to flex at the hip as the femoral neck impinges on the anterior acetabulum.[28]

It is important to understand that the literature regarding femoral acetabular impingement conditions is still in its development stages. Abnormal morphology in the pediatric age group may not reflect the fully formed pathologic abnormalities evident in adults. Certainly, although labral tears are commonly seen in adolescents and are in themselves frequently related to impingement conditions, degenerative changes are fortunately not usually seen. Even the femoral waist deficiency may be more subtle in the adolescent age group. The osseous irregularity and protuberance of the anterior femoral neck may enlarge as symptomatology progresses and may not be well apparent in children, although this is speculative. Here the pediatric radiologist is in the vanguard. He or she is in a unique position possibly to diagnose subtle osseous abnormalities that interdict what is thought to be an inexorable course to end-stage degenerative disease and early hip arthroplasty.

TRAUMATIC APOPHYSEAL ABNORMALITIES

Another point of weakness at the pelvis is the various apophyses about the pelvis all of which are vulnerable to acute and chronic traction abnormalities. The anterior-superior and inferior iliac spines serve as the origin of the sartorius and the straight head of the rectus femoris, respectively. The hamstring complex arises along the inferior and lateral surface of the ischium, whereas the iliac crest apophysis takes the insertion of tensor fascia lata (**Fig. 14**).

As is frequently the case in the skeleton, apophyseal changes may be solely acute but is more commonly a mixture of acute on chronic changes. Frank separation of the apophysis from the pelvic bones is diagnosed by displacement of the

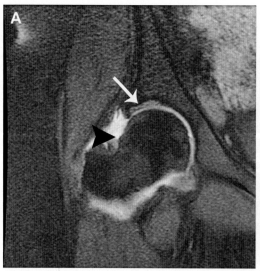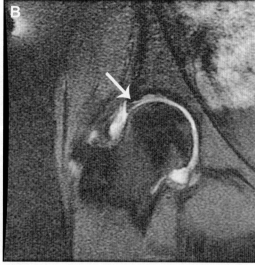

Fig. 12. (*A*) Coronal T1 fat-saturated MR arthrographic image. The joint is distended with dilute gadolinium contrast. Chondral abnormality is seen at superolateral acetabulum (*arrow*). Note bump on lateral aspect of femoral neck (*arrowhead*) causing impingement during abduction. (*B*) Coronal T1 fat-saturated MR arthrographic image. Note gadolinium extending into labral tear (*arrow*). Chondral defect is seen adjacent.

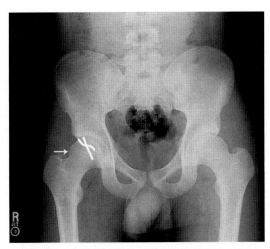

Fig. 13. Anteroposterior view of the pelvis in 15-year-old boy with acetabular impingement and hip pain on flexion. Note bilateral acetabular crossover findings are present. Right hip has anterior and posterior walls of the acetabulum outlined. Note pistol grip deformity bilaterally (*arrow*).

apophyseal ossific center from its normal site with bright T2 edema signal present. Chronic avulsive changes are recognized by slight widening of the physis again with T2 bright signal abnormality. Some bright signal is normal on T2 fat-saturated images at the apophysis because it is an area of active growth like any metaphysis so that comparison of one side with its contralateral side is very helpful, although changes can be frequently bilateral.

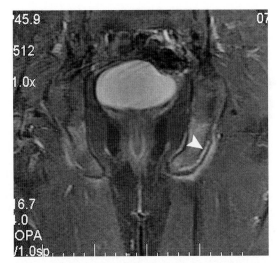

Fig. 14. Coronal T1-weighted postcontrast fat-saturated MR image. Bilateral hamstring avulsions are present. Note bright line of the physeal separation on left (*arrowhead*).

SUMMARY

MR imaging is uniquely suited to the diagnosis and evaluation of multiple disease processes about the hip ranging from DDH in infancy, LCP in the child, and SCFE and FAI in the adolescent. It provides a clear picture without the use of ionizing radiation of geometric abnormalities in the pelvis that cause or contribute short- and long-term deficiencies and pain. Use of fluid-sensitive sequences allows an accurate depiction of progressive disease processes at the time of the examination, whereas the use of gadolinium intravenous enhancement adds the ability to assess for tissue viability and adds significant conspicuity to active disease processes. It should be understood that the use of MR imaging in pediatric hip abnormalities is an active area of investigation and changes in its use are to be expected as research and understanding of the various disease processes discussed evolves and matures.

REFERENCES

1. Ramsey PL, Lasser S, MacEwen GD. Congenital dislocation of the hip: use of the Pavlik harness in the child during the first six months of life. J Bone Joint Surg Am 1976;58:1000–4.
2. Haines RW. Cartilage canals. J Anat 1933;68:45–64.
3. Hurrell DJ. The vascularisation of cartilage. J Anat 1934;69:47–61.
4. Tucker FR. Arterial supply to the femoral head and its clinical importance. J Bone Joint Surg Am 1949; 31B(1):82–93.
5. Jaramillo D, Villegas-Medina OL, Doty DK, et al. Gadolinium-enhanced MR imaging demonstrates abduction-caused hip ischemia and its reversal in piglets. Pediatr Radiol 1995;25(8):578–87.
6. Sebag G, Ducou Le Pointe H, Klein I, et al. Dynamic gadolinium-enhanced subtraction MR imaging: a simple technique for the early diagnosis of Legg-Calve-Perthes disease: preliminary results. Pediatr Radiol 1997;27(3):216–20.
7. Jaramillo D, Connolly SA, Vajapeyam S, et al. Normal and ischemic epiphysis of the femur: diffusion MR imaging study in piglets. Radiology 2003; 227(3):825–32.
8. Menezes NM, Connolly SA, Shapiro F, et al. Early ischemia in growing piglet skeleton: MR diffusion and perfusion imaging. Radiology 2007;242(1): 129–36.
9. Ha AS, Wells L, Jaramillo D. Importance of sagittal MR imaging in nontraumatic femoral head osteonecrosis in children. Pediatr Radiol 2008;38(11): 1195–200.
10. Salter RB, Thompson GH. Legg-Calve-Perthes disease: the prognostic significance of the

subchondral fracture and a two-group classification of the femoral head involvement. J Bone Joint Surg Am 1984;66(4):479–89.

11. Bos CF, Bloem JL, Bloem RM. Sequential magnetic resonance imaging in Perthes' disease. J Bone Joint Surg Br 1991;73(2):219–24.

12. Czerny C, Hofmann S, Urban M, et al. MR arthrography of the adult acetabular capsular-labral complex: correlation with surgery and anatomy. AJR Am J Roentgenol 1999;173(2):345–9.

13. Petersilge CA, Haque MA, Petersilge WJ, et al. Acetabular labral tears: evaluation with MR arthrography. Radiology 1996;200(1):231–5.

14. Jaramillo D, Kasser JR, Villegas-Medina OL, et al. Cartilaginous abnormalities and growth disturbances in Legg-Calve-Perthes disease: evaluation with MR imaging. Radiology 1995; 197(3):767–73.

15. Bashir A, Gray ML, Boutin RD, et al. Glycosaminoglycan in articular cartilage: in vivo assessment with delayed Gd(DTPA)(2-)-enhanced MR imaging. Radiology 1997;205(2):551–8.

16. Bashir A, Gray ML, Burstein D. Gd-DTPA2- as a measure of cartilage degradation. Magn Reson Med 1996;36(5):665–73.

17. Burstein D, Bashir A, Gray ML. MRI techniques in early stages of cartilage disease. Invest Radiol 2000;35(10):622–38.

18. Menezes NM, Olear EA, Li X, et al. Gadolinium-enhanced MR images of the growing piglet skeleton: ionic versus nonionic contrast agent. Radiology 2006;239(2):406–14.

19. Pritchett JW, Perdue KD. Mechanical factors in slipped capital femoral epiphysis. J Pediatr Orthop 1988;8(4):385–8.

20. Pritchett JW, Perdue KD, Dona GA. The neck shaft-plate shaft angle in slipped capital femoral epiphysis. Orthop Rev 1989;18(11):1187–92.

21. Ganz R, Parvizi J, Beck M, et al. Femoroacetabular impingement: a cause for osteoarthritis of the hip. Clin Orthop Relat Res 2003;417:112–20.

22. Fraitzl CR, Kafer W, Nelitz M, et al. Radiological evidence of femoroacetabular impingement in mild slipped capital femoral epiphysis: a mean follow-up of 14.4 years after pinning in situ. J Bone Joint Surg Br 2007;89(12):1592–6.

23. Notzli HP, Wyss TF, Stoecklin CH, et al. The contour of the femoral head-neck junction as a predictor for the risk of anterior impingement. J Bone Joint Surg Br 2002;84(4):556–60.

24. Pfirrmann CW, Mengiardi B, Dora C, et al. Cam and pincer femoroacetabular impingement: characteristic MR arthrographic findings in 50 patients. Radiology 2006;240(3):778–85.

25. Leunig M, Beck M, Kalhor M, et al. Fibrocystic changes at anterosuperior femoral neck: prevalence in hips with femoroacetabular impingement. Radiology 2005;236(1):237–46.

26. Jamali AA, Mladenov K, Meyer DC, et al. Anteroposterior pelvic radiographs to assess acetabular retroversion: high validity of the cross-over-sign. J Orthop Res 2007;25(6):758–65.

27. Kalberer F, Sierra RJ, Madan SS, et al. Ischial spine projection into the pelvis: a new sign for acetabular retroversion. Clin Orthop Relat Res 2008;466(3): 677–83.

28. Siebenrock KA, Schoeniger R, Ganz R. Anterior femoro-acetabular impingement due to acetabular retroversion: treatment with periacetabular osteotomy. J Bone Joint Surg Am 2003;85A(2):278–86.

The Knee: MR Imaging of Uniquely Pediatric Disorders

Ramon Sanchez, MD*, Peter J. Strouse, MD

KEYWORDS

- Pediatric • MR imaging • Knee • Ligaments • Menisci
- Sport related injuries

Skeleton immaturity and intense physical activity render the pediatric population prone to musculoskeletal injury. Knee pain due to trauma is one of the most common musculoskeletal complaints. Injury patterns seen in children vary from those in adults. Clinical assessment of knee injuries may be difficult owing to severe pain, swelling, and joint effusion. Conventional radiology remains the primary imaging modality for children with knee pain, but many serious injuries will not be shown. In particular, most soft tissue abnormalities will not be seen; therefore, the value of radiography is often limited.

MR imaging is an excellent modality for pediatric knee disorders because of its lack of ionizing radiation, multiplanar capabilities, soft tissue contrast, and high resolution providing accurate assessment of bone, cartilage, menisci, ligaments, and adjacent soft tissues. MR imaging should not be used as a routine test because it carries significant additional cost, is associated with a potential delay in diagnosis and treatment, and, for younger children, is not exempt of risks attendant to selection or anesthesia. The main indications to perform MR imaging of the knee are clinical suspicion of suspected internal derangement or an occult fracture, persistent pain, refusal to bear weight, or hemarthrosis.

TECHNIQUE

Regardless of the pediatric knee protocol used, it should at least include the three planes with marrow-, fluid-, and cartilage-sensitive sequences. Proton density images are the primary sequence in most knee MR imaging protocols. T1-weighted images may be useful to differentiate between bone contusions and fractures. Cartilaginous structures are well delineated on fat-saturated proton density, spoiled gradient recalled echo (SPGR), or three-dimensional, T1-weighted gradient echo images. Either conventional or fast/turbo proton density imaging is ideal for showing ligamentous and meniscal derangements and can also show subtle articular cartilage injuries.[1,2] Some investigators have shown that fast spin echo images are less reliable in showing meniscal pathology. Fluid-sensitive short tau inversion recovery (STIR) and fat-suppressed fast/turbo spin echo T2-weighted imaging can be used; however, marrow and soft tissue edema are usually sufficiently seen on fat-saturated proton density images.

At the authors' center, two different pediatric knee protocols are used depending on the MR unit and patient's age. For younger patients, the following protocol and sequences are used: axial T1-weighted fast spin echo (FSE) localizer (repetition time [TR] 300 ms, echo time [TE] 17 ms, 10 mm with 2 mm gap), sagittal proton density spine echo (SE) (TR 1000 ms, TE 12 ms, 3 mm with 1 mm gap), sagittal three-dimensional gradient-recalled echo (GRE) (TR 650 ms, minimum TE, flip angle 30 degrees, 3 mm with 1 mm gap), coronal proton density FSE (TR 4500 ms, TE 17 ms, 4 mm with 0.5 mm gap), coronal proton density FSE with fat saturation (TR 4000 ms, TE 16 ms, 4 mm with 0.5 mm gap), and axial proton density FSE with fat saturation (TR 4000 ms, TE 16 ms, 4 mm with 0.5 mm gap). The second

Section of Pediatric Radiology, C.S. Mott Children's Hospital, University of Michigan Health System, F3503A Mott SPC5252, 500 E. Medical Center Drive, Ann Arbor, MI 48109-5252, USA
* Corresponding author.
E-mail address: ramonsan@umich.edu (R. Sanchez).

Magn Reson Imaging Clin N Am 17 (2009) 521–537
doi:10.1016/j.mric.2009.03.008

protocol is mainly used for older patients and includes these sequences: axial T1-weighted FSE localizer (TR 300 ms, TE 17 ms, 10 mm with 2 mm gap), sagittal proton density SE (TR 1000 ms, TE 12 ms, 3 mm with 1 mm gap), sagittal proton density FSE with fat saturation (TR 3000 ms, TE 17 ms, 3 mm with 1 mm gap), coronal proton density FSE with fat saturation (TR 3000 ms, TE 17 ms, 3 mm with 1 mm gap), and axial proton density FSE with fat saturation (TR 3000 ms, TE 17 ms, 3 mm with 1 mm gap).

ACUTE INJURIES
Ligamentous Injuries

Ligamentous injuries are more frequent in adolescents than in preadolescent children. In children, ligaments are protected by relative weakness of the physis and by physiologic ligamentous laxity; however, with increasing participation in high level and competitive sports at a younger age, ligamentous injuries are now more common. The most frequent ligamentous injury in the knee is a tear of the anterior cruciate ligament (ACL), more frequent in girls. The predisposition of ACL injuries in girls is multifactorial and related to hormonal influence, relative valgus alignment, increased joint laxity, and intercondylar notch morphology.[3]

In young patients, stretching of the ACL may result in avulsion of the tibial insertion (described later). MR imaging findings of ACL injuries in children do not differ from those in adult patients; however, in children, the pattern of bone marrow edema in the lateral femoral condyle, posteromedial tibial plateau, and posterolateral corner of the tibia can occasionally be seen without ACL tear, presumably due to physiologic ligamentous laxity.[4]

MR imaging of an ACL tear will show increased signal intensity with a disrupted pattern (**Fig. 1**). As is true in adults, ACL injury is commonly associated with collateral ligamentous tears and meniscal tears. Surgical repair of ACL tears in children may require special surgical techniques to avoid growth plate transgression.[5]

Collateral ligament injuries are not as common in children as in adults. Again, this observation may be due to the fact that severe valgus or varus stress will more likely result in a physeal fracture than a ligamentous injury in a skeletally immature patient.

MENISCUS INJURIES

Meniscal tears are also rare in children with an open physis. With advancing age, the incidence of internal knee derangement increases

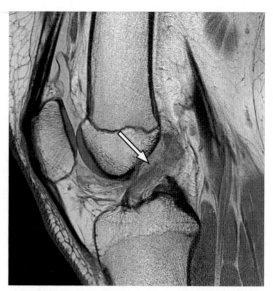

Fig. 1. ACL tear in a 15-year-old boy who injured his right knee while playing football. Sagittal proton density turbo spin echo (TR 3613 ms, TE 30 ms) shows that the ACL is markedly thickened and demonstrates increased signal intensity (*arrow*). Some fibers are intact. At surgery, a partial ACL tear was found.

dramatically. Pediatric meniscal injuries have a similar MR imaging appearance and distribution to those in adults, although there are a few unique characteristics of the pediatric menisci that are worth mentioning.

The medial and lateral menisci are equally vulnerable to injury in the immature patient; however, most meniscal injuries in patients before 10 years of age are due to a discoid meniscus. This defect accounts for a slightly higher prevalence of lateral (versus medial) meniscus injuries in the younger pediatric population.

Longitudinal tears and peripheral detachment are the most common meniscal lesions in younger patients. The posterior horns of the menisci are most commonly involved. Bucket-handle tears are more frequent in older teens.

The menisci are richly vascularized during infancy, and intrameniscal vessels are seen as areas of peripheral high signal intensity and should not be confused with tear. The vascular tissue is identified as central, horizontal-oriented linear or globular areas (**Fig. 2**), whereas meniscal tears tend to be less peripheral, more linear, well defined, and vertical.[6]

Discoid Meniscus

A discoid meniscus is a large, dysplastic meniscus lacking the normal semilunar shape. The prevalence of this anatomic variant is 1.5% to 4.5% of the population. Discoid menisci are almost always

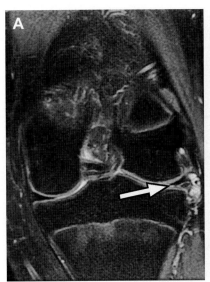
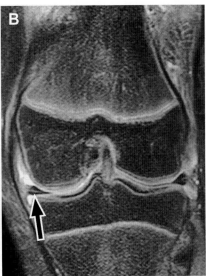

Fig. 2. Meniscal tear versus normal intrameniscal vessels. (*A*) Image of a 15-year-old boy with left knee pain hit by a sled on the lateral side of his knee. Coronal proton density fat saturation (TR 4666 ms, TE 28 ms) shows high linear signal intensity extending to the articular surface of the lateral meniscus, which represents a tear (*arrow*) with an adjacent parameniscal cyst. (*B*) Image of a 13-year-old boy with knee pain after trauma. Coronal proton density fat saturation (TR 2000 ms, TE 15 ms) shows linear, horizontal-oriented, high signal intensity within the body of the medial meniscus (*arrow*), which represents intrameniscal vascular tissue and should not be confused with a tear.

lateral; however, medial discoid menisci have been reported.[7]

The aberrant meniscal configuration probably results from deficiency in the normal meniscofemoral attachments and lack of involution of the central portion of the fetal meniscus. The abnormal configuration allows repetitive drawing and stress during knee extension and increases the incidence of degeneration and tears.[8] Several types of discoid meniscus have been described.[9]

A discoid meniscus may be asymptomatic. If symptoms occur, the patient may present in early childhood (even infancy); however, symptoms may not develop until adolescence or early adulthood. The most common symptoms are pain, clicking, snapping, and locking of the joint.

On MR imaging, a discoid meniscus is identified as large (more than 13 mm in cross section and usually 2 mm greater than the opposite meniscus). On sagittal images, discoid meniscus continuity of the anterior and posterior horns is seen on three or more 4- to 5-mm thick images.[7] Coronal views show abnormal medial extension of the body of the meniscus toward the intercondylar notch (**Fig. 3**). A discoid meniscus often covers more than 50% of the lateral tibial plateau on sagittal and coronal views.

Symptomatic discoid menisci usually show diffusely increased high signal intensity on all sequences due to mucinous degeneration. These areas of high signal may or may not extend into

the joint surface. Intrameniscal cysts, horizontal tears, and a large extruded posterior horn may also be seen (**Fig. 4**). When a discoid meniscus is torn and displaced, it may be difficult to identify it as discoid.

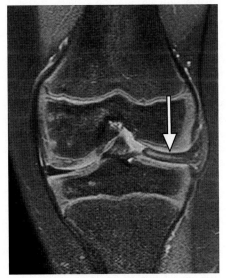

Fig. 3. Discoid meniscus in an 8-year-old boy with left knee popping. Coronal proton density with fat saturation (TR 1524 ms, TE 8 ms) shows discoid lateral meniscus (*arrow*) extending into the intercondylar notch with high signal consistent with degeneration.

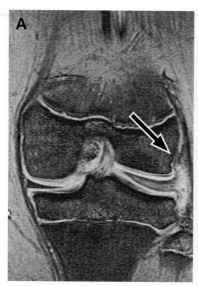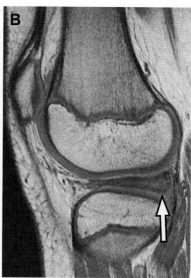

Fig. 4. Images of a 10-year-old patient with a discoid lateral meniscus. (*A*) Coronal GRE (TR 32 ms, TE 11 ms, flip angle 30 degrees) shows a discoid configuration of the lateral meniscus with a large intrameniscal cyst (*arrow*). (*B*) Sagittal proton density (TR 1524 ms, TE 8 ms) demonstrates a large extruded posterior horn (*arrow*).

SALTER-HARRIS FRACTURES

Physeal fractures account for almost 20% of all fractures of the extremities in children. The physeal cartilage represents the weakest portion of the immature skeleton. The ligaments and capsular attachments are up to five times stronger than the physis.[10]

The Salter-Harris classification of physeal fractures classifies fractures according to the course of the fracture through the physis, metaphysis, and epiphysis.[11] The incidence of subsequent growth disturbance is less with lower grade Salter-Harris fractures.

Although distal femoral and proximal tibial physeal fractures are uncommon, accounting for 1.4% and 0.8%, respectively, of physeal fractures,[11,12] these sites are responsible for approximately 40% and 16%, respectively, of physeal bridges requiring surgical management.[13] Physeal fractures at the knee are considered at high risk for causing abnormal growth. The higher incidence of bridge formation is partially explained by the fact that the knee is often subject to violent injury mechanisms. Another contributing factor is involvement of the central physeal undulation of the distal femur.[14]

Most physeal fractures at the knee are obvious on radiography; however, occasionally, fractures may be very subtle or frankly occult on radiography.[15] Interpretation of knee MR imaging in skeletally immature patients must include a careful search for physeal fracture. MR imaging has an important role not only for the initial accurate

diagnosis when plain films are negative or equivocal but also for delineating the extent of the fracture.

Salter II fractures of the distal femur are the most common type diagnosed by MR imaging. Fractures are seen as a linear signal abnormality within the metaphysis (low on T1-weighting, high on fluid-sensitive sequences) extending to the physis, widening with increased signal of the involved physis, adjacent bone marrow and soft tissue edema, and disruption and elevation of the periosteum (**Fig. 5**).[15] MR imaging may detect interposed soft tissue or periosteum within the fracture which may prevent reduction and lead to open surgical reduction (**Fig. 6**).[16]

MR imaging can also be used to detect and delineate premature physeal fusion. Cartilage-sensitive sequences such as fat-saturated proton density and three-dimensional SPGR are used. Discontinuity of the normal physeal signal is seen (**Fig. 7**). The location and size of bone bridges have important prognostic and surgical implications.

AVULSION FRACTURES
Anterior Tibial Spine

The anterior tibial spine is the site of insertion of the ACL. Avulsion fractures of the anterior tibial spine are a common sport-related preadolescent injury, whereas ACL tears become more common after physeal closure.[17] In the skeletally immature patient, the chondro-osseous tibial spine is the weakest aspect of the ACL complex. The

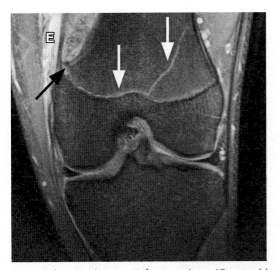

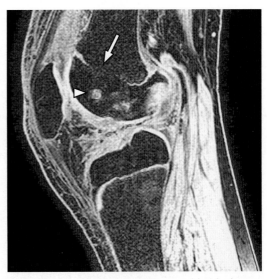

Fig. 5. Salter-Harris type II fracture in a 15-year-old patient who sustained an injury while playing football. Coronal proton density with fat suppression (TR 1524 ms, TE 8 ms) demonstrates a line of fracture (*white arrows*) extending from the lateral aspect of the distal femoral metaphysis through the medial physis, consistent with a nondisplaced Salter II fracture. E = associated soft tissue swelling. Periosteum is disrupted medially (*black arrow*).

Fig. 7. Premature closure in a 12-year-old girl who sustained a Salter-Harris type IV fracture of the right distal femur when hit by a motor boat. Sagittal water selective excitation T1 (TR 20 ms, TE 7.5 ms) shows discontinuity of the high signal along the distal femoral condyle physis, consistent with premature closure and a bone bridge (*arrow*). A tract from prior screw fixation through the distal femoral epiphysis is also seen (*arrowhead*).

intercondylar notch width index also seems to have a role in determining the type of injury. Children with wide intercondylar notches tend to sustain avulsion fractures of the anterior spine, whereas patients with narrow notches are more prone to ACL intrasubstance tears.[3]

Tibial spine avulsions are often subtle radiographically, particularly to the untrained observer. Addition of oblique and tunnel view projections may be helpful.[18] Joint effusion (with or without lipohemarthrosis) may be the only radiographic finding. MR imaging allows visualization of the avulsed fragment in different planes. The fracture line can be appreciated on different sequences as a low signal intensity line (**Fig. 8**). ACL fibers are usually seen inserting onto the fragment. Additional intrasubstance high signal intensity signal may be seen along the ACL ligament, representing associated partial ACL tears.[19] Treatment is based on the degree of displacement. Nondisplaced fractures (type 1) may be treated conservatively, whereas hinged (type 2) and displaced (type 3) fractures may require reduction and fixation of the avulsed fragment.

Transient Patellar Dislocation

Transient patellar dislocation occurs due to lateral dislocation of the patella from the femoral trochlea as a result of trauma. It usually occurs in adolescent patients during sport-related activities with direct trauma, valgus stress, or twisting injury of the knee. Patients present with anterior knee

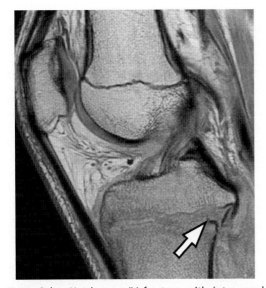

Fig. 6. Salter-Harris type IV fracture with interposed periosteum in a 15-year-old soccer player who sustained a proximal tibial fracture. Sagittal proton density turbo spin echo (2136/30) reveals the presence of periosteum (*arrow*) within the fracture line which may be responsible for failure to reduction.

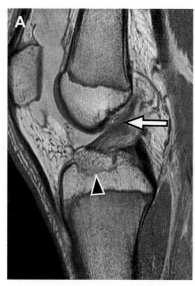
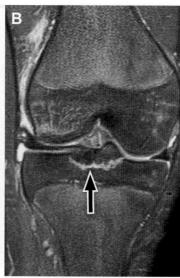

Fig. 8. Anterior tibial spine fracture in a 14-year-old boy. (*A*) Sagittal proton density image (TR 2137 ms, TE 9 ms) demonstrates a tibial spine fracture (*arrowhead*) with preserved ACL (*white arrow*). (*B*) Coronal proton density with fat suppression (TR 2137 ms, TE 9 ms) shows the fracture line (*arrow*) extending through the tibia at the base of the tibial spine.

pain and swelling. Clinical assessment and differentiation from other entities is often difficult.[20–22] Spontaneous patellar relocation occurs in 50% to 75% of patients. Often, the patient is unaware that the patella was dislocated. Radiologic findings may be subtle and include small fractures of the medial patella of the lateral femoral condyle, soft tissue swelling, joint effusion, and underlying patellofemoral dysmorphology.

MR imaging findings include joint effusion, bone marrow edema involving the inferomedial patella and lateral femoral condyle (**Fig. 9**), cartilage injuries, and partial disruption of the medial retinaculum.[23] Osteochondral fragments or intra-articular loose bodies are seen in 42% of patients. Concomitant ligamentous or meniscal injuries have been reported to occur in 23% of pediatric patients.

MR imaging is useful to evaluate predisposing factors for transient patellar dislocation, including patellar tilt, patellar subluxation, femoral trochlear dysplasia, and patella alta. MR imaging may show some degree of lateral subluxation in otherwise asymptomatic patients when the knee is imaged in the extended position.

CHRONIC OR OVERUSE INJURIES

Approximately 30% to 50% of sport-related injuries in the pediatric population are due to overuse. Sport-related activities in which repetitive microtrauma is common include jumping, running, and dancing.[24]

Stress Fractures

Stress fractures occur after repetitive trauma on a normal bone. In skeletally immature patients,

the tibia is the most common site (at the proximal posteromedial metadiaphyseal junction), followed by the fibula (21%) and femur (12%).[25] These fractures usually occur in teenagers. Stress fractures have also been reported in teenage female athletes with osteoporosis, amenorrhea, and eating disorders, the so-called "female athlete triad."[26] Only 10% to 25% of stress fractures are radiographically detected at presentation.[27] Early in the course of a stress fracture, MR imaging shows nonspecific soft tissue and bone marrow

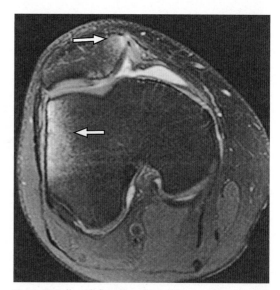

Fig. 9. Patellar dislocation in a 16-year-old girl with medial knee pain after injury. Axial proton density FSE with fat saturation (TR 3000 ms, TE 18 ms) shows bone marrow edema involving the lateral condyle and the medial aspect of the patella (*arrows*).

edema. Subsequently, the fracture line can be appreciated on different sequences as a low signal intensity. T2-weighted images, STIR, and post-contrast sequences reveal an area of high signal involving both cortex and marrow, indicating edema surrounding a linear area of low signal intensity that corresponds to the fracture line and callus (**Fig. 10**). Adjacent soft tissues show high signal due to edema. MR imaging has an important role not only for early detection but also for differential diagnosis from other entities which may present similar radiologic findings, including osteoid osteoma, infection, and shin splints.[28]

Physeal widening in the knee due to stress injury in high-level child athletes has also been reported (**Fig. 11**).[29]

Osgood-Schlatter Disease

Osgood-Schlatter disease is defined as a traction apophysitis at the insertion of the patellar tendon on the anterior tibial tubercle secondary to repetitive forces and traction microtrauma. The entity is most common in active adolescent boys between 10 and 15 years of age participating in jumping activities such as basketball, gymnastics, or volleyball. Patients present with unilateral or bilateral disease (20% to 30%) with an insidious onset, low-grade knee pain, and soft tissue swelling at the level of the anterior tibial tubercle.

Osgood-Schlatter disease is usually a self-limited entity with a good prognosis, and the diagnosis is usually established clinically. MR imaging is performed to exclude other pathologies when the diagnosis is doubt or to clarify equivocal conventional radiographic findings. MR imaging findings include the presence of hypertrophy or fragmentation of the tibial tubercle with possible heterotopic ossification within the distal patellar tendon. Fluid-sensitive sequences may show high signal intensity in the tibial tubercle and thickening and edema of the adjacent patellar tendon and surrounding soft tissues (**Fig. 12**). An infrapatellar bursa may be seen.[30,31]

The normal tibial tubercle may show irregularity and fragmentation. In the absence of symptoms and without associated inflammatory changes (ie, edema), this appearance should be considered a normal variant.

Sinding-Larsen-Johansson Disease

In 1921, Sinding, Larsen, and Johansson independently described a syndrome in adolescents consisting of tenderness at the level of the inferior pole of the patella associated with radiologic evidence of fragmentation. The abnormality is thought to result from persistent or repetitive traction microtrauma on the patellar tendon as a result of running, stair climbing, or kneeling activities.[32]

The condition is most common among boys 10 to 12 years of age. The chief complaint is anterior knee pain, which increases with activity and decreases at rest, and focal tenderness at the patella-tendon junction. Sinding-Larsen-Johansson disease is usually a self-limited entity. Resolution occurs in 6 to 12 months with rest and quadriceps flexibility exercises. The diagnosis is usually is made based on physical examination and conventional radiology findings. Conventional radiography and MR imaging demonstrate the presence of fragmentation of the inferior pole of the patella with or without ossification at the proximal aspect of the patellar tendon, as well as

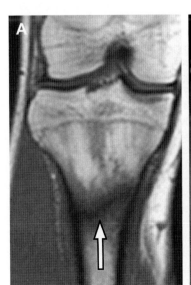 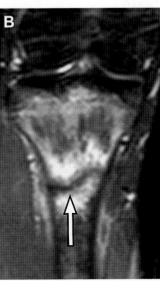

Fig. 10. Stress fracture in a 17-year-old cross country runner with left proximal tibial pain for the last 2 weeks. (*A*) Coronal T1 (TR 478 ms, TE 9 ms) and (*B*) coronal STIR (TR 4730 ms, TE 30 ms) show a line of fracture across the proximal tibia metaphysis (*arrows*) with adjacent soft tissue swelling and bone marrow edema.

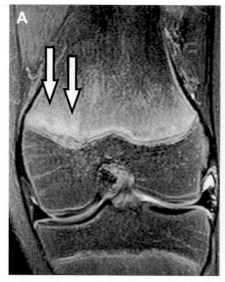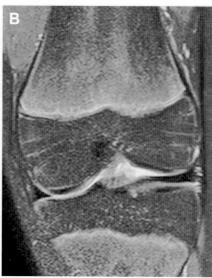

Fig. 11. Physeal stress fracture in an 11-year-old female, high-level softball player with long history of left knee pain. (A) Image (TR 2200 ms, TE 40 ms) demonstrates lateral femoral physeal widening and irregularity within adjacent metaphyseal bone marrow edema (*arrows*). (B) Same patient 3 months later after rest. Coronal proton density with fat saturation (TR 3000 ms, TE 30 ms) shows normal appearance of the distal femoral physis with resolution of metaphyseal edema.

inflammatory changes and thickening of the patellar tendon (**Fig. 13**).

MR imaging is important for the correct diagnosis of other entities that present with similar or equivocal radiologic findings, such as patellar sleeve fracture (acute osteocartilaginous avulsion of the lower pole of the patella), infrapatellar tendinopathy or "jumper's knee" (in skeletally mature athletes), patellar fractures, irregular ossification of the inferior pole of the patella, and type I bipartite patella.[33,34]

Osteochondritis Dissecans

Osteochondritis dissecans is thought to be an osteochondral fracture secondary to avascular necrosis of an area of the subchondral bone and cartilage. The etiology of osteochondritis dissecans remains controversial, but repetitive trauma, ischemia, and familial tendency are common predisposing factors.[35] A recent history of trauma is found in approximately 50% of cases.

In the knee, 75% of cases involve the posterolateral aspect of the medial femoral condyle, often extending to the intercondylar region. The lateral condyle is involved in 20% of patients. Osteochondritis dissecans is bilateral in one third of the patients but often with asymmetric severity. The peak incidence is around 12 to 13 years of age. The most common symptom of femoral osteochondritis dissecans is insidious onset of activity-related knee pain and locking when an unstable or loose fragment forms.

The role of MR imaging is to determine the size and location of the osteochondral fragment, to evaluate extension into the articular cartilage, to

Fig. 12. Osgood-Schlatter disease in a 12-year-old male basketball player with right anterior knee pain. Sagittal proton density FSE with fat saturation (TR 3000 ms, TE 21 ms) demonstrates high signal intensity involving the tibial tubercle (*white arrow*), the distal aspect of the patellar tendon (*black arrow*), and Hoffa's fat pad (*asterisk*).

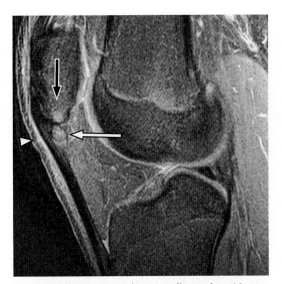

Fig. 13. Sinding-Larsen-Johansson disease in a 14-year-old tennis player with knee pain for months. Sagittal proton density with fat saturation (TR 2000 ms, TE 30 ms) demonstrates bone marrow edema involving the inferior pole of the patella (*black arrow*), ossification at the proximal aspect of the patellar tendon with edema (*white arrow*), thickening of the patellar tendon, and prepatellar edema (*arrowhead*).

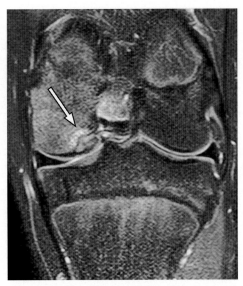

Fig. 14. Osteochondritis dissecans, stable fragment in a 16-year-old boy with an osteochondral defect of the medial left femoral condyle. Coronal proton density fat saturation (TR 3000 ms, TE 30 ms) shows a defect in the medial aspect of the medial femoral condyle with adjacent marrow edema (*arrow*). There is no fluid between the defect and the medial femoral condyle to suggest instability.

establish the degree of stability of the fragment, and to determine the presence of loose intra-articular fragments. Findings that suggest stability on MR imaging are a fragment size of less than 1 cm and continuity of the fragment with the parent bone with no high signal intensity interface (**Fig. 14**). Findings that suggest instability are a larger size of the fragment (>1 cm), the presence of cystic areas larger than 5 mm within the donor site (**Fig. 15**), the presence of T2-weighted high signal intensity fluid between the donor site and the fragment (even if the adjacent cartilage appears intact),[36] and the evidence of loose bodies within the joint. Small loose fragments may be subtle on MR imaging and should be carefully looked for, particularly in recesses of the joint space. MR arthrography may be performed to assess the stability of an osteochondritis dissecans fragment. Extension of intra-articular contrast between the donor site and the fragment suggests instability. Intra-articular gadolinium is not used routinely but may be of benefit in problematic cases when determination of fragment stability will alter therapy.

Good prognostic factors are the presence of an open physis, small sized lesions, and evidence of stability on serial MR imaging.[37] Recently, Kijowski and colleagues[38] described different sensitivity and specificity of MR imaging criteria for instability in juvenile versus adult osteochondritis dissecans.

Findings indicating instability in adults may not hold true in children due to a greater ability to heal or to later presentation of lesions in adults than in children.[38] The clinical outcome of osteochondritis dissecans in children is better than in adults. The better prognosis in children can be partially explained by the erroneous diagnosis of some normal variants of ossification as osteochondritis dissecans. Distal femoral epiphyseal irregularity is usually seen on MR imaging as areas of irregular ossification of the femoral epiphysis involving the posterior aspect of the lateral condyle (**Fig. 16**). The overlying cartilage remains intact, and there are no areas of high signal intensity on T2-weighted images in the adjacent bone marrow.[39,40]

TUMORS AND INCIDENTAL OSSEOUS LESIONS

The knee is the most common joint imaged with MR, and osseous tumors and tumorlike lesions are common incidental imaging findings. Most of these incidental findings are benign conditions with no relation to the patient's symptoms. The lesions are often incompletely evaluated because the study is not specifically tailored to evaluate a mass; therefore, they may become diagnostically challenging. Correlation with conventional radiography of bone is often helpful in further defining these incidental lesions.[41]

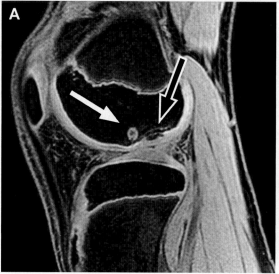
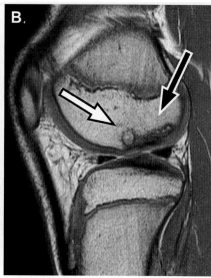

Fig. 15. Unstable osteochondritis dissecans in a 13-year-old male baseball player with a history of recurrent knee pain. (*A*) Sagittal water selective excitation T1 (TR 20 ms, TE 7.5 ms) and (*B*) sagittal proton density turbo spin echo (TR 3146 ms, TE 30 ms) show cortical irregularity involving the posteromedial aspect of the lateral femoral condyle (*black arrows*). The presence of a 6-mm subchondral cyst suggests instability (*white arrows*).

Nonossifying Fibroma/Fibrous Cortical Defect

Benign fibrous cortical defects and nonossifying fibromas are common lesions found in the metadiaphysis of the distal femur of children. Arbitrarily, lesions smaller than 2 cm are called fibrous cortical defects, whereas larger lesions are called nonossifying fibromas.

The MR imaging appearance of fibrous cortical defects/nonossifying fibromas usually parallels their radiographic appearance, with a well-defined, eccentric, scalloped geographic lesion. The signal intensity of MR imaging varies depending on the degree of maturation. On T1-weighted images, the lesions have low signal intensity compared with that of skeletal muscle (**Fig. 17**). Early in development, these lesions are bright on T2-weighted images. As the lesions heal and mature, they show low signal intensity on T2-weighted images. Heterogeneity of signal usually implies an intermediate stage of development.[42]

Osteochondromas

Osteochondromas, or exostoses, are benign cartilaginous lesions commonly found about the knee.

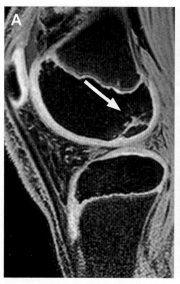
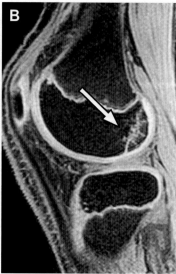

Fig. 16. Normal variant that mimics osteochondritis dissecans in an 11-year-old boy with a 2-year history of bilateral intermittent knee pain and abnormal cortical irregularity of the distal femoral epiphysis on plain films. Sagittal water selective excitation T1 (TR 20 ms, TE 7.4 ms) of the left (*A*) and right (*B*) knee demonstrates osseous irregularity involving the posterior aspect of the lateral femoral condyles (*arrows*). There is complete cartilaginous coverage with no bone marrow signal abnormality.

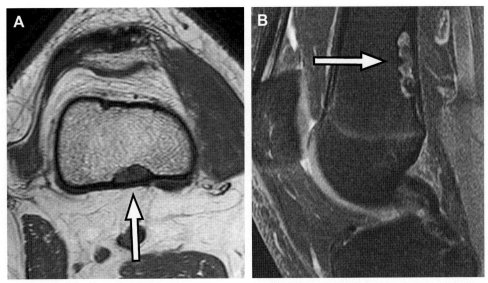

Fig. 17. Incidental fibrous cortical defect in an 18-year-old man. (*A*) Axial T1 (TR 420 ms, TE 8 ms) and (*B*) sagittal proton density with fat saturation (TR 2000 ms, TE 30 ms) demonstrate a lobulated, well-circumscribed cortically based lesion in the posterior distal femur, which is low signal on T1 and heterogeneous on T2 and consistent with a fibrous cortical defect (*arrows*).

Many of these lesions are solitary, asymptomatic, and discovered incidentally. Radiographic findings are characteristic. When symptomatic, complications are usually due to mechanical impingement on adjacent structures. Malignant transformation is extremely rare, particularly from a solitary lesion.[43]

Osteochondromas are classified as pedunculated or sessile based on morphology. The lesions are contiguous with the cortex of the underlying bone and project outward from the metaphysis, pointing away from the adjacent physis. Continuity of the medullary space is seen on radiography and MR imaging. The cartilage cap of the osteochondroma is best seen on MR imaging and shows signal intensity similar to that of muscle on T1-weighted images and fluidlike signal on T2-weighted images (**Fig. 18**). The overlying

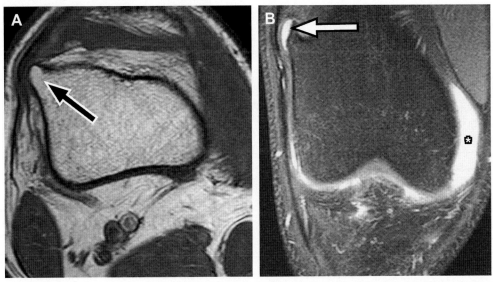

Fig. 18. Osteochondroma in an 18-year-old patient who sustained knee injury and was referred to rule out a meniscal tear. (*A*) Axial T1 (TR 420 ms, TE 8 ms) and (*B*) coronal proton density fat saturation (TR 2000 ms, TE 30 ms) show lateral femoral exostosis (*black arrow*) with a cartilage cap (*white arrow*) and joint effusion (*asterisk*).

perichondrium is seen as a thin peripheral area of decreased signal intensity on T2-weighted images.

Trevor's disease, or dysplasia epiphysialis hemimelica, is characterized by ostechondroma-like lesions involving the epiphysis. The lesion is predominantly cartilaginous in younger patients, and MR imaging is especially useful for delineation of the abnormality.[44]

Distal Femoral Cortical Irregularity

Distal femoral cortical irregularity (also referred as a cortical desmoid or distal femoral metaphyseal irregularity) represents a common finding that occurs along the posterior aspect of the medial femoral condyle cortex approximately 1 to 2 cm proximal to the physis. The finding is closely approximated to the site of attachment of tendinous fibers of the adductor magnus muscle. The pathogenesis of this lesion is controversial; some investigators postulate a traumatic origin related to the muscle insertion, whereas others consider it to have a developmental origin.[45]

On MR imaging, low signal is seen on T1-weighted images and high signal on T2-weighted images (**Fig. 19**). The defect often slightly enhances after the administration of contrast, but no adjacent soft tissue component is seen.[46] Plain radiographs may show an ill-defined or scalloped appearance and occasionally may mimic an aggressive lesion.

INFLAMMATORY CONDITIONS
Juvenile Rheumatoid Arthritis

Juvenile rheumatoid arthritis is defined as a systemic idiopathic inflammatory arthritis affecting patients younger than 16 years of age and with symptoms persisting for more than 6 weeks. It represents one the most common forms of arthritis in the pediatric population. When the knee is involved, patients may present with a swollen, warm, painful joint and occasionally with contracture. Presentation may mimic other pathology of the knee. MR imaging can have an important role in establishing a correct diagnosis, determining the degree of activity and extent of the disease, and monitoring the response to treatment.

The most common findings of juvenile rheumatoid arthritis on MR imaging are joint effusion, synovial proliferation, and the presence of pannus and infrapatellar fat pad changes.[47] Synovial proliferation with increased thickness (more than 3 mm) is usually seen in the suprapatellar bursa. Synovial proliferation is seen as low-to-intermediate signal to muscle on T1-weighted images and low-to-intermediate signal on T2-weighted

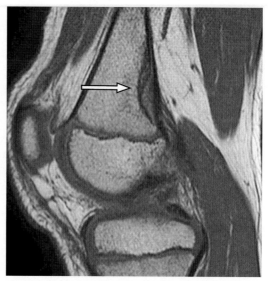

Fig. 19. Distal femoral cortical irregularity in a 9-year-old boy with a stable osteochondral defect of the medial femoral condyle (not shown). Sagittal proton density fat saturation (TR 2229 ms, TE 9 ms) demonstrates a cortical irregularity along the distal femur metaphysis (*arrow*).

images when compared with the joint effusion. The proliferative tissue enhances after the administration of gadolinium (**Fig. 20**). The pannus is

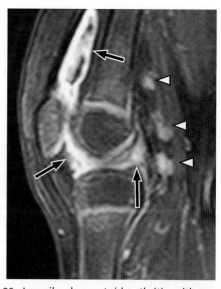

Fig. 20. Juvenile rheumatoid arthritis with synovial proliferation in a 2-year-old girl with a history of left knee morning stiffness and flexion contracture. Sagittal T1 fat saturation three-dimensional postcontrast sequence (TR 13 ms, TE 6.6 ms) demonstrates synovial proliferation with diffuse enhancement in the suprapatellar bursa, infrapatellar fat pad, and posterior recess (*arrows*). A few small popliteal lymph nodes are noted (*arrowheads*).

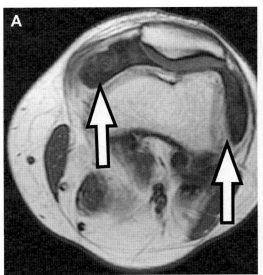

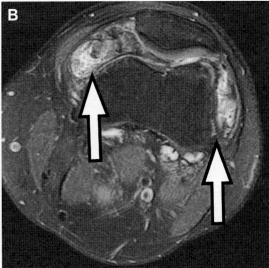

Fig. 21. Pigmented villonodular synovitis in a 16-year-old boy involving the left knee. (*A*) Axial T1 (TR 300 ms, TE 14 ms) identifies multiple nodular (*arrows*) and (*B*) axial T2 FSE fat saturation (TR 3900 ms, TE 41 ms) hypointense lesions (*arrows*) through the joint, representing synovial proliferation.

usually seen as low signal on T1- and T2-weighted images with minimal enhancement after contrast administration. Hypointense "rice" bodies may be seen, representing detached fragments of synovium. Other less common but useful findings are the presence of cartilage and bone changes, meniscal hypoplasia, popliteal synovial cysts, and popliteal lymph node enlargement.

Pigmented Villonodular Synovitis

Pigmented villonodular synovitis is a rare proliferative disease of unknown etiology that affects synovium, bursae, and tendon sheaths. It is considered a neoplastic condition characterized by significant synovial hyperplasia, hypervascularity, and accumulation of hemosiderin-laden macrophages.

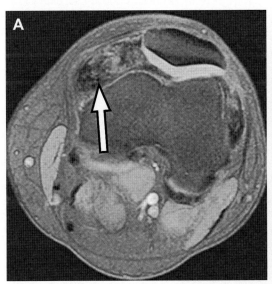

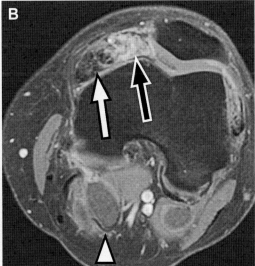

Fig. 22. Pigmented villonodular synovitis in a 16-year-old boy involving the left knee. Axial SPGR fat-saturated (TR 160 ms, TE 3.5 ms) images pre- (*A*) and post gadolinium (*B*). Low T1 signal intensity areas represent hemosiderin deposits within the intra-articular masses and synovium (*white arrows*). Heterogeneous enhancement of the intra-articular masses and synovium is noted (*black arrow*). Synovial enhancement also extends into a loculated Baker cyst (*arrowhead*).

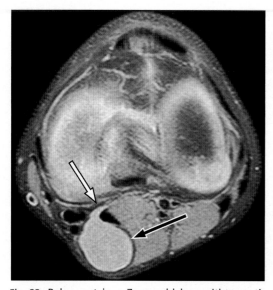

Fig. 23. Baker cyst in a 7-year-old boy with a cystic mass involving the left posterior knee. Axial T2 fat saturation (TR 1500 ms, TE 15 ms) shows a high signal intensity structure (*black arrow*) with a small neck between the gastrocnemius and semimembranous muscles (*white arrow*).

Although pigmented villonodular synovitis is mainly found in adults, a recent series with childhood presentation has been reported.[48]

In the knee, pigmented villonodular synovitis usually presents with similar symptoms as juvenile rheumatoid arthritis, that is, insidious onset of pain, decreased range of motion, and swelling with increased skin temperature. Joint effusion and a noncalcified but dense soft tissue mass representing hemosiderin deposits are common

nonspecific early findings on conventional radiography. MR imaging has an important role in making the diagnosis and evaluating the extent of the disease.

The chief findings of MR imaging are a large joint effusion with synovial proliferation in the form of frondlike septations and masses and thickened synovium (**Fig. 21**). An associated Baker cyst is common, whereas bony changes of edema and erosion are uncommon. The paramagnetic effects of hemosiderin deposits create the low signal intensity on all sequences within the synovium, intra-articular masses, and septations. GRE sequences are more sensitive to the paramagnetic effect (**Fig. 22**). With gadolinium, there is diffuse enhancement of the thickened synovium, masses, and septations.

Venous malformation involving the synovium may mimic pigmented villonodular synovitis, especially when repeated episodes of bleeding lead to intra-articular hemosiderin deposits.

DEVELOPMENTAL/CONGENITAL CONDITIONS
Baker Cyst

A Baker cyst, or popliteal cyst, is a fluid collection resulting from distention of the gastrocnemius–semimembranous bursa. These cysts develop at any age and usually resolve spontaneously. In children, most Baker cysts are isolated, although they may be associated with intra-articular pathology.[49] In young children, Baker cysts are thought to arise from local irritation as opposed to extension of fluid from the joint as is believed to occur in adults.

On MR imaging, Baker cysts are seen as a fluid-filled structure located at the posteromedial

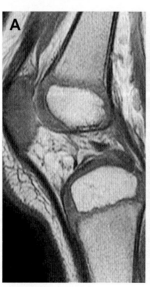
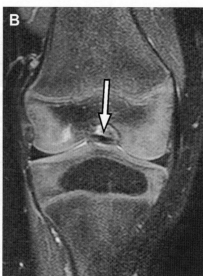

Fig. 24. A 4-year-old boy with a loose right knee on examination and absent ACL and posterior cruciate ligament (PCL). (*A*) Sagittal turbo spin echo proton density (TR 3000 ms, TE 30 ms) shows absent ACL and PCL. (*B*) Coronal proton density with fat suppression (TR 3000 ms, TE 30 ms) shows prominent meniscofemoral ligament extending from the lateral meniscus to the femoral condyle (*arrow*).

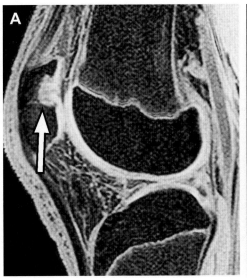
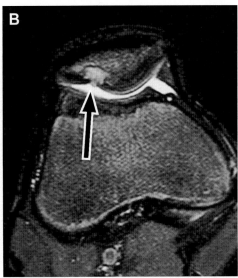

Fig. 25. Dorsal defect of the patella in a 14-year-old boy with an abnormal right patellar ovoid lesion on radiography. (*A*) Sagittal water selective excitation T1 (TR 20 ms, TE 7.5 ms) shows intermediate signal, well-defined lesion located within the posterior, lateral, and superior aspect of the patella (*white arrow*). (*B*) Axial proton density fat saturation (TR 3849 ms, TE 30 ms) shows a small cartilage defect adjacent to the patellar defect (*black arrow*).

aspect of the knee, with a neck or beak between the gastrocnemius and semimembranous muscles (**Fig. 23**). Fine septations may be seen. Rupture and infection are uncommon.

Congenital Absence of the Cruciate Ligaments

Congenital absence of the cruciate ligaments is a rare condition. Most cases are sporadic, bilateral, and combined with other malformations such as fibular hemimelia, or a congenital short femur, or occur in association with a skeletal dysplasia.[50] The most common presentation is knee laxity and pain. MR imaging demonstrates an abnormal shape of the tibial spines and dysplastic femoral condyles, absent (**Fig. 24**) or sometimes rudimentary ligaments, and hypertrophy of the meniscofemoral ligament of Humphrey.[50]

The differential diagnosis of congenital absence of the cruciate ligaments is chronic posttraumatic ligamentous injury. A prior undiagnosed injury is suggested by a history of prior trauma, the presence of secondary signs such as associated meniscal lesions, avulsion injuries of the intercondylar eminence of the tibia,[51] and the earlier progression of degenerative changes.

Dorsal Defect of the Patella

A dorsal defect of the patella is present in 1% of the population. Although considered a normal variant, it may cause patellofemoral symptoms and knee pain. Dorsal defect of the patella may be associated with a multipartite patella.[52,53] The

defect is usually located at the superolateral aspect of the articular surface of the patella and measures 1 to 2 cm.[54] MR imaging of a dorsal defect of the patella shows the lucent area with intact overlying cartilage and adjacent bone marrow edema (**Fig. 25**).[55] Occasionally, articular cartilage over a dorsal defect of the patella is indented or thinned. Cartilage irregularities of the

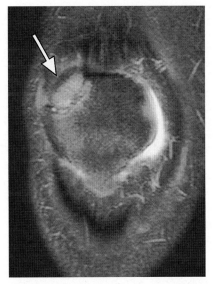

Fig. 26. A 15-year-old boy with a symptomatic type III bipartite patella. Coronal proton density with fat suppression (TR 3000 ms, TE 30 ms) shows a linear increased signal intensity involving the superior lateral aspect of the patella (*arrow*). Bone marrow edema is also noted.

lateral patellar facet, chondral defects, and sub-chondral bone changes are more consistent with chondromalacia patella or patellar osteochondral fractures, uncommon injury findings that may result from chronic patellar dislocation or acute patellar trauma.

Bipartite Patella

A bipartite patella represents the failure of fusion of a secondary ossification center of the patella, usually at the superolateral aspect of the patella. Although considered a normal variant, a bipartite patella can cause anterior knee pain. Chronic or direct trauma can cause disruption of the syn-chondrosis between the ossification centers, causing symptoms.[56] On MR imaging, the pres-ence of edema within the bipartite fragment, abnormal signal across the synchondrosis, and cartilage discontinuity are suggestive of a symp-tomatic bipartite patella (**Fig. 26**); in the absence of edema, an alternative explanation for knee pain should be sought.

SUMMARY

MR imaging is a superb imaging modality for pedi-atric knee disorders. Familiarity with common injury patterns and disease processes, develop-mental abnormalities, and incidental findings unique to the pediatric population is necessary for optimal diagnostic accuracy of MR imaging of the pediatric knee.

REFERENCES

1. Jaramillo D, Laor T. Pediatric musculoskeletal MRI: basic principles to optimize success. Pediatr Radiol 2008;38(4):379–91.
2. Oeppen RS, Connolly SA, Bencardino JT, et al. Acute injury of the articular cartilage and subchon-dral bone: a common but unrecognized lesion in the immature knee. AJR Am J Roentgenol 2004; 182(1):111–7.
3. Kocher MS, Mandiga R, Klingele K, et al. Anterior cruciate ligament injury versus tibial spine fracture in the skeletally immature knee: a comparison of skeletal maturation and notch width index. J Pediatr Orthop 2004;24(2):185–8.
4. Snearly WN, Kaplan PA, Dussault RG. Lateral compartment bone contusions in adolescents with intact anterior cruciate ligaments. Radiology 1996; 198(1):205–8.
5. Schachter AK, Rokito AS. ACL injuries in the skele-tally immature patient. Orthopedics 2007;30(5): 365–70 [quiz: 371–362].
6. Busch MT. Meniscal injuries in children and adoles-cents. Clin Sports Med 1990;9(3):661–80.
7. Silverman JM, Mink JH, Deutsch AL. Discoid menisci of the knee: MR imaging appearance. Radi-ology 1989;173(2):351–4.
8. Resnick D, Kang HS. Knee. In: Resnick D, editor. Internal derangements of joints: emphasis on MR imaging. Philadelphia: WB Saunders; 1997. p. 551–758.
9. Stark JE, Siegel MJ, Weinberger E, et al. Discoid menisci in children: MR features. J Comput Assist Tomogr 1995;19(4):608–11.
10. Rogers LF, Poznanski AK. Imaging of epiphyseal injuries. Radiology 1994;191(2):297–308.
11. Riseborough EJ, Barrett IR, Shapiro F. Growth distur-bances following distal femoral physeal fracture-sepa-rations. J Bone Joint Surg Am 1983;65(7):885–93.
12. Mizuta T, Benson WM, Foster BK, et al. Statistical anal-ysis of the incidence of physeal injuries. J Pediatr Orthop 1987;7(5):518–23.
13. Peterson HA. Physeal and apophyseal injuries. In: Rockwood CA Jr, Wilkins KE, Beaty JH, editors. Fractures in children. Philadelphia: Lippincott-Raven; 1996. p. 103–65.
14. Harcke HT, Synder M, Caro PA, et al. Growth plate of the normal knee: evaluation with MR imaging. Radi-ology 1992;183(1):119–23.
15. Close BJ, Strouse PJ. MR of physeal fractures of the adolescent knee. Pediatr Radiol 2000;30(11): 756–62.
16. Whan A, Breidahl W, Janes G. MRI of trapped perios-teum in a proximal tibial physeal injury of a pediatric patient. AJR Am J Roentgenol 2003;181(5):1397–9.
17. Johnston DR, Ganley TJ, Flynn JM, et al. Anterior cruciate ligament injuries in skeletally immature patients. Orthopedics 2002;25(8):864–71 [quiz: 872–63].
18. Stevens MA, El-Khoury GY, Kathol MH, et al. Imaging features of avulsion injuries. Radiographics 1999;19(3):655–72.
19. Accousti WK, Willis RB. Tibial eminence fractures. Orthop Clin North Am 2003;34(3):365–75.
20. Jacobsen K, Metz P. Occult traumatic dislocation of the patella. J Trauma 1976;16(10):829–35.
21. Kirsch MD, Fitzgerald SW, Friedman H, et al. Tran-sient lateral patellar dislocation: diagnosis with MR imaging. AJR Am J Roentgenol 1993;161(1): 109–13.
22. Lance E, Deutsch AL, Mink JH. Prior lateral patellar dislocation: MR imaging findings. Radiology 1993; 189(3):905–7.
23. Zaidi A, Babyn P, Astori I, et al. MRI of traumatic patellar dislocation in children. Pediatr Radiol 2006;36(11):1163–70.
24. Dalton SE. Overuse injuries in adolescent athletes. Sports Med 1992;13(1):58–70.
25. Walker RN, Green NE, Spindler KP. Stress fractures in skeletally immature patients. J Pediatr Orthop 1996;16(5):578–84.

26. Hoch AZ, Pepper M, Akuthota V. Stress fractures and knee injuries in runners. Phys Med Rehabil Clin N Am 2005;16(3):749–77.

27. Connolly SA, Connolly LP, Jaramillo D. Imaging of sports injuries in children and adolescents. Radiol Clin North Am 2001;39(4):773–90.

28. Aoki Y, Yasuda K, Tohyama H, et al. Magnetic resonance imaging in stress fractures and shin splints. Clin Orthop Relat Res 2004;421:260–7.

29. Laor T, Wall EJ, Vu LP. Physeal widening in the knee due to stress injury in child athletes. AJR Am J Roentgenol 2006;186(5):1260–4.

30. Bodne D, Quinn SF, Murray WT, et al. Magnetic resonance images of chronic patellar tendinitis. Skeletal Radiol 1988;17(1):24–8.

31. Rosenberg ZS, Kawelblum M, Cheung YY, et al. Osgood-Schlatter lesion: fracture or tendinitis? Scintigraphic, CT, and MR imaging features. Radiology 1992;185(3):853–8.

32. Medlar RC, Lyne ED. Sinding-Larsen-Johansson disease: its etiology and natural history. J Bone Joint Surg Am 1978;60(8):1113–6.

33. Bates DG, Hresko MT, Jaramillo D. Patellar sleeve fracture: demonstration with MR imaging. Radiology 1994;193(3):825–7.

34. Mellado JM, Ramos A, Salvado E, et al. Avulsion fractures and chronic avulsion injuries of the knee: role of MR imaging. Eur Radiol 2002;12(10):2463–73.

35. Kozlowski K, Middleton R. Familial osteochondritis dissecans: a dysplasia of articular cartilage? Skeletal Radiol 1985;13(3):207–10.

36. De Smet AA, Fisher DR, Graf BK, et al. Osteochondritis dissecans of the knee: value of MR imaging in determining lesion stability and the presence of articular cartilage defects. AJR Am J Roentgenol 1990;155(3):549–53.

37. De Smet AA, Ilahi OA, Graf BK. Untreated osteochondritis dissecans of the femoral condyles: prediction of patient outcome using radiographic and MR findings. Skeletal Radiol 1997;26(8):463–7.

38. Kijowski R, Blankenbaker DG, Shinki K, et al. Juvenile versus adult osteochondritis dissecans of the knee: appropriate MR imaging criteria for instability. Radiology 2008;248(2):571–8.

39. Nawata K, Teshima R, Morio Y, et al. Anomalies of ossification in the posterolateral femoral condyle: assessment by MRI. Pediatr Radiol 1999;29(10):781–4.

40. Gebarski K, Hernandez RJ. Stage I osteochondritis dissecans versus normal variants of ossification in the knee in children. Pediatr Radiol 2005;35(9):880–6.

41. Kransdorf MJ, Peterson JJ, Bancroft LW. MR imaging of the knee: incidental osseous lesions. Radiol Clin North Am 2007;45(6):943–54.

42. Jee WH, Choe BY, Kang HS, et al. Nonossifying fibroma: characteristics at MR imaging with pathologic correlation. Radiology 1998;209(1):197–202.

43. Lee KC, Davies AM, Cassar-Pullicino VN. Imaging the complications of osteochondromas. Clin Radiol 2002;57(1):18–28.

44. Lang IM, Azouz EM. MRI appearances of dysplasia epiphysealis hemimelica of the knee. Skeletal Radiol 1997;26(4):226–9.

45. Resnick D, Greenway G. Distal femoral cortical defects, irregularities, and excavations. Radiology 1982;143(2):345–54.

46. Stacy GS. Contour irregularities of the distal femur caused by developmental, traumatic, and benign cortically based neoplastic conditions: radiographic and MRI correlation. Clin Radiol 2004;59(9):793–802.

47. Gylys-Morin VM, Graham TB, Blebea JS, et al. Knee in early juvenile rheumatoid arthritis: MR imaging findings. Radiology 2001;220(3):696–706.

48. Pannier S, Odent T, Milet A, et al. [Pigmented villonodular synovitis in children: review of six cases]. Rev Chir Orthop Reparatrice Appar Mot 2008; 94(1):64–72 [in French].

49. De Maeseneer M, Debaere C, Desprechins B, et al. Popliteal cysts in children: prevalence, appearance and associated findings at MR imaging. Pediatr Radiol 1999;29(8):605–9.

50. Gabos PG, El Rassi G, Pahys J. Knee reconstruction in syndromes with congenital absence of the anterior cruciate ligament. J Pediatr Orthop 2005;25(2):210–4.

51. DeLee JC, Curtis R. Anterior cruciate ligament insufficiency in children. Clin Orthop Relat Res 1983;172:112–8.

52. Mellado JM, Salvado E, Ramos A, et al. Dorsal defect on a multipartite patella: imaging findings. Eur Radiol 2001;11(7):1136–9.

53. Monu JU, De Smet AA. Case report 789: dorsal defect of the left patella. Skeletal Radiol 1993; 22(7):528–31.

54. De Wilde V, De Maeseneer M, Lenchik L, et al. Normal osseous variants presenting as cystic or lucent areas on radiography and CT imaging: a pictorial overview. Eur J Radiol 2004;51(1):77–84.

55. Ho VB, Kransdorf MJ, Jelinek JS, et al. Dorsal defect of the patella: MR features. J Comput Assist Tomogr 1991;15(3):474–6.

56. Elias DA, White LM. Imaging of patellofemoral disorders. Clin Radiol 2004;59(7):543–57.

The Foot and Ankle: MR Imaging of Uniquely Pediatric Disorders

Chirag V. Patel, MD

KEYWORDS

• MR imaging • Pediatric • Foot • Ankle • Musculoskeletal

Although the primary imaging modality for ankle- and foot-related problems in children is plain radiographs, MR imaging becomes useful for specific indications, such as evaluating osteo-chondral abnormalities, preoperative assessment of tumors and infection, evaluating occult osseous trauma and soft tissue injury, and less commonly evaluating the cartilaginous anlagen in clubfoot.

TECHNICAL CONSIDERATIONS

The most important technical factor for consideration is coil selection. This depends on patient size. Although extremity, knee, or head coil are appropriate for most children, smaller surface coils are needed for evaluating babies and smaller children and for high-resolution imaging in older children. Rarely, torso coils are needed to evaluate more extensive abnormalities involving the calf and the foot. Almost all the studies are performed in supine position. On occasion, however, prone position is used to advantage in older patients for imaging the midfoot and forefoot for such indications as metatarsal and sesamoid stress fracture. Other considerations of sedation and immobilization are the same as in other MR imaging examinations.[1,2]

Selection of sequence is tailored to individual examination but routine imaging includes T1 fast spin echo proton density images with and without fat saturation and fluid-sensitive sequence (short tau inversion recovery or T2 fast spin echo with fat saturation) in at least one plane, usually sagittal. Intravenous gadolinium-based contrast is used in cases of suspected infection, evaluation of mass, and differentiating solid from cystic abnormality.

OSTEOCHONDRAL LESIONS
Osteochondritis Dissecans

Osteochondritis dissecans most commonly involves the talar dome in the ankle and foot. The postulated mechanism is repetitive microtrauma. The common locations for this abnormality are the posterior one third of the medial margin and middle one third of the lateral margin and less commonly the central talar dome. MR imaging is useful in assessing stability of the lesions, which significantly influences management.[3,4] Features that indicate instability include loose body, focal cartilage defect greater than 5 mm, subchondral cyst, and linear high T2 signal abnormality tracking at the donor-fragment interface for at least 5 mm or circumferentially around the osteochondral fragment (**Fig. 1**).[3,5–7]

Routine imaging includes proton density spin echo and T2-weighted fat-suppressed fast spin echo sequences. Cartilage-sensitive sequences, however, such as three-dimensional T1-weighted fat-suppressed spoiled gradient recalled, have been found helpful in assessing cartilage integrity. Use of gadolinium to distinguish granulation tissue from fluid at the linear high T2 signal at the donor fragment interface has been reported. Intra-articular use of gadolinium has not been shown to improve accuracy of articular cartilage damage.[8–11]

On occasions osteochondritis dissecans may be encountered incidentally in a child evaluated for acute or subacute ankle injury. Osteochondritis dissecans can be differentiated from acute osteo-chondral fracture by the presence of adjacent focal marrow edema and kissing contusion in the tibial plafond. Both represent parts of a spectrum,

Division of Pediatric Imaging, Department of Radiology, University of California, Davis, Medical Center and UC Davis Children's Hospital, 4860 Y Street, Suite 300, Sacramento, CA 95817, USA
E-mail address: chiragv.patel@ucdmc.ucdavis.edu

Magn Reson Imaging Clin N Am 17 (2009) 539–547
doi:10.1016/j.mric.2009.03.005
1064-9689/09/$ – see front matter © 2009 Elsevier Inc. All rights reserved.

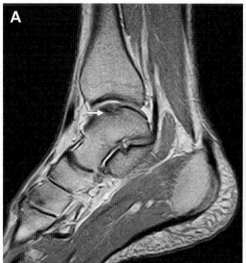
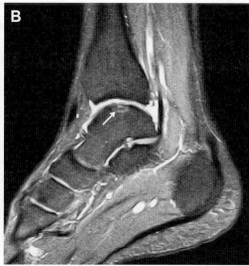

Fig. 1. Osteochondritis dissecans. (*A*) Sagittal T1-weighted image shows osteochondral defect in the central talar dome (*arrow*). (*B*) Sagittal T2 fat-suppressed image shows a rim of high signal (*arrow*) encircling the osteochondral fragment suggesting unstable osteochondritis dissecans.

however, and as such do not differ from management perspective.

Osteonecrosis of talar dome can mimic osteochondritis dissecans on MR imaging. The presence, however, of a predisposing condition, such as talar neck fracture, corticosteroids, or vasculitis, and the presence of characteristic double-rim sign on MR imaging with hyperintense inner rim and hypointense outer rim on T2-weighted images makes differentiation easier (**Fig. 2**).[12]

Focal subchondral edema is seen in both acute and chronic injury and following high-intensity exercise. They present as ill-defined areas of high signal on T2-weighted sequences. These findings may persist for months after resolution of symptoms. In contrast to lesions with ill-defined reticular margin, well-defined subchondral lesions have about 50% likelihood of progressing to focal cartilage loss.[13,14]

OTHER OSTEOCHONDROSES AND OSTEONECROSES

Other common locations for osteochondroses and osteonecrosis in the foot include the tarsal navicular or Köhler disease and head of second or third metatarsal or Freiberg infraction.

Köhler disease is an abnormality of endochondral ossification. Clinical presentation includes swelling, erythema, and tenderness along the medial foot. It is more commonly seen in boys between 3 and 10 years if age and may be bilateral in up to 25%. Diagnosis is based on clinical and radiographic findings, which shows sclerosis and fragmentation of the navicular ossification center.

MR imaging is usually not indicated unless either of these is atypical or there is concern of other etiologies of foot pain. MR imaging features include diffuse increase in T2 signal in the

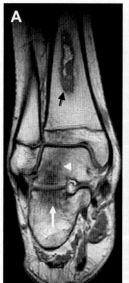
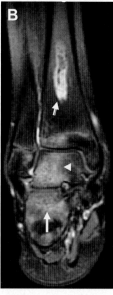

Fig. 2. Multifocal osteonecrosis. (*A*) Coronal T1-weighted image in patient status posttherapy for leukemia, showing focal ill-defined loss of normal marrow signal in talus (*arrow*) and calcaneus (*white arrow*) adjacent to the posterior subtalar facet. Bone infarct is seen in the distal tibia (*black arrow*). (*B*) Coronal T2-weighted fat-suppressed image shows increased signal at those areas in talus (*arrow*) and calcaneus (*long arrow*) and infarct in the distal tibia (*short arrow*).

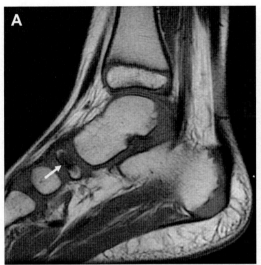
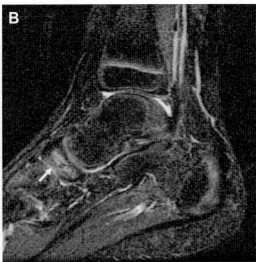

Fig. 3. Köhler disease. (A) Sagittal T1-weighted image showing focal loss of normal marrow signal in the ossification center of navicular (arrow). (B) Sagittal short tau inversion recovery (STIR) image shows diffuse hyperintensity within this ossification center (arrow) with normal appearance of the surrounding cartilage.

navicular ossification center with preservation of surrounding cartilage (Fig. 3).[15,16]

Freiberg infraction is postulated to be osteonecrosis from repetitive trauma. The head of second metatarsal is most commonly involved followed by third metatarsal. It affects adolescent girls more commonly presenting as focal pain and tenderness. Plain radiographs are used for diagnoses, which show sclerosis and flattening of the metatarsal head with increase in the metatarsophalangeal joint space. MR imaging is used when radiographs are atypical or alternate etiologies, such as osteomyelitis or stress fracture, are considered. The MR imaging features depend on the degree of avascular sclerotic bone, which shows low signal on both T1- and T2-weighted images. There is usually associated joint effusion at the metatarsophalangeal joint with edema in surrounding soft tissues (Fig. 4).[17–19]

TARSAL COALITION

Tarsal coalition is an anomaly of segmentation. Coalition can be osseous, cartilaginous, or fibrous and is bilateral in approximately half of the cases.

Talocalcaneal and calcaneonavicular coalition constitute 90% of the cases. Talonavicular, calcaneocuboid, and calcaneonavicular coalition are less common. Clinical presentation is with painful stiff foot. Although all cases are congenital, patients present when the tarsal bones ossify and the age at presentation is 8 to 16 years.[20–23]

Plain film and CT are the preferred modalities of imaging; however, on occasion MR imaging may be requested in cases of negative or equivocal CT but strong clinical suspicion. Alternately, tarsal coalition may be encountered incidentally during evaluation of adolescent foot for other indications.

Osseous coalition can be easily diagnosed by noting the continuity of the marrow space between two tarsal bones. Incomplete coalitions can be diagnosed by diffuse decrease and irregularity in the intertarsal joint space. Fibrous coalitions show low signal in all sequences and may sometimes be indistinguishable from osseous coalition if the bridging bone is sclerotic. Cartilaginous coalition follows signal of cartilage as in the rest of the foot (Fig. 5).[23–25] Additional MR imaging findings include marrow edema in the juxta-articular aspects of the tarsal bones, and soft tissue edema

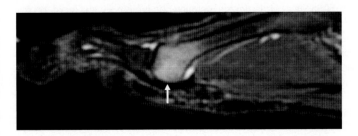

Fig. 4. Freiberg infraction. Sagittal STIR image through the first metatarsophalangeal joint shows diffuse increased signal in the head of the first metatarsal (arrow), seen in early Freiberg infraction.

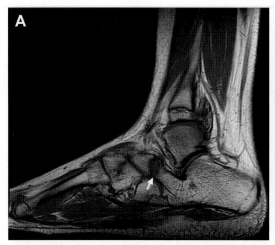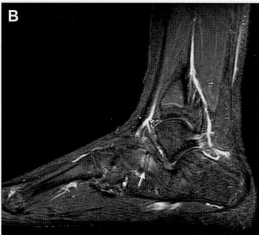

Fig. 5. Cartilagenous calcaneonavicular coalition. (*A*) Sagittal T1-weighted image shows enlarged anterior process of the calcaneus (*arrow*). (*B*) Sagittal STIR image shows focal hyperintensity in the juxta-articular aspects of this joint (*arrow*). The coalition follows signal corresponding to cartilage in the rest of the foot.

in mid foot and hind foot. Adaptive shortening of the peroneal tendons may produce changes of tendinitis or tenosynovitis with associated hind foot valgus alignment.[26]

NEOPLASMS
Soft Tissue Tumors

Soft tissue tumors of the foot are rare, and although the spectrum of pathologies is wide, most of them are benign. Tumor-like lesions, such as ganglion cyst and plantar fibromatosis, outnumber neoplasms, such as hemangioma, nerve sheath tumors, lipoma, pigmented villonodular synovitis, and synovial chondromatoses.[27] Although the imaging appearance of the rest of the soft tissue tumors is the same as in other locations, plantar fibromatosis is unique to the foot and deserves specific discussion.

Plantar fibromatosis begins as painless single or multiple infiltrative nodules in the plantar fascia with well-defined inferior margin and infiltrative superior margin, which can grow into deeper soft tissues. Symptoms develop when the lesion attains a large size or as a result of local infiltration into adjacent soft tissues and neurovascular bundle. Bilateral lesions occur in 20% to 50% of cases (tumor and tumor-like lesions).[28,29] A subset of plantar fibromatosis found in children younger than 16 years of age and limited to the plantar surface of the heel has been described as less aggressive variant. MR imaging features include low or intermediate signal intensity on both T1- and T2-weighted sequences, and postcontrast enhancement is variable. Surgical resection when

indicated in large or symptomatic lesions can be difficult and the lesion may recur.[30,31]

Synovial sarcoma is the most common malignant soft tissue tumor of the foot. It affects children in the second decade of life and adults up to 45 years of age. Contradictory to the name, only 10% lesions are intra-articular. The tumors are intimately related to the tendons, tendon sheaths, and bursae and are deep seated.[32] Apart from scattered calcification, which is present in approximately half of the cases, imaging appearance on MR imaging is nonspecific, often mimicking a benign looking well-defined lobulated lesion or can be cystic.[33,34] Necrosis and hemorrhage may be present, along with destruction of adjacent bones.[35] Rhabdomyosarcoma (**Fig. 6**) and fibrosarcoma are other rare soft tissue malignant neoplasms reported in the foot without any distinct MR imaging features.

Bone Tumors

Most bone tumors of the foot in children are benign and include simple or aneurysmal bone cyst (**Fig. 7**), intraosseous lipoma, enchondroma, osteochondroma, osteoblastoma, chondroblastoma (**Fig. 8**), osteoid osteoma, and fibrous dysplasia.[36–38] MR imaging is usually not indicated for most of the lesions unless the presentation is atypical and for larger tumors before surgery. Imaging features are not different from the same tumors at other anatomic sites.

Among the malignant tumors Ewing sarcoma is the second most common malignant neoplasm of the foot after synovial sarcoma. It occurs in the second decade of life, more common in boys

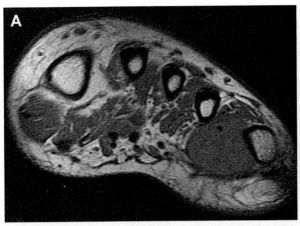

Fig. 6. Rhabdomyosarcoma of the foot. (A) Coronal T1-weighted image of the foot shows a low signal well-defined soft tissue mass in the plantar aspect at fourth and fifth intermetatarsal space. (B) Coronal T2-weighted fat-suppressed image at the same level show diffuse increased but heterogeneous signal pattern. This lesion was diagnosed as rhabdomyosarcoma on biopsy.

and most frequently involving the calcaneus and the metatarsal bones.[39] MR imaging features are nonspecific and indistinguishable at times from osteomyelitis. MR imaging is, however, helpful in delineating the extent of the tumor with respect to adjacent structures, especially the neurovascular bundle.[40]

Osteosarcoma rarely involves foot bones, accounting for less than 2% of the overall incidence, but nonetheless should be considered in the differential diagnosis for aggressive-appearing

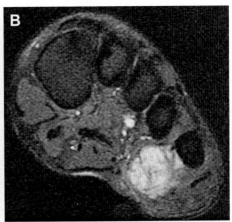

Fig. 7. Aneurysmal bone cyst. (A) Coronal T1 contrast-enhanced image shows enhancing septae (arrow) in a multiloculated expansile lesion in distal tibia. (B) Coronal T2-weighted image at the same level shows fluid within the multiloculated lesion (arrow).

osseous lesions.[41] Presentation is in the second decade of life. Plain radiographs are useful in depicting mineralized osteoid. MR imaging features are nonspecific but helpful for determining local extent and preoperative evaluation. Insufficiency fractures can sometimes mimic infiltrative bone tumor (Fig. 9).

INFECTION

Osteomyelitis or soft tissue infection of the foot is not very common in children as compared with adults, especially with predispositions like diabetes or peripheral vascular disease (Fig. 10).

Infection is more commonly acquired by direct inoculation by foreign body puncture wound or open fracture. If left untreated it may result in necrotizing fasciitis. Although ultrasound and CT are more commonly used for radiolucent foreign body localization, MR imaging may be used on occasion to detect small foreign bodies and associated inflammatory response. The MR imaging appearance of most foreign bodies is low signal intensity on both T1- and T2-weighted sequences with surrounding soft tissue edema, abscess, or osteomyelitis.[42,43]

Hematogenous spread of infection is uncommon in immunocompetent children; however, those with sickle cell disease and chronic granulomatous disease are prone to hematogenous seeding of infection in the bones of foot apart from other sites.

In sickle cell disease osteomyelitis is accompanied and preceded by bone infarctions. There is no appropriate reference standard for diagnosing sickle cell osteomyelitis, given that

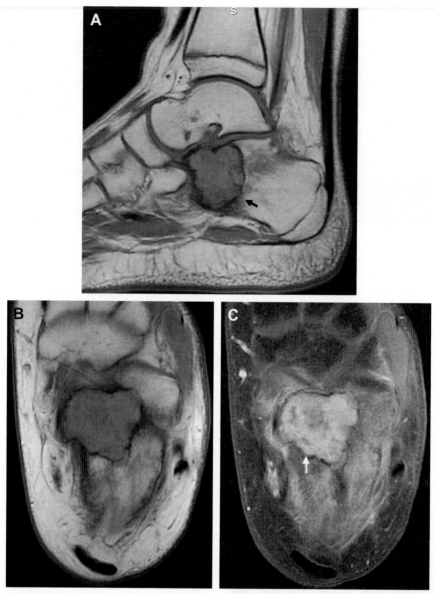

Fig. 8. Chondroblastoma of the calcaneus. (*A*) Sagittal T1-weighted image showing low signal focal calcaneal lesion with well-demarcated hypointense rim (*arrow*). (*B*) Axial T1-weighted image shows the same characteristics. (*C*) Axial T1-weighted fat-suppressed contrast enhanced image show heterogeneous but significant enhancement of the lesion (*arrow*). The lesion was diagnosed as chondroblastoma on histopathology.

cultures of biopsies too have been considered unreliable. The sensitivity and specificity of MR imaging has not been adequately evaluated for differentiating these two entities.[30,44]

Chronic granulomatous disease is an immunodeficiency disorder with phagocyte dysfunction. Affected children are susceptible to catalase-positive organisms. Hematogenous infection involves metatarsal bones apart from vertebral bodies and ribs, which are other common sites.[45]

CONGENITAL
Clubfoot

Clubfoot is the most common congenital foot abnormality with an incidence of 1:1000 in North America. It can be classified as postural or positional and fixed. The fixed form, also known as "congenital clubfoot," is the most common type and requires correction. Imaging is generally done before surgical correction after 4 to 12 weeks of conservative treatment involving

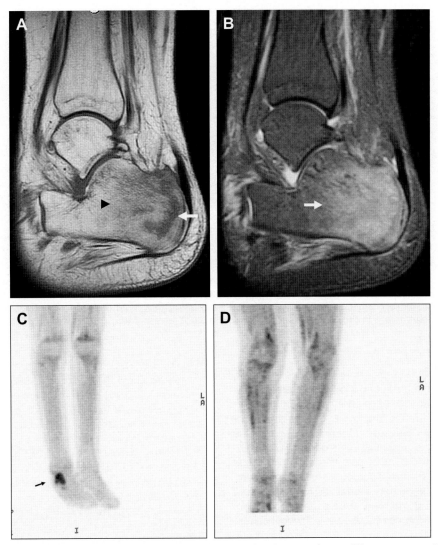

Fig. 9. Insufficiency fracture of calcaneus. (*A*) Sagittal T1-weighted image shows diffuse marrow edema in the posterior calcaneus (*arrowhead*) with focal linear area of low signal oriented perpendicularly, diagnosed as insufficiency fracture (*arrow*). (*B*) Sagittal STIR image at the same level shows diffuse marrow edema (*arrow*). (*C*) Positron emission tomography (PET) CT image shows increased fluorodeoxyglucose activity at the site of fracture (*arrow*). (*D*) Follow-up PET CT at 6 weeks showed resolution of abnormal increased activity. Patient was off therapy after complete remission of acute lymphoblastic lymphoma at the time of MR imaging and first PET CT.

passive serial manipulation and casting.[46] Radiographs are the mainstay for evaluating residual deformity before surgery.[31] MR imaging is not used routinely; however, there has been an interest in using MR imaging because of its ability to elaborate the relationships of the cartilage anlagen rather than the ossification center of the tarsal bones. Although the components of malalignment producing clubfoot are the same in all cases (forefoot adduction, hindfoot varus, medial subluxation of navicular, and elevation of heel), the differing extent of these makes each clubfoot different from the other. Wang and colleagues[47]

have sought to classify clubfoot on the basis of MR imaging findings of relationship of talus and calcaneus using multiplanar reconstruction from three-dimensional gradient echo sequences. Saito and colleagues[48] evaluated calcaneal malposition with respect to the lower leg axis. Kamegaya and colleagues[49] described the relationship of talonavicular cartilage and its usefulness in predicting the severity of clubfoot. MR imaging is, however, significantly limited by scan time, requirement for sedation, and inconclusive evidence regarding its impact on surgical management.[47,48,50,51]

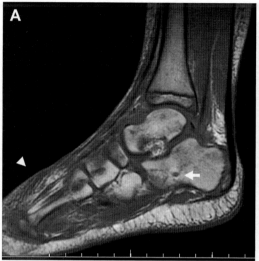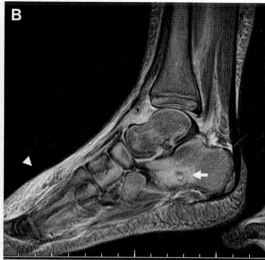

Fig. 10. Osteomyelitis of calcaneus. (*A*) Sagittal T1-weighted image show well-defined low signal area (*arrow*) in the calcaneus. Note soft tissue edema (*arrowhead*). (*B*) Sagittal T1-weighted fat-suppressed postcontrast image shows diffuse marrow enhancement adjacent to the focal lesion (*arrow*) and also in the other tarsal bones. Also note enhancement in the soft tissue at the dorsum of foot (*arrowhead*).

SUMMARY

MR imaging of ankle and foot in children is useful especially because of its ability to depict the cartilage anlagen of tarsal and metatarsals and articular cartilage. Because of excellent soft tissue depiction it is essential in preoperative assessment and follow-up of soft tissue and osseous neoplasms. Plain radiographs and CT, however, do remain the primary modalities for several foot and ankle abnormalities, such as tarsal coalition, and MR imaging can be used in equivocal cases.

REFERENCES

1. Spouge AR, Pope TL. Practical MRI of the foot and ankle. Boca Raton (FL): CRC Press; 2001.
2. Schreibman K. Computed tomography and magnetic resonance imaging of the foot and ankle. 4th edition. In: CT and MR imaging of the whole body. vol. 2. Missouri: Mosby Inc.; 2003. p. 1825–68.
3. Mosher TJ. MRI of osteochondral injuries of the knee and ankle in the athlete. Clin Sports Med 2006;25(4): 843–66.
4. Letts M, Davidson D, Ahmer A. Osteochondritis dissecans of the talus in children. J Pediatr Orthop 2003;23(5):617–25.
5. Winalski CS, Gupta KB. Magnetic resonance imaging of focal articular cartilage lesions. Top Magn Reson Imaging 2003;14(2):131–44.
6. McCauley TR. MR imaging of chondral and osteochondral injuries of the knee. Radiol Clin North Am 2002;40(5):1095–107.
7. Nelson DW, DiPaola J, Colville M, et al. Osteochondritis dissecans of the talus and knee: prospective comparison of MR and arthroscopic classifications. J Comput Assist Tomogr 1990;14(5):804–8.
8. Bohndorf K. Imaging of acute injuries of the articular surfaces (chondral, osteochondral and subchondral fractures). Skeletal Radiol 1999;28(10):545–60.
9. Bohndorf K. Osteochondritis (osteochondrosis) dissecans: a review and new MRI classification. Eur Radiol 1998;8(1):103–12.
10. Disler DG, McCauley TR, Kelman CG, et al. Fat-suppressed three-dimensional spoiled gradient-echo MR imaging of hyaline cartilage defects in the knee: comparison with standard MR imaging and arthroscopy. AJR Am J Roentgenol 1996;167(1): 127–32.
11. McCauley TR, Disler DG. MR imaging of articular cartilage. Radiology 1998;209(3):629–40.
12. Adelaar RS, Madrian JR. Avascular necrosis of the talus. Orthop Clin North Am 2004;35(3):383–95, xi.
13. Boks SS, Vroegindeweij D, Koes BW, et al. Follow-up of occult bone lesions detected at MR imaging: systematic review. Radiology 2006;238(3):853–62.
14. Vellet AD, et al. Occult posttraumatic osteochondral lesions of the knee: prevalence, classification, and short-term sequelae evaluated with MR imaging. Radiology 1991;178(1):271–6.
15. Harty MP, Hubbard AM. MR imaging of pediatric abnormalities in the ankle and foot. Magn Reson Imaging Clin N Am 2001;9(3):579–602, xi.
16. Borges JL, Guille JT, Bowen JR. Köhler's bone disease of the tarsal navicular. J Pediatr Orthop 1995;15(5):596–8.

17. Chowchuen P, Resnick D. Stress fractures of the metatarsal heads. Skeletal Radiol 1998;27(1):22–5.

18. Lechevalier D, Fournier B, Leleu T, et al. Stress fractures of the heads of the metatarsals: a new cause of metatarsal pain. Rev Rhum Engl Ed 1995;62(4): 255–9.

19. Torriani M, Thomas BJ, Bredella MA, et al. MRI of metatarsal head subchondral fractures in patients with forefoot pain. AJR Am J Roentgenol 2008; 190(3):570–5.

20. Gessner AJ, Kumar SJ, Gross GW. Tarsal coalition in pediatric patients. Semin Musculoskelet Radiol 1999;3(3):239–46.

21. Bohne WH. Tarsal coalition. Curr Opin Pediatr 2001; 13(1):29–35.

22. Schoenberg NY, Lehman WB. Magnetic resonance imaging of pediatric disorders of the ankle and foot. Magn Reson Imaging Clin N Am 1994;2(1): 109–22.

23. Pachuda NM, Lasday SD, Jay RM. Tarsal coalition: etiology, diagnosis, and treatment. J Foot Surg 1990;29(5):474–88.

24. Emery KH, Bisset GS, Johnson ND, et al. Tarsal coalition: a blinded comparison of MRI and CT. Pediatr Radiol 1998;28(8):612–6.

25. Nalaboff KM, Schweitzer ME. MRI of tarsal coalition: frequency, distribution, and innovative signs. Bull NYU Hosp Jt Dis 2008;66(1):14–21.

26. Agostinelli JR. Tarsal coalition and its relation to peroneal spastic flatfoot. J Am Podiatr Med Assoc 1986;76(2):76–80.

27. Kier R. MR imaging of foot and ankle tumors. Magn Reson Imaging 1993;11(2):149–62.

28. Godette GA, O'Sullivan M, Menelaus MB. Plantar fibromatosis of the heel in children: a report of 14 cases. J Pediatr Orthop 1997;17(1):16–7.

29. Wetzel LH, Levine E. Soft-tissue tumors of the foot: value of MR imaging for specific diagnosis. AJR Am J Roentgenol 1990;155(5):1025–30.

30. Rosenberg ZS, Beltran J, Bencardino JT. From the RSNA Refresher Courses. Radiological Society of North America. MR imaging of the ankle and foot. Radiographics 2000;20(Spec No):S153–79.

31. Harty MP. Imaging of pediatric foot disorders. Radiol Clin North Am 2001;39(4):733–48.

32. Waldt S, Rechl H, Rummeny EJ, et al. Imaging of benign and malignant soft tissue masses of the foot. Eur Radiol 2003;13(5):1125–36.

33. Blacksin MF, Siegel JR, Benevenia J, et al. Synovial sarcoma: frequency of nonaggressive MR characteristics. J Comput Assist Tomogr 1997;21(5):785–9.

34. Nakanishi H, Araki N, Sawai Y, et al. Cystic synovial sarcomas: imaging features with clinical and histopathologic correlation. Skeletal Radiol 2003;32(12): 701–7.

35. Berthoty D, Haghighi P, Sartoris DJ, et al. Osseous invasion by soft-tissue sarcoma seen better on MR than on CT. AJR Am J Roentgenol 1989;152(5): 1131.

36. Nomikos GC, Murphey MD, Kransdorf MJ, et al. Primary bone tumors of the lower extremities. Radiol Clin North Am 2002;40(5):971–90.

37. Ashman CJ, Klecker RJ, Yu JS. Forefoot pain involving the metatarsal region: differential diagnosis with MR imaging. Radiographics 2001;21(6): 1425–40.

38. Keigley BA, Haggar AM, Gaba A, et al. Primary tumors of the foot: MR imaging. Radiology 1989; 171(3):755–9.

39. Rammal H, Ghanem I, Torbey PH, et al. Multifocal Ewing sarcoma of the foot. J Pediatr Hematol Oncol 2008;30(4):298–300.

40. Baraga JJ, Amrami KK, Swee RG, et al. Radiographic features of Ewing's sarcoma of the bones of the hands and feet. Skeletal Radiol 2001;30(3): 121–6.

41. Biscaglia R, Gasbarrini A, Bohling T, et al. Osteosarcoma of the bones of the foot: an easily misdiagnosed malignant tumor. Mayo Clin Proc 1998;73(9): 842–7.

42. Imoisili MA, Bonwit AM, Bulas DI. Toothpick puncture injuries of the foot in children. Pediatr Infect Dis J 2004;23(1):80–2.

43. Peterson JJ, Bancroft LW, Kransdorf MJ. Wooden foreign bodies: imaging appearance. AJR Am J Roentgenol 2002;178(3):557–62.

44. Wong AL, Sakamoto KM, Johnson EE. Differentiating osteomyelitis from bone infarction in sickle cell disease. Pediatr Emerg Care 2001;17(1):60–3 [quiz 64].

45. Fisher RG, Boyce TG, et al. Moffet's pediatric infectious diseases: a problem-oriented approach. Philadelphia: Lippincott Williams and Wilkins; 2005.

46. Ponseti IV. Treatment of congenital club foot. J Bone Joint Surg Am 1992;74(3):448–54.

47. Wang C, Petursdottir S, Leifsdottir I, et al. MRI multiplanar reconstruction in the assessment of congenital talipes equinovarus. Pediatr Radiol 1999;29(4): 262–7.

48. Saito S, Hatori M, Kokubun S, et al. Evaluation of calcaneal malposition by magnetic resonance imaging in the infantile clubfoot. J Pediatr Orthop B 2004;13(2):99–102.

49. Kamegaya M, Shinohara Y, Kokuji Y, et al. Evaluation of pathologic abnormalities of clubfoot by magnetic resonance imaging. Clin Orthop Relat Res 2000;(379):218–23.

50. Downey DJ, Drennan JC, Garcia JF. Magnetic resonance image findings in congenital talipes equinovarus. J Pediatr Orthop 1992;12(2):224–8.

51. Grayhack JJ, Zawin JK, Shore RM, et al. Assessment of calcaneocuboid joint deformity by magnetic resonance imaging in talipes equinovarus. J Pediatr Orthop B 1995;4(1):36–8.

MR Imaging in Congenital and Acquired Disorders of the Pediatric Upper Extremity

Kathleen H. Emery, MD[a,b,*]

KEYWORDS
- Pediatric • Musculoskeletal • Congenital
- Sports-related injury • Upper extremity

Various congenital and acquired disorders can affect the upper extremity in pediatric and adolescent patients. Other articles in this issue have discussed the unique role that MR imaging can play in evaluating inflammatory, infectious, arthritic, and neoplastic disorders of the pediatric musculoskeletal system. The focus of this article is unique congenital and traumatic conditions (mainly sports-related injuries) that affect the shoulder, elbow, and wrist in children for which MR imaging plays a role in diagnosis and management.

With regard to traumatic conditions, chronic repetitive stress injuries seen commonly in skeletally immature athletes are a recurring theme. The frequency of these repetitive microtraumatic injuries increases during the mid to late teen years. During this period of life, not only is the growing skeleton subjected to the ever increasing forces generated by normal progressive muscular development and strength but also the physis becomes particularly vulnerable. It is responsive to hormonal influences, decreasing in strength with exposure to increasing levels of testosterone[1] that typify the adolescent stage of development. This is further intensified by the often progressively demanding training schedules placed on athletes during this stage. Many upper extremity injuries occur with sports that use a repetitive overhead throwing motion (eg, baseball, football, tennis) or sports in which the upper extremity is subjected to excessive weight or simulated weight bearing (eg, gymnastics and weightlifting).

SHOULDER
Congenital Disorders

Neonatal brachial plexus palsy
Neonatal brachial plexus palsy is defined as injury to one or more nerve roots of the brachial plexus (C5-T1) that occurs around the time of birth. The incidence of this injury in the United States is currently 1.5 per 1000 live births.[2] This number represents a significant decrease in incidence over time and may be attributed to an increase in cesarean section rates, increasing multiple birth rates, and wider use of preterm labor induction for macrosomic infants.[2] Risk factors for this injury include shoulder dystocia, macrosomia, and breech delivery, although slightly less than 50% of affected infants have an identifiable risk factor, which suggests lack of full understanding of the etiology.[2]

[a] Department of Radiology, Cincinnati Children's Hospital Medical Center, 3333 Burnet Avenue MLC 5031, Cincinnati, OH 45229-3039, USA
[b] Department of Pediatrics, Cincinnati Children's Hospital Medical Center, 3333 Burnet Avenue MLC 5031, Cincinnati, OH 45229-3039, USA
* Department of Radiology, Cincinnati Children's Hospital Medical Center, 3333 Burnet Avenue MLC 5031, Cincinnati, OH 45229-3039.
E-mail address: kathleen.emery@cchmc.org

Magn Reson Imaging Clin N Am 17 (2009) 549–570
doi:10.1016/j.mric.2009.03.004
1064-9689/09/$ – see front matter © 2009 Elsevier Inc. All rights reserved.

Although spontaneous recovery rates of 60% to 90% are reported,[3] the remainder have a persistent deficit. The most common deficit involves weakness of the external rotators of the shoulder (mainly the infraspinatus and teres minor muscles), which are innervated by the suprascapular and axillary nerves, respectively, both of which originate from the C5-6 nerve roots. Functionally, this deficit results in an internal rotation contracture with limitation of shoulder abduction and secondary progressive glenohumeral deformity.[4,5] An internal rotation contracture tightens the anterior soft tissues and applies a posteriorly directed force on the humeral head, which leads to posterior humeral head displacement.[5,6] Over time, this displacement affects development of the normally symmetric, concave cartilaginous glenoid and leads to flattening and possible pseudoglenoid formation, analogous to pseudoacetabulum formation in congenital hip dysplasia (**Fig. 1**).[6]

Early nerve grafting surgery (within 3 months of injury) may improve functional outcome in patients with isolated rupture of the upper brachial plexus.[7] Later surgical options involve anterior capsular release, tendon transfers, and osteotomies to address the functional deformities and allow remodeling of the glenohumeral articulation. The decision to surgically intervene is a clinical one based on the severity of the internal rotation contracture and external rotation weakness.[5] Because the presence of an internal rotation contracture alone does not necessarily imply glenoid deformity,[6] preoperative imaging evaluation of the glenohumeral deformity is helpful in surgical planning. Because the humeral head and glenoid are largely cartilaginous in young children, they are not adequately evaluated on conventional radiographs. Arthrography and MR imaging have been shown to accurately depict the cartilaginous structures of the glenoid and humeral head.[5,6,8] MR imaging accomplishes this in noninvasive fashion and can provide additional information about scapular deformity and muscle atrophy. There is a significant association between the severity of the contracture and the severity of the deformity on arthrography and MR imaging.[5,6]

At our institution, we use an eight-channel phased array cardiac coil to image both shoulders with coronal T1, axial proton density without fat saturation, and coronal multiplanar gradient recalled (MPGR) images to obtain a comparison of glenohumeral morphology and muscle asymmetry with the normal shoulder. Using the same

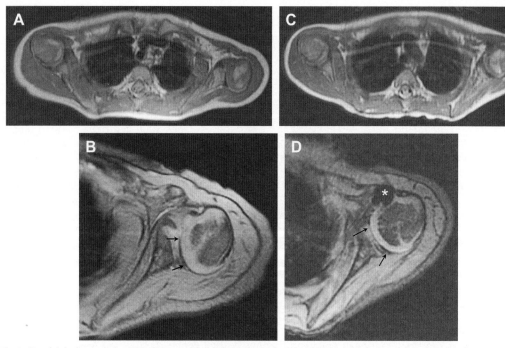

Fig. 1. Brachial plexus palsy. This 3-year-old child presented with a left brachial plexus injury at birth. Preoperative MR imaging, including bilateral axial proton density (*A*) and axial MPGR images of the left shoulder (*B*), show posterior subluxation of the left humeral head, an internal rotation contraction, and pseudoglenoid formation (*arrows*). At age 5 after subscapularis and capsular release, bilateral axial proton density (*C*) and axial MPGR images of the left shoulder (*D*) show normal positioning of the left humeral head and normal glenoid development (*arrows*). Metal artifact postoperatively (***).

coil, dedicated axial MPGR and oblique coronal proton density or intermediate-weighted images are then obtained using a smaller field-of-view offset to only the affected shoulder to evaluate glenoid and humeral head morphology and humeral head subluxation and to measure the glenoscapular angle (scapular retroversion angle).[8] MR imaging also can be used to monitor the structural effect of a surgical intervention (see **Fig. 1**).

Acute Traumatic Injuries

Fractures

Acute fractures in the shoulder region in children are not infrequent and most commonly involve the clavicle as a result of a direct blow or a fall on an outstretched hand.[9] Proximal humeral and scapular fractures are less common. Most of these acute fractures are readily diagnosed by conventional radiographs. Coracoid and glenoid growth center avulsion fractures can be more challenging

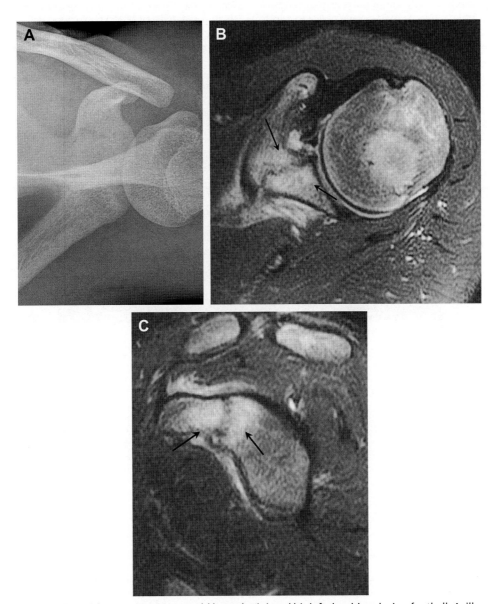

Fig. 2. Coracoid physeal fracture in a 14-year-old boy who injured his left shoulder playing football. Axillary radiograph (*A*) shows questionable widening of the coracoid growth plate. Axial (*B*) and oblique sagittal (*C*) T2-weighted images with fat saturation show increased signal (*arrows*) consistent with marrow edema surrounding the widened coracoid growth plate.

to detect on conventional radiographs, and CT or MR imaging may be necessary to diagnose these injuries (**Fig. 2**).

Dislocation

The glenohumeral joint is highly mobile and inherently unstable, which makes it prone to dislocation. Dislocation tends to be a disorder of adolescence and young adults, with approximately 40% of patients who experience dislocation being younger than age 22,[10] yet it is uncommon in younger children, with only 1.6% seen in patients under the age of 10 years (8 patients in a series of 500).[11] Athletic events, particularly collision sports such as football and hockey, are a frequent cause for shoulder dislocation.

Most glenohumeral dislocations occur anteriorly with the humerus abducted and externally rotated at the time of impact, which results in anterior and inferior displacement of the humeral head. During this injury, the anteroinferior labroligamentous complex may be avulsed from the glenoid (classic Bankart lesion) with or without disruption of the adjacent scapular periosteum or a fracture of the bony glenoid (**Fig. 3**). Posterior dislocation is much less common (1%–4%)[11] and usually results from axial loading of an adducted internally rotated arm, violent muscle contraction (electric shock or seizure disorder), or posterior glenoid deficiency, as in the setting of brachial plexus palsy.[12]

Recurrent dislocation and glenohumeral instability are common after a first-time dislocation.

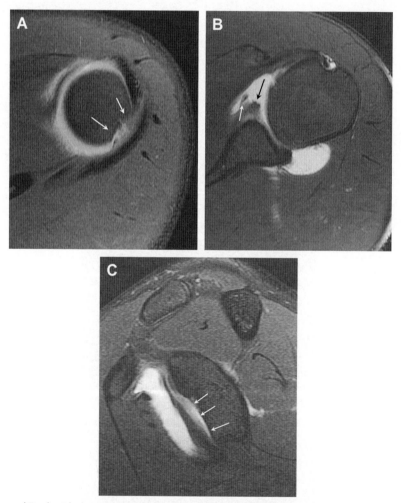

Fig. 3. Hill-Sachs and Bankart lesions on shoulder MR arthrogram of a 17-year-old boy with recent shoulder dislocation. Axial fat saturated T1-weighted images more superiorly (*A*) show the Hill-Sachs lesion in the posterolateral humeral head (*arrows*), with the more inferior image (*B*) below the subscapularis tendon showing the torn anterior labrum (*black arrow*) and the partially avulsed anterior band of the inferior glenohumeral ligament (*white arrow*). The oblique sagittal image (*C*) shows the extent of the anterior labral disruption involving the anterior inferior quadrant (*arrows*).

Recurrent dislocation rates of 48% to 100% are reported in the literature, with the highest incidence seen in athletes who resume sports activities and in patients with open physes.[11,13–15] The presence of a superolateral humeral head defect (Hill-Sach's lesion) on radiography is also associated with a higher incidence of recurrent dislocation;[16] 82% versus 50% without a Hill-Sach's lesion.[11] First time dislocators have a high incidence of capsular and labral injuries based on arthroscopy[17] and MR arthrography studies.[18] In a recent study of 66 first-time dislocators, patients in the younger age group (34 patients < 30 years, including patients as young as 12 years) had a labral injury that was more likely to be an extensive labral injury on MR arthrography than the older group (> 30 years).[18] This increased incidence of extensive labral injuries may partly explain the higher rate of recurrent dislocation in young patients. Patients older than 30 years had a relatively lower incidence of labral injury (72%) that tended to be less extensive, but these patients were more likely to have large rotator cuff tears (53% versus 3% in patients younger than age 30).[18]

Imaging diagnosis of soft tissue capsulolabral injuries associated with acute and/or chronic, recurrent dislocation or instability is best provided by MR imaging. Many agree that direct MR arthrography is the most accurate method[19] with the greatest efficacy in the younger, athletic population.[20] A wide variety of capsulolabral injuries can be seen with shoulder dislocation or instability. A full discussion of these injuries and the known labral variants and pitfalls is beyond the scope of this article, although those injuries are covered in detail in other publications.[19,21–23]

Despite activity and sports restriction for 6 to 12 weeks, surgical treatment is ultimately necessary in 40% to 50% of children and adolescents to improve functional outcome.[13,16,24] One randomized, prospective study with arthroscopically diagnosed anterior labral injuries in 76 younger patients (95%) with first-time dislocation (many age 15–24) found that the rate of recurrent dislocation at 2 years was significantly higher in patients treated conservatively compared to patients treated with primary open Bankart repair (54% versus 3%, $P = .0011$).[25] Results such as these are leading many surgeons to recommend primary surgical repair of labral injuries in active patients to reduce the likelihood of recurrent dislocation.

Chronic Repetitive Trauma

Little Leaguer's shoulder
Little Leaguer's shoulder is a descriptive term for a stress-related injury of the proximal humeral physis originally described by Dotter[26] in a Little League pitcher. The inciting force is rotational stress applied to the physis with overhead throwing as the shoulder is forced into an adducted, internally rotated position from the abducted, externally rotated (cocked) position.[27] The injury is characteristically seen in 13- to 16-year-old baseball players (most frequently pitchers). The typical presentation is gradual onset of dominant arm shoulder pain aggravated by throwing and tenderness to palpation over the proximal humerus laterally.[28] The condition is a benign, self-limited one that responds well to conservative management with cessation of throwing activities for an average of 3 months.[28]

Proximal humeral growth plate widening laterally is the most common radiographic finding in Little Leaguer's shoulder, although it may be subtle, and comparison views of the contralateral shoulder may be necessary for detection of associated fragmentation, sclerosis, and cystic change as the physeal injury becomes more chronic. The physeal widening is well seen on T1- and T2-weighted MR imaging sequences with abnormal ill-defined physeal signal extending into the metaphysis (**Fig. 4**).[29,30] Physeal widening in the setting of trauma has been shown to occur experimentally with disruption of metaphyseal blood vessels.[31] The resultant disordered endochondral bone formation causes extension of hypertrophic chondrocytes into the metaphysis correlating with the imaging finding of growth plate widening.[31] Although MR imaging is not used routinely to make the diagnosis, which often can be made clinically, the findings should be recognizable if MR imaging is obtained to evaluate other suspected shoulder injuries.

Rotator cuff injuries
Rotator cuff tears tend to be encountered in older individuals, with fewer than 1% of cases occurring in patients younger than age 20.[32,33] The rotator cuff in young patients is more elastic and stronger and generally lacks the degenerative changes that are a frequent finding in an older population.[34] Rotator cuff injury in skeletally immature patients more commonly manifests as tendonitis or strain in response to repetitive microtrauma.[9] Sports that require overhead arm motion, such as swimming, tennis, and baseball, put patients at risk for injury to the rotator cuff. The repeated mechanical contact of the supraspinatus tendon, greater tuberosity, long head of the biceps, and subacromial bursa with the coracoacromial arch that occurs with these activities can lead to inflammation of the rotator cuff that may progress to tendinopathy and possible tear.[9] In children and

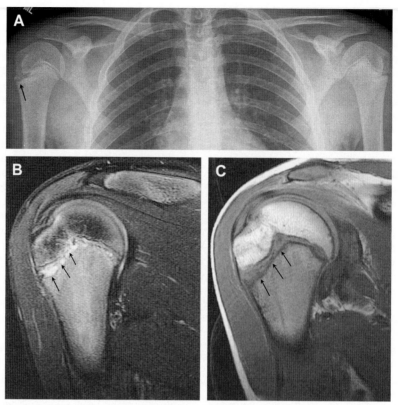

Fig. 4. Little Leaguer's shoulder in a 13-year-old, right-handed baseball pitcher with right shoulder pain. (*A*) Anteroposterior radiograph of both shoulders shows the widened right proximal humeral growth plate laterally (*arrow*). Coronal oblique T2-weighted image with fat saturation (*B*) and T1-weighted image (*C*) show irregular widening of the proximal humeral physis laterally with cartilage signal (*arrows*) and normal marrow signal in the epiphysis and metaphysis.

adolescents, rotator cuff inury is frequently associated with joint instability.

Normal joint stability requires intact static and dynamic stabilizers. The static stabilizers (the joint capsule, glenohumeral ligaments, and labrum) function at extreme ranges of motion with the dynamic stabilizers (rotator cuff muscles, deltoid and scapulothoracic muscles) to provide joint stability at the midrange of motion.[35] Given the inherent laxity of the static stabilizers in children, greater demand is placed on the dynamic shoulder stabilizers to provide glenohumeral stability through all ranges of motion. With repetitive stress, the muscles become fatigued, and rotator cuff impingement can result secondary to multidirectional instability and humeral head migration. In young athletes with shoulder pain that suggests impingement, clinical assessment for instability is necessary so that both issues are addressed with treatment.[9]

Rotator cuff impingement as the result of a tight coracoacromial arch is often referred to as external or outlet impingement. It is usually seen in the adult population because of variation in shape or sloping of the acromion or pathologic spurring at the acromioclavicular joint. Younger patients with a normal coracoacromial arch may develop external impingement usually as a result of repetitive microtrauma from instability that leads to structural changes in the tendon, ligament, and capsule.[36] These changes result in secondary rotator cuff muscle weakness and further biomechanical imbalance of the glenohumeral joint. Internal impingement refers to impingement of the undersurface of the supraspinatus and infraspinatus by the posterosuperior glenoid labrum. This condition is typically seen with maximal abduction and external rotation of the shoulder, as encountered during the late cocking phase of throwing.[37,38]

MR imaging is the modality of choice for imaging the rotator cuff.[39,40] The normal rotator cuff tendons are dark on all pulse sequences. With tendinopathy, intermediate T2 signal (less than fluid) is present within the tendon, which itself may be thickened. Full-thickness rotator cuff tears (uncommon in children) appear as fluid signal extending completely through the tendon. A partial-thickness tear appears as fluid signal on T2-weighted images along the bursal or, more commonly, the articular surface. A rim-rent tear is a partial articular-sided tear of the insertional fibers of the rotator cuff at the greater tuberosity.[41–43] This tear, which is recognized as a common form of partial rotator cuff tear, may involve either the supraspinatus or infraspinatus insertion and tends to occur in younger patients.[42,43] Careful examination of the anterior-most fibers of the supraspinatus and infraspinatus at the greater tuberosity footprint insertion is necessary to avoid missing a rim-rent

tear.[43] Some believe that if left untreated, this injury may progress to a full-thickness tear.[43]

Internal impingement has a unique constellation of imaging findings. In overhead sports characterized by overhead motion with extreme abduction and external rotation, the undersurface of the posterior supraspinatus tendon or anterior infraspinatus tendon becomes entrapped between the humeral head and posterior glenoid. Undersurface tears of one or both tendons associated with cystic changes in the posterior humeral head and posterosuperior labral pathology are believed to be diagnostic of internal impingement (**Fig. 5**).[44]

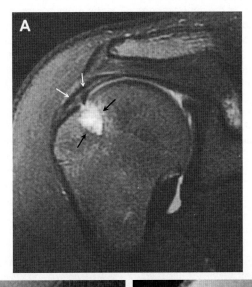

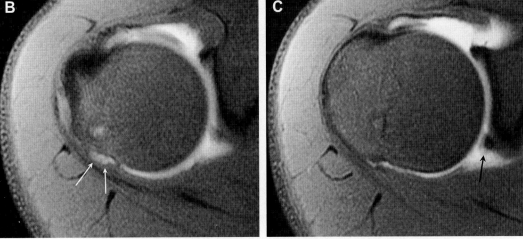

Fig. 5. Posterior impingement in a 16-year-old baseball pitcher with clinical findings of posterior impingement. On shoulder MR arthrogram, coronal oblique T2-weighted image with fat saturation (A) shows high signal cystic change in the posterior humeral head (*black arrows*) and abnormal increased signal in the infraspinatus portion of the rotator cuff (*white arrows*), which is also seen as fraying of the undersurface of the posterior rotator cuff on the axial fat saturated T1-weighted image (B). On the same sequence just inferior (C), the posterior labrum is frayed and irregular (*arrow*).

The overall reported sensitivity and specificity of MR imaging for rotator cuff tear detection varies from 84% to100%.[39,45,46] Direct MR arthrography with use of the abducted, externally rotated position enhances detection of articular side partial-thickness tears.[45,47,48]

ELBOW
Congenital Disorders

Congenital radial head dislocation is the most common congenital anomaly of the elbow.[49] The deformity may be unilateral or bilateral and is thought to have an autosomal dominant inheritance pattern.[50] The prime insult is believed by many to be failure of normal formation of the capitellum, which secondarily affects the development of the radial head and radiocapitellar joint. The ulna is often bowed and short compared to the radius in response to the altered dynamics.[50] Although it may be an isolated anomaly, more than half of the cases are associated with other conditions such as anomalies of the lower extremities, scoliosis, and various syndromes, including arthrogryposis and Klippel-Feil and Nail patella syndromes. In childhood, functional limitation is usually limited and significant pain does not develop until adulthood. It is treated with radial head excision.[51]

Congenital radioulnar synostosis is a much less common anomaly than congenital radial head dislocation. It may present in a unilateral or bilateral fashion and has a male predominance. Failure of longitudinal segmentation between the radius and ulna—likely caused by an insult during early in utero development—is the proposed cause, with the resulting fusion being fibrous or bony.[49,52] It may be associated with other disorders, including Apert syndrome, Carpenter syndrome, and other upper extremity anomalies such as syndactyly, polydactyly, and carpal coalition.[49] Radiographs are the mainstay for evaluating these congenital elbow anomalies, with MR imaging being reserved for problem solving in difficult cases (Fig. 6).

Acute Traumatic Injury: Medial Epicondyle

Acute injuries of the elbow are a frequent occurrence in children and may occur in the setting of sports participation. Medial epicondyle avulsion is the most common fracture encountered in skeletally immature throwing athletes. The mechanism is medial traction secondary to acute valgus stress in conjunction with violent contraction of the flexor-pronator muscle groups that attach on the medial epicondyle. The onset of medial pain is acute after a hard pitch or throw, is occasionally accompanied by a crack or pop, and renders the patient unable to continue throwing.[53] There may be acute ulnar nerve parasthesia. Associated ulnar collateral ligament (UCL) rupture is unlikely.[53]

Radiographs show variable physeal widening with or without rotation of the medial epicondyle. If the force is sufficient, as is more common with an elbow dislocation, the epicondyle may be displaced into the joint. Medial epicondylar fractures are classified into three types base on patient age and fragment size as proposed by Woods and Tullos.[54] Type I injuries involve the entire

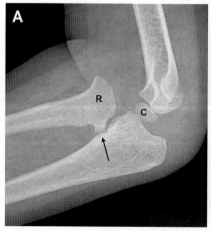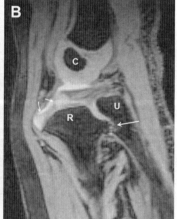

Fig. 6. Radial head dislocation and radioulnar synchondrosis in a 5-year-old child who presented with elbow pain and decreased range of motion. (*A*) The lateral radiograph shows the superior dislocation of the proximal radius (R) relative to the capitellum (C) and the developing proximal radioulnar synchondrosis (*arrow*). (*B*) On sagittal three-dimensional gradient echo imaging the cartilaginous radial head (*small arrows*) has a normal concave appearance, and cartilage signal is present in the radioulnar synchondrosis (*large arrow*). U, ulna.

apophysis and occur in children younger than age 14 in whom the physis is completely unfused. Type II and III injuries occur in patients aged 15 and older as the growth plate is fusing or is fused. The fragment involves only a portion of the apophysis, with type II fragments being larger than type III fragments.

Treatment with immobilization is adequate for nondisplaced fractures. A displaced fragment in the joint is treated surgically if not reducible nonoperatively. A lack of agreement about acceptable fragment displacement (2 mm versus 3–5 mm) has led to controversy regarding conservative versus surgical therapy of less displaced fragments. Associated valgus instability, ulnar nerve dysfunction, and future functional demands on the elbow are factors that must be considered in management of these athletes.[53] MR imaging is not indicated in most patients with a medial epicondylar avulsion fracture but may be helpful in select cases to clarify radiographic findings (**Fig. 7**).

Chronic Traumatic Injury

Elbow injuries occur with greater frequency than shoulder injuries in adolescent athletes.[55] The elbow is subjected to various forces that have been described in detail with the overhead throwing motion common to baseball, the tennis serve, the football pass, and the javelin throw. During the cocking portion of the throwing motion with the elbow flexed, there is tension overload on the medial elbow restraints (medial epicondyle, common flexor tendon, and UCL) and compression overload on the lateral articular surfaces of the capitellum and radial head. Posteromedial shear forces on the olecranon fossa occur during

this phase, with additional force placed on the olecranon and anterior capsule during the follow-through phase when there is prominent hyperextension of the elbow.[56] Given this knowledge, one can predict the injury patterns that may be encountered in these patients.

Medial Epicondyle Apophyseal Injury

In throwing athletes with medial elbow pain, tenderness over the medial epicondyle with soft tissue swelling is common.[56] The type of injury depends on the skeletal maturity of the patient. For skeletally immature patients, the physeal growth plate of the medial epicondyle is the weakest link. Radiographic results may be normal or show physeal widening with overgrowth or fragmentation of the medial epicondyle when compared to the nondominant arm, a condition often termed Little Leaguer's elbow.[57] The radiographic features represent a physiologic response to repetitive traction stress and can be seen in asymptomatic throwing athletes (nearly 50% in one study).[58] MR imaging is usually not necessary for diagnosis but would show physeal widening (**Fig. 8**). Treatment is conservative. If this injury is not treated, nonunion of the medial epicondyle may result.

Ulnar Collateral Ligament Injury

In athletes approaching skeletal maturity, MR imaging is more helpful for identifying other causes of medial elbow pain. The UCL and common flexor tendon (the conjoined tendon of the flexor carpi radialis, flexor carpi ulnaris, flexor digitorum superficialis, palmaris longus, and pronator teres muscles) insert on the medial epicondyle. The

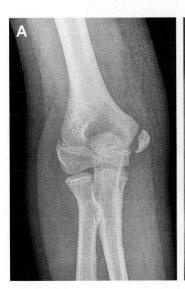
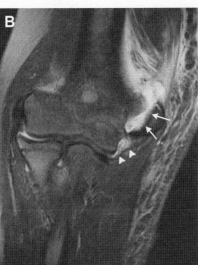

Fig. 7. Acute medial epicondyle avulsion in a 13-year-old, right-handed boy who suffered acute right elbow pain while pitching in a game. (*A*) The anteroposterior radiograph shows the widened medial epicondylar physis and medial soft tissue swelling. (*B*) Coronal T2-weighted image with fat saturation shows the abnormally widened growth plate (*arrows*) with an intact UCL (*arrowheads*).

UCL is composed of three bands: anterior, posterior, and transverse. The anterior band, which inserts on the sublime tubercle of the coronoid process of the ulna, is functionally the most important of the three bands and acts as the primary stabilizer to valgus stress.[59]

Patients with UCL injury complain of pain medially that is accentuated during the late cocking and acceleration stages of throwing.[55] Physical examination may show valgus instability. Radiographic results are typically normal but can show heterotopic calcification in the ligament.[60] Tears of the UCL are seen on MR imaging as laxity, irregularity, and increased T1 and T2 signal within and around the ligament.[61] Repetitive microtears weaken or disrupt the ligament with hemorrhage or edema that is visible at arthroscopy, correlating with the MR signal alterations.[61] The normal UCL epicondylar insertion before physeal fusion has been noted to have slightly higher T2 and T1 signal than the normal mature ligament, which is thought to be caused by high elastin and low type I collagen content at the enthesis.[62] This factor must be taken into consideration when evaluating skeletally immature athletes' elbows, bearing in mind the rarity of UCL injuries in this age group.

Full-thickness UCL tears show discontinuity of the ligament and usually involve the mid-substance of the anterior band.[63] Partial tears are more challenging (see **Fig. 8**). One older study

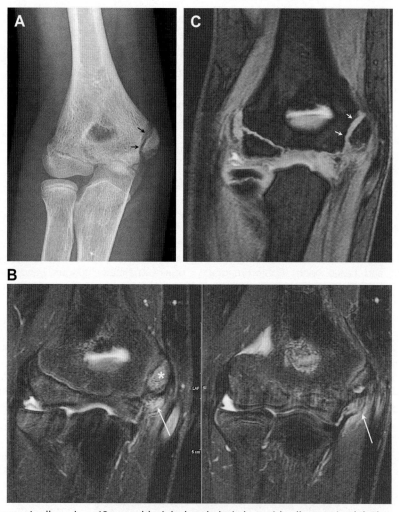

Fig. 8. Little Leaguer's elbow in a 12-year-old, right-handed pitcher with elbow pain. (*A*) The anteroposterior radiograph shows widening of the medial epicondylar physis (*arrows*) and fragmentary irregularity of the inferior portion of the epicondylar growth center. (*B*) Coronal T2-weighted images with fat saturation show edema in the epicondyle (*) and abnormal increased signal in a partially torn UCL (*arrows*). (*C*) The abnormal widening of the chronically stressed medial epicondylar growth plate (*arrows*) is best seen on the coronal three-dimensional gradient echo image.

found only 57% sensitivity and 100% specificity of MR for surgically proven partial-thickness UCL tears.[64] The use of MR arthrography may have helped increase sensitivity up to 86% in one study.[65] One should look for the characteristic "T sign" originally described by Timmerman and colleagues.[64] This sign is created by contrast leaking around the detached deep distal fibers of the UCL but remaining contained within the intact superficial fibers and joint capsule.[64] Much less commonly, the ligament may be partially avulsed at the distal attachment, which results in an avulsion fracture of the sublime tubercle of the ulna, a condition that may be more apparent on conventional radiographs.[66]

Medial Epicondylitis

Medial epicondylitis is a much less common cause of chronic medial elbow pain in throwing athletes. Microscopic or macroscopic avulsion of the common flexor tendon at the medial epicondylar insertion is the pathologic condition termed "medial epicondylitis." This condition is sometimes seen in late adolescence when the medial epicondylar apophyseal growth plate is fusing or has fused. MR imaging shows thickening of the tendon with increased T1 and T2 signal and peritendinous edema.[67,68]

Nerve Compression Syndromes

Nerve compression syndromes of the median and ulnar nerves are seen about the elbow in throwing athletes. There are several sites at which these nerves can be compressed. The ulnar nerve is the most common site of compression, with the most frequent site of compression being the cubital tunnel as it passes behind the medial epicondyle.[69] Repetitive elbow flexion causes compromise of the size of the cubital tunnel as the arcuate ligament dorsally is stretched tightly and there is medial bulging of the UCL and joint capsule. The cubital tunnel also can be compromised by an accessory muscle, the anconeus epitrochlearis, as it traverses the tunnel. The nerve is stretched against the medial epicondyle and may sublux.[69] Patients may have ulnar-sided paresthesias. The ulnar nerve is surrounded by fat, which adds to its conspicuity in the cubital tunnel on MR images. With ulnar neuritis, the nerve is usually thickened and of increased T2 signal. There may be associated edema in the denervated flexor carpi ulnaris and flexor digitorum profundus muscles.

Pronator syndrome refers to compression of the median nerve at the elbow and proximal forearm.[69] It most frequently occurs between the superficial and deep heads of the pronator teres muscle 2 to 4 cm distal to the medial epicondyle during protracted pronation when the space between the two heads is compromised.[69] The symptoms can mimic carpal tunnel syndrome but are usually absent at night and are aggravated by forceful pronation of the forearm. Besides increased T2 signal in the nerve, abnormal muscle signal or atrophy in the pronator flexor muscles may be seen on MR imaging.[69]

LATERAL ELBOW
Panner's Disease and Osteochondritis Dissecans

In the late cocking phase of throwing, in addition to the tension overload on the medial elbow restraints, there is lateral compression overload on the capitellum and radial head. Panner's disease and osteochondritis dissecans (OCD) are the most recognized lateral compression injuries of the elbow. They may represent different stages of the same pathophysiologic process, namely disordered endochondral ossification of the capitellum,[70] but they affect different age groups and have different clinical outcomes.[56,71,72]

Panner's disease—osteochondrosis of the capitellum—was first described in 1927, and its resemblance to Legg-Calvé-Perthes disease was recognized.[73] The condition affects predominately the dominant elbow of boys between the ages of 7 and 12 years during the active phase of capitellar ossification. The blood supply of the capitellum in the skeletally immature elbow is mainly from posterior vessels that function as end arteries. Repetitive trauma may compromise this tenuous vascular supply within the chondroephiphysis of the capitellum and lead to the disordered endochondral ossification.[74,75] Patients complain of dull elbow pain and stiffness aggravated by activity and there is tenderness directly over the capitellum.[70,71] Radiographs show fragmentation with intermixed areas of rarefaction and sclerosis that may affect all or part of the capitellum. MR imaging, although not generally necessary, shows replacement of the normal fatty marrow with decreased T1 and increased T2 signal.[76] The overlying cartilage should be unaffected and there should be no loose body formation. Healing with conservative management is the rule.

OCD of the capitellum also occurs in the dominant elbow but is generally seen in slightly older patients, aged 12 to 15, when capitellar ossification is nearly complete, affecting the anterolateral aspect of the capitellum. Baseball players and gymnasts are vulnerable to this condition. In addition to the tenuous blood supply of the capitellum, the central aspect of the radial head is considerably stiffer than the capitellum.[77] The combination of ischemia with articular cartilage biomechanical differences may explain the propensity for development of capitellar OCD with repetitive lateral compression force. Trochlear osteochondral injuries have been described but are much less common.[56]

The typical patient with capitellar OCD is an adolescent athlete who presents with lateral elbow pain and swelling. Locking and mechanical symptoms are late findings. In the early stages, standard radiographic results often are normal or may have subtle subchondral flattening that may be more apparent on an anteroposterior radiograph with 45° elbow flexion[78] or by comparing to the asymptomatic elbow. Over time with repeated trauma, findings progress to focal cystic rarefaction, fragment formation, and eventual articular cartilage defect with loose body formation (**Fig. 9**).[72,78] Conventional radiographs are unreliable for assessing lesion stability and detecting intra-articular loose bodies, which are key features for determining clinical management.[71,78–80]

MR imaging is exquisitely sensitive for detecting OCD lesions, even in the earliest stages when radiographic results are normal. At that time, only diminished T1 signal is seen at the surface of the capitellum, without any T2 signal changes.[81] With more advanced stage lesions, associated increased T2 signal is seen uniformly throughout the lesion or as a peripheral ring, not infrequently with cyst formation at the bone–fragment interface as the lesion becomes loose in situ.[82] The presence of a surrounding high signal intensity rim or fluid-filled cyst on T2-weighted images has been shown to correlate with unstable fragments.[83] Early stage, stable lesions in patients with an open capitellar growth plate and good elbow motion are likely to heal with elbow rest.[84] Long-term elbow symptoms even with activities of daily living occur in approximately 50% of patients regardless of therapy and are associated with advanced, larger lesions and osteoarthritic change.[85] This finding implies that identifying early, smaller lesions may offer a better prognosis.

To that end, assessing integrity of the articular cartilage, determining fragment viability, and identifying loose bodies in the joint are critical to determine whether the lesion is stable or unstable. Assessment of elbow articular cartilage is more challenging than in larger joints such as the knee, but use of dedicated surface coils and high-resolution three-dimensional gradient echo sequences may help. The well-known pseudodefect of the capitellum may create a pitfall in diagnosis, but identification of this normal groove in the articular cartilage between the rounded capitellum and the lateral epicondyle—not a usual site for OCD—should help distinguish between the two.[86] Fragment viability is difficult to assess. Early experience in a small group of patients (n = 3) with intravenous gadolinium suggested it may be useful by showing fragment enhancement as a sign of

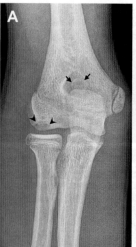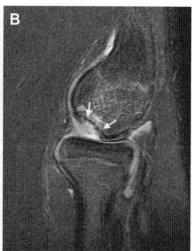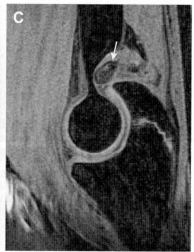

Fig. 9. (*A–C*) Capitellar OCD and loose body in a 13-year-old boy with pain and locking of the right elbow. (*A*) Anteroposterior radiograph of the right elbow shows a lucent defect near the articular surface of the capitellum (*arrowheads*) and an ossified loose body overlying the olecranon fossa (*arrows*). (*B*) Sagittal T2-weighted image with fat saturation shows the osteochondral defect in the capitellum (*arrows*) with loss of the overlying articular cartilage. The sagittal three-dimensional gradient echo sequence clearly shows the ossified loose body in the olecranon fossa (*arrow*).

viability.[87] No subsequent reports have confirmed this finding, and our own experience with intravenous gadolinium in OCD of the knee did not find it helpful in determining fragment viability.[88]

For detecting intra-articular loose bodies, MR imaging has been shown to be more sensitive than radiography in one study of 13 children with a total of three loose bodies (see **Fig. 9**).[82] In another study of 26 skeletally mature adults with OCD and mechanical elbow symptoms (locking or catching), neither CT arthrography nor MR imaging was better than radiography for loose body detection.[89] These contradictory results may be caused by differences in the bony content of the loose bodies, which were not described fully in either study. Certainly intracapsular fat pads and synovial folds can mimic loose bodies on MR imaging

and pose challenges.[86] Gadolinium MR arthrography has shown similar sensitivity and specificity when compared to CT arthrography for detecting articular cartilage lesions of the elbow in a study of 26 cadaver joints,[90] but no controlled studies in patients have evaluated the relative value of this technique in patients with OCD of the elbow.

WRIST
Congenital

Madelung deformity
Madelung deformity is a congenital deformity of the wrist that usually becomes apparent in late childhood or adolescence and is characterized clinically by palmar tilt of the wrist, shortening of the forearm with bayonet-wrist deformity, and diminished forearm rotation.[91,92] Patients present

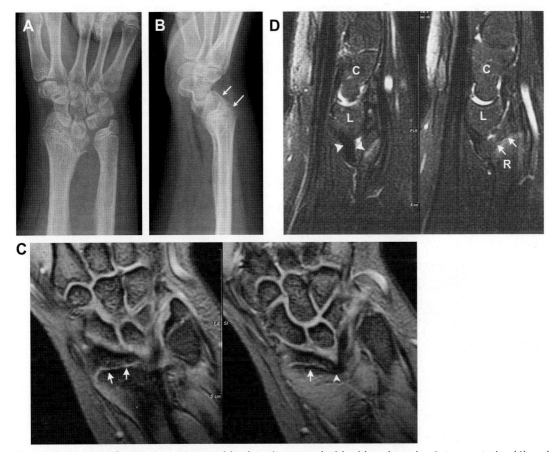

Fig. 10. Madelung deformity in a 12-year-old otherwise normal girl with wrist pain. Anteroposterior (*A*) and lateral (*B*) radiographs show the marked ulnar and volar tilt of the distal radius (*arrows*). Sequential coronal MPGR images (*C*) show the abnormal ulnar tilt of the radial growth plate (*arrows*) and focal growth plate fusion medially (*arrowhead*). Sagittal T2-weighted fat saturated images (*D*) illustrate the abnormally thickened anomalous Vicker's ligament (*arrowheads*) and the volar tilt of the radial growth plate (*arrows*). C, capitellum, L, lunate.

with pain, deformity, or limited motion. The condition is more frequent in girls and may be isolated but has been associated with prior trauma or infection and syndromes such as dyschondrosteosis (Léri-Weill syndrome), in which it is frequently bilateral. Although a precise genetic origin remains under investigation, a growth disturbance of the volar and ulnar aspect of the distal radial physis has been identified as the primary disorder leading to the deformity. An anomalous ligament tethering the lunate to the radius proximal to the physis (Vickers ligament) also has been observed clinically and on MR imaging (Fig. 10).[92–94]

The characteristic radiographic features of Madelung deformity include dorsal bowing of the radius, marked ulnar and volar tilt of the distal radius, radial tilt of the distal ulna, and triangular appearance of the distal radial epiphysis.[92,94,95] The proximal carpal row is pyramidal or wedge shaped in appearance. The severity of the abnormalities is not absolute and represents a spectrum.[96] Although MR imaging is not necessary in all cases, it can further document the anticipated small physeal bar on the volar aspect of the distal radial growth plate that may be bony or fibrous and detect hypertrophy of the short radiolunate ligament and the anomalous Vickers ligament (see Fig. 10).[92,94]

Acute Trauma

Most acute traumatic injuries of the pediatric wrist result in fractures of the distal radius that may involve the growth plate.[97] These injuries usually occur as the result of a fall on an outstretched hand.[97] Uneventful healing is the general rule, but in rare cases, there can be associated injury of the triangular fibrocartilage (TFC) or

scapholunate ligament, both of which are uncommon injuries in children.[98,99] Patients with TFC tears have ulnar-sided wrist pain and may have an ulnar click or distal radioulnar joint instability.[100] Patients with scapholunate ligament tears generally have localized persistent pain over the dorsal scapholunate region with pain on weight bearing on the dorsiflexed wrist (Fig. 11). Not all patients have an associated fracture with these injuries, which can be either acute or caused by chronic repetitive trauma.

A retrospective review of 29 skeletally immature patients with surgically proven TFC tears noted that 15 patients (52%) had a history of a distal radial fracture at the time of the original injury and that 12 patients (41%) had an ununited ulnar styloid fracture. Given the peripheral attachments of the TFC at the base of the ulnar styloid, it is not surprising that patients with ununited ulnar styloid fractures seem to be at some increased risk for TFC tears (Fig. 12).[101] Coexisting pathologic conditions include distal radioulnar joint instability, ulnocarpal impaction, and intercarpal ligament tears.[99] With scapholunate ligament tears, the incidence of prior radial fractures varies from 22% (7 of 32 patients) in one study[102] to 100% (3 of 3 patients) in a smaller study.[98] Isolated ligament injury without associated chondral injury, TFC tear, or other intercarpal ligament abnormality is the exception and was reported in only 1 of 32 patients.[102]

No published series have evaluated the efficacy of MR imaging in children for diagnosing TFC and scapholunate ligament injuries. Most traumatic TFC tears are peripheral, with central tears tending to be degenerative in nature and not seen in younger patients (see Fig. 12).[103] These peripheral

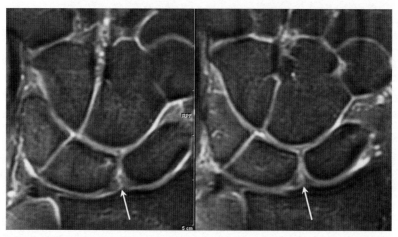

Fig. 11. Scapholunate ligament tear in a 17-year-old boy who hit his wrist dunking a basketball. Coronal intermediate-weighted images with fat saturation show abnormal signal in the membranous portion of the scapholunate ligament (arrows). This was debrided arthroscopically.

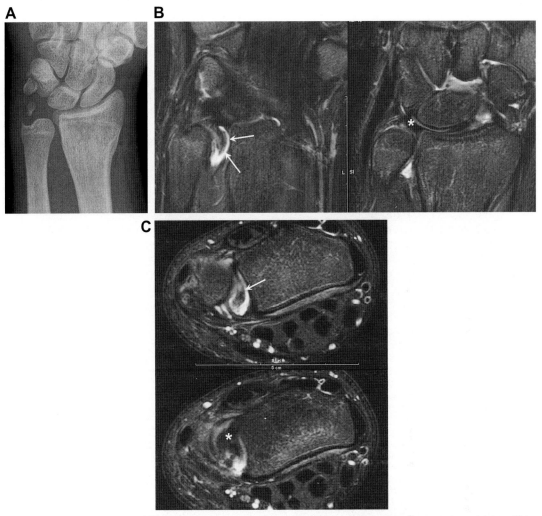

Fig. 12. TFC tear in a 13-year-old boy with pain, popping, and instability of the wrist after a motor vehicle collision 6 months earlier. The anteroposterior radiograph (*A*) illustrates findings of a healed radius fracture and ununited ulnar styloid and a probable old pisiform fracture. Coronal (*B*) and axial (*C*) T2-weighted images with fat saturation show fluid in the distal radioulnar joint surrounding fragments of the ulnar-sided TFC tear (*arrows*). More normal TFC dorsally is seen (*).

tears can be difficult to diagnose on MR imaging. One study that involved 86 predominately adult patients evaluated MR imaging (both unenhanced studies and indirect arthrograms) for diagnosing peripheral TFC tears and found it to be only 17% sensitive, 79% specific, and 64% accurate with no significant difference between the conventional MR and indirect MR arthrograms.[104] The same authors compared the two techniques in this same group of patients for scapholunate ligament tears and found significantly improved sensitivity (94% versus 41%) for indirect MR arthrography over conventional MR imaging with diagnostic accuracy of 89%.[105] Adding two- or three-compartment direct MR arthrography to

conventional MR imaging may improve diagnostic performance.[106]

Carpal bone fractures in children are relatively uncommon, but of the carpal bones, the scaphoid is the most frequently fractured.[107] Initial radiographs may not reveal a fracture, but one should be suspected if tenderness is localized to the anatomic snuff box. The secondary radiographic features (dorsal soft tissue swelling and obliteration of the scaphoid fat stripe) may not be visible in children.[108] As in adults, scaphoid fractures must be immobilized to minimize the risk of nonunion and avascular necrosis. Obtaining repeat radiographs after 1 to 2 weeks of immobilization is the standard in patients with suggestive

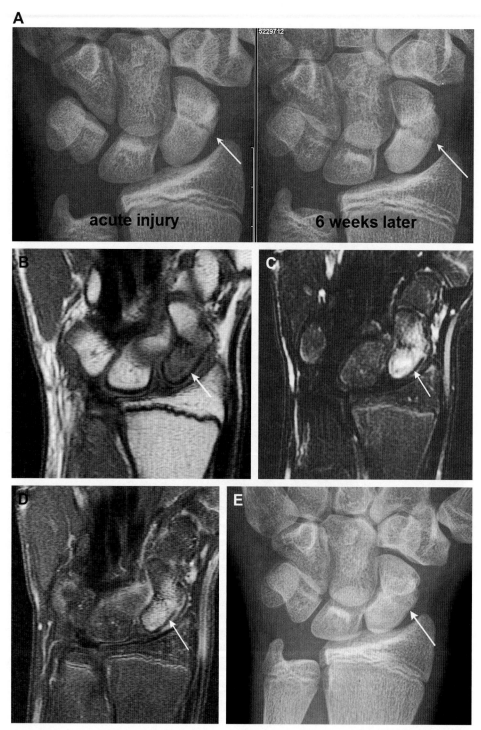

Fig.13. Scaphoid fracture with suspected avascular necrosis in a 15-year-old boy who fell while skateboarding. (*A*) Initial anteroposterior radiograph and comparison 6 weeks later show a nondisplaced scaphoid waist fracture (*arrow*) with concern for increasing sclerosis in the proximal pole on the 6-week follow-up. MR imaging coronal T1-weighted (*B*) and T2-weighted (*C*) images show nonspecific abnormal marrow signal (*arrows*). (*D*) Coronal fat-suppressed T1-weighted image after gadolinium administration shows symmetric enhancement of the scaphoid on both sides of the fracture, which indicates viability of the fragment. Two months later (*E*), the radiograph showed interval fracture healing and no features of avascular necrosis.

physical findings in the absence of radiographic abnormality.[109]

Early MR imaging was evaluated in skeletally immature patients with suspected scaphoid fractures. Of 18 patients, 10 had abnormal increased T2 marrow signal in the scaphoid with a low signal intensity fracture line in 6 of the 10 patients, and only 2 of those fractures were visible on the initial radiographs. The other 4 patients with a marrow contusion pattern and the remaining 8 patients with normal scaphoid marrow signal never developed a fracture on follow-up.[109] These results indicate a 100% negative predictive value for MR imaging for diagnosing scaphoid fractures in children.[109] It is not clear whether the information influences patient management, and MR imaging has not become a standard part of the diagnostic algorithm for suspected scaphoid fractures in children.

In children, nondisplaced scaphoid distal pole and waist fractures diagnosed promptly will usually heal with cast immobilization.[110] Nonunions and avascular necrosis are relatively rare complications that are often attributed to missed or delayed diagnosis of a proximal pole or displaced fracture.[111] Avascular necrosis of the proximal fragment of a scaphoid fracture is a critical issue that affects the outcome of ununited scaphoid fractures. Operative evaluation is the gold standard for diagnosing scaphoid avascular necrosis. MR imaging with intravenous gadolinium has been shown to have 66% sensitivity, 88% specificity, and 83% accuracy compared with operative findings for diagnosing this condition in an adult population of 30

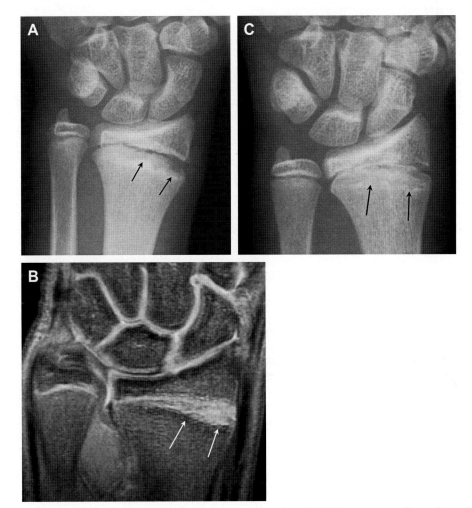

Fig. 14. Gymnast's wrist in a 14-year-old female gymnast with wrist pain. (*A*) Anteroposterior radiograph shows asymmetric abnormal widening of the lateral aspect of the distal radial growth plate with adjacent metaphyseal irregularity (*arrows*). Coronal proton density image with fat saturation (*B*) shows cartilage signal within the widened physis (*arrows*) consistent with growth plate stress injury and disruption of endochondral ossification. The follow-up radiograph 1 month later (*C*) after bracing and rest showed evidence of healing (*arrows*).

patients and is considered the most helpful noninvasive imaging modality (**Fig. 13**).[112]

Chronic Repetitive Trauma

Gymnast's wrist

Wrist pain is a common complaint that reportedly occurs in approximately two thirds of gymnasts.[113,114] Stress injury of the distal radial physis, also called "gymnast's wrist," has become a well-recognized cause of wrist pain in skeletally immature gymnasts and weightlifters whose wrists are subjected to excessive axial compression loading in dorsiflexion.[115,116] There may be focal tenderness over the radial condyle, and wrist pain is aggravated with weight bearing and wrist dorsiflexion.[116]

Radiographic results may be normal in symptomatic patients but can show findings that overlap with features described in rickets, including varying degrees of partial or complete growth plate widening sometimes with osseous fragmentation within the widened growth plate and metaphyseal flaring and sclerosis.[113,116] The similarity has prompted one author to render the name "pseudorickets" for the radiographic appearance.[117] In one large study of 261 adolescent Chinese gymnasts, an abnormal radiographic appearance of the growth plate was seen in approximately 25% of symptomatic and 10% of asymptomatic gymnasts.[113] Similar changes can occasionally be seen in the distal ulna, but positive ulnar variance is much more common and seems to increase in frequency with increased duration of training.[113,115] It is likely secondary to the localized growth disturbance in the distal radius. The positive ulnar variance can result in ulnocarpal impingement and TFC pathology.[118]

On MR imaging, the growth plate widening can vary from subtle and localized to pronounced and diffuse. Cartilage signal paralleling that of the growth plate (intermediate on T1- and high on T2-weighted images) can be seen extending into the distal radial metaphysis and may be band-like paralleling the physis or run perpendicular to the physis and appear as focal tongues (**Fig. 14**).[119] Similar changes have been described in other stressed growth plates, including the shoulder[29] and the knee.[120] The findings have been attributed to disrupted endochondral ossification and extension of hypertrophic cartilage cells into the metaphysis.[120,121] MR imaging is more sensitive than radiography for detecting this growth plate stress injury. In one study of 47 skeletally immature gymnasts with wrist pain who had radiographs and MR imaging, 12 of 17 wrists that were normal on radiography had visible growth plate abnormalities on MR imaging.[119] As with other physeal stress injuries, most patients respond to a regimen of rest (with or without immobilization) and later rehabilitation.[116] Premature growth plate fusion is a rare complication.[116]

REFERENCES

1. Bright RW, Burstein AH, Elmore SM. Epiphyseal-plate cartilage: a biomechanical and histological analysis of failure modes. J Bone Joint Surg Am 1974;56(4):688–703.

2. Foad SL, Mehlman CT, Ying J. The epidemiology of neonatal brachial plexus palsy in the United States. J Bone Joint Surg Am 2008;90(6):1258–64.

3. Greenwald AG, Schute PC, Shiveley JL. Brachial plexus birth palsy: a 10-year report on the incidence and prognosis. J Pediatr Orthop 1984;4(6):689–92.

4. Pearl ML, Edgerton BW, Kazimiroff PA, et al. Arthroscopic release and latissimus dorsi transfer for shoulder internal rotation contractures and glenohumeral deformity secondary to brachial plexus birth palsy. J Bone Joint Surg Am 2006;88(3):564–74.

5. Pearl ML, Edgerton BW, Kon DS, et al. Comparison of arthroscopic findings with magnetic resonance imaging and arthrography in children with glenohumeral deformities secondary to brachial plexus birth palsy. J Bone Joint Surg Am 2003;85(5):890–8.

6. Kon DS, Darakjian AB, Pearl ML, et al. Glenohumeral deformity in children with internal rotation contractures secondary to brachial plexus birth palsy: intraoperative arthrographic classification. Radiology 2004;231(3):791–5.

7. Chuang DC, Mardini S, Ma HS. Surgical strategy for infant obstetrical brachial plexus palsy: experiences at Chang Gung Memorial Hospital. Plast Reconstr Surg 2005;116(1):132–42 [discussion: 143–34].

8. Waters PM, Smith GR, Jaramillo D. Glenohumeral deformity secondary to brachial plexus birth palsy. J Bone Joint Surg Am 1998;80(5):668–77.

9. Curtis R. Shoulder Injuries: anatomy, biomechanics and physiology. In: Stanitski CL, DeLee JC, Drez D, editors. Pediatric and adolescent sports medicine. Philadelphia: WB Saunders Co.; 1994. p. 183–90.

10. Cleeman E, Flatow EL. Shoulder dislocations in the young patient. Orthop Clin North Am 2000;31(2):217–29.

11. Rowe CR. Prognosis in dislocations of the shoulder. J Bone Joint Surg Am 1956;38(5):957–77.

12. Dahlin LB, Erichs K, Andersson C, et al. Incidence of early posterior shoulder dislocation in brachial

plexus birth palsy. J Brachial Plex Peripher Nerve Inj 2007;2:24.

13. Deitch J, Mehlman CT, Foad SL, et al. Traumatic anterior shoulder dislocation in adolescents. Am J Sports Med 2003;31(5):758–63.

14. Marans HJ, Angel KR, Schemitsch EH, et al. The fate of traumatic anterior dislocation of the shoulder in children. J Bone Joint Surg Am 1992;74(8):1242–4.

15. Simonet WT, Cofield RH. Prognosis in anterior shoulder dislocation. Am J Sports Med 1984; 12(1):19–24.

16. Hovelius L, Augustini BG, Fredin H, et al. Primary anterior dislocation of the shoulder in young patients: a ten-year prospective study. J Bone Joint Surg Am 1996;78(11):1677–84.

17. Baker CL, Uribe JW, Whitman C. Arthroscopic evaluation of acute initial anterior shoulder dislocations. Am J Sports Med 1990;18(1):25–8.

18. Antonio GE, Griffith JF, Yu AB, et al. First-time shoulder dislocation: high prevalence of labral injury and age-related differences revealed by MR arthrography. J Magn Reson Imaging 2007;26(4):983–91.

19. Waldt S, Burkart A, Imhoff AB, et al. Anterior shoulder instability: accuracy of MR arthrography in the classification of anteroinferior labroligamentous injuries. Radiology 2005;237(2):578–83.

20. Magee T, Williams D, Mani N. Shoulder MR arthrography: which patient group benefits most? AJR Am J Roentgenol 2004;183(4):969–74.

21. Beltran J, Rosenberg ZS, Chandnani VP, et al. Glenohumeral instability: evaluation with MR arthrography. Radiographics 1997;17(3):657–73.

22. Beltran J, Bencardino J, Mellado J, et al. MR arthrography of the shoulder: variants and pitfalls. Radiographics 1997;17(6):1403–12 [discussion: 1412–05].

23. Harish S, Nagar A, Moro J, et al. Imaging findings in posterior instability of the shoulder. Skeletal Radiol 2008;37(8):693–707.

24. Lawton RL, Choudhury S, Mansat P, et al. Pediatric shoulder instability: presentation, findings, treatment, and outcomes. J Pediatr Orthop 2002; 22(1):52–61.

25. Jakobsen BW, Johannsen HV, Suder P, et al. Primary repair versus conservative treatment of first-time traumatic anterior dislocation of the shoulder: a randomized study with 10-year follow-up. Arthroscopy 2007;23(2):118–23.

26. Dotter WE. Little leaguer's shoulder: a fracture of the proximal epiphyseal cartilage of the humerus due to baseball pitching. Guthrie Clin Bull 1953; 23(1):68–72.

27. Gainor BJ, Piotrowski G, Puhl J, et al. The throw: biomechanics and acute injury. Am J Sports Med 1980;8(2):114–8.

28. Carson WG Jr, Gasser SI. Little Leaguer's shoulder: a report of 23 cases. Am J Sports Med 1998;26(4): 575–80.

29. Obembe OO, Gaskin CM, Taffoni MJ, et al. Little Leaguer's shoulder (proximal humeral epiphysiolysis): MRI findings in four boys. Pediatr Radiol 2007;37(9):885–9.

30. Song JC, Lazarus ML, Song AP. MRI findings in Little Leaguer's shoulder. Skeletal Radiol 2006; 35(2):107–9.

31. Jaramillo D, Laor T, Zaleske DJ. Indirect trauma to the growth plate: results of MR imaging after epiphyseal and metaphyseal injury in rabbits. Radiology 1993;187(1):171–8.

32. Itoi E, Tabata S. Rotator cuff tears in the adolescent. Orthopedics 1993;16(1):78–81.

33. Tarkin IS, Morganti CM, Zillmer DA, et al. Rotator cuff tears in adolescent athletes. Am J Sports Med 2005;33(4):596–601.

34. Wasserlauf BL, Paletta GA Jr. Shoulder disorders in the skeletally immature throwing athlete. Orthop Clin North Am 2003;34(3):427–37.

35. Cole B, Warner J. Anatomy, biomechanics, and pathophysiology of glenohumeral instability. In: Iannotti J, Williams G, editors. Disorders of the shoulder: diagnosis and management. New York: Lippincott, Williams & Wilkins; 1999. p. 207–32.

36. Jobe FW, Kvitne RS, Giangarra CE. Shoulder pain in the overhand or throwing athlete: the relationship of anterior instability and rotator cuff impingement. Orthop Rev 1989;18(9):963–75.

37. Liu SH, Boynton E. Posterior superior impingement of the rotator cuff on the glenoid rim as a cause of shoulder pain in the overhead athlete. Arthroscopy 1993;9(6):697–9.

38. Paley KJ, Jobe FW, Pink MM, et al. Arthroscopic findings in the overhand throwing athlete: evidence for posterior internal impingement of the rotator cuff. Arthroscopy 2000;16(1):35–40.

39. Burk DL Jr, Karasick D, Kurtz AB, et al. Rotator cuff tears: prospective comparison of MR imaging with arthrography, sonography, and surgery. AJR Am J Roentgenol 1989;153(1):87–92.

40. Sanders TG, Morrison WB, Miller MD. Imaging techniques for the evaluation of glenohumeral instability. Am J Sports Med 2000;28(3):414–34.

41. Codman EA. Rupture of the supraspinatus tendon: 1911. Clin Orthop Relat Res 1990;(254):3–26.

42. Tuite MJ, Turnbull JR, Orwin JF. Anterior versus posterior, and rim-rent rotator cuff tears: prevalence and MR sensitivity. Skeletal Radiol 1998;27(5):237–43.

43. Vinson EN, Helms CA, Higgins LD. Rim-rent tear of the rotator cuff: a common and easily overlooked partial tear. AJR Am J Roentgenol 2007;189(4): 943–6.

44. Giaroli EL, Major NM, Higgins LD. MRI of internal impingement of the shoulder. AJR Am J Roentgenol 2005;185(4):925–9.

45. Meister K, Thesing J, Montgomery WJ, et al. MR arthrography of partial thickness tears of the

undersurface of the rotator cuff: an arthroscopic correlation. Skeletal Radiol 2004;33(3):136–41.

46. Quinn SF, Sheley RC, Demlow TA, et al. Rotator cuff tendon tears: evaluation with fat-suppressed MR imaging with arthroscopic correlation in 100 patients. Radiology 1995;195(2):497–500.

47. Tirman PF, Bost FW, Steinbach LS, et al. MR arthrographic depiction of tears of the rotator cuff: benefit of abduction and external rotation of the arm. Radiology 1994;192(3):851–6.

48. Lee SY, Lee JK. Horizontal component of partial-thickness tears of rotator cuff: imaging characteristics and comparison of ABER view with oblique coronal view at MR arthrography initial results. Radiology 2002;224(2):470–6.

49. Laor T. Congenital malformations of bone. In: Slovis TL, editor. Caffey's pediatric diagnostic imaging. 11th edition. Philadelphia: Mosby Elsevier; 2008. p. 2594–612.

50. Sachar K, Mih AD. Congenital radial head dislocations. Hand Clin 1998;14(1):39–47.

51. Kelly DW. Congenital dislocation of the radial head: spectrum and natural history. J Pediatr Orthop 1981;1(3):295–8.

52. Cleary JE, Omer GE Jr. Congenital proximal radioulnar synostosis: natural history and functional assessment. J Bone Joint Surg Am 1985;67(4):539–45.

53. Rudzki JR, Paletta GA Jr. Juvenile and adolescent elbow injuries in sports. Clin Sports Med 2004;23(4):581–608, ix.

54. Woods GW, Tullos HS. Elbow instability and medial epicondyle fractures. Am J Sports Med 1977;5(1):23–30.

55. Chen FS, Diaz VA, Loebenberg M, et al. Shoulder and elbow injuries in the skeletally immature athlete. J Am Acad Orthop Surg 2005;13(3):172–85.

56. Bradley JP. Upper extremity: elbow injuries in children and adolescents. In: Stanitski CL, DeLee JC, David Drez J, editors. Pediatric and adolescent sports medicine. Philadelphia: WB Saunders Co.; 1994. p. 242–61.

57. Brogdon BG, Crow NE. Little leaguer's elbow. Am J Roentgenol Radium Ther Nucl Med 1960;83:671–5.

58. Hang DW, Chao CM, Hang YS. A clinical and roentgenographic study of Little League elbow. Am J Sports Med 2004;32(1):79–84.

59. Schwab GH, Bennett JB, Woods GW, et al. Biomechanics of elbow instability: the role of the medial collateral ligament. Clin Orthop Relat Res 1980;146:42–52.

60. Mulligan SA, Schwartz ML, Broussard MF, et al. Heterotopic calcification and tears of the ulnar collateral ligament: radiographic and MR imaging findings. AJR Am J Roentgenol 2000;175(4):1099–102.

61. Mirowitz SA, London SL. Ulnar collateral ligament injury in baseball pitchers: MR imaging evaluation. Radiology 1992;185(2):573–6.

62. Sugimoto H, Ohsawa T. Ulnar collateral ligament in the growing elbow: MR imaging of normal development and throwing injuries. Radiology 1994;192(2):417–22.

63. Carrino JA, Morrison WB, Zou KH, et al. Noncontrast MR imaging and MR arthrography of the ulnar collateral ligament of the elbow: prospective evaluation of two-dimensional pulse sequences for detection of complete tears. Skeletal Radiol 2001;30(11):625–32.

64. Timmerman LA, Schwartz ML, Andrews JR. Preoperative evaluation of the ulnar collateral ligament by magnetic resonance imaging and computed tomography arthrography: evaluation in 25 baseball players with surgical confirmation. Am J Sports Med 1994;22(1):26–31 [discussion: 32].

65. Schwartz ML, al-Zahrani S, Morwessel RM, et al. Ulnar collateral ligament injury in the throwing athlete: evaluation with saline-enhanced MR arthrography. Radiology 1995;197(1):297–9.

66. Glajchen N, Schwartz ML, Andrews JR, et al. Avulsion fracture of the sublime tubercle of the ulna: a newly recognized injury in the throwing athlete. AJR Am J Roentgenol 1998;170(3):627–8.

67. Kijowski R, De Smet AA. Magnetic resonance imaging findings in patients with medial epicondylitis. Skeletal Radiol 2005;34(4):196–202.

68. Martin CE, Schweitzer ME. MR imaging of epicondylitis. Skeletal Radiol 1998;27(3):133–8.

69. Bordalo-Rodrigues M, Rosenberg ZS. MR imaging of entrapment neuropathies at the elbow. Magn Reson Imaging Clin N Am 2004;12(2):247–63.

70. Kobayashi K, Burton KJ, Rodner C, et al. Lateral compression injuries in the pediatric elbow: Panner's disease and osteochondritis dissecans of the capitellum. J Am Acad Orthop Surg 2004;12(4):246–54.

71. Bradley JP, Petrie RS. Osteochondritis dissecans of the humeral capitellum: diagnosis and treatment. Clin Sports Med 2001;20(3):565–90.

72. Kijowski R, Tuite M, Sanford M. Magnetic resonance imaging of the elbow. Part I: normal anatomy, imaging technique, and osseous abnormalities. Skeletal Radiol 2004;33(12):685–97.

73. Panner H. An affection of the capitulum humeri resembling Calve-Perthes disease of the hip. Acta Radiol 1927;8:617–8.

74. Haraldsson S. On osteochondrosis deformas juvenilis capituli humeri including investigation of intraosseous vasculature in distal humerus. Acta Orthop Scand Suppl 1959;38:1–232.

75. Douglas G, Rang M. The role of trauma in the pathogenesis of the osteochondroses. Clin Orthop Relat Res 1981;158:28–32.

76. Stoane JM, Poplausky MR, Haller JO, et al. Panner's disease: X-ray, MR imaging findings and review of the literature. Comput Med Imaging Graph 1995;19(6):473–6.

77. Schenck RC Jr, Athanasiou KA, Constantinides G, et al. A biomechanical analysis of articular cartilage of the human elbow and a potential relationship to osteochondritis dissecans. Clin Orthop Relat Res 1994;299:305–12.

78. Takahara M, Ogino T, Takagi M, et al. Natural progression of osteochondritis dissecans of the humeral capitellum: initial observations. Radiology 2000;216(1):207–12.

79. Takahara M, Ogino T, Fukushima S, et al. Nonoperative treatment of osteochondritis dissecans of the humeral capitellum. Am J Sports Med 1999;27(6):728–32.

80. Kijowski R, De Smet AA. Radiography of the elbow for evaluation of patients with osteochondritis dissecans of the capitellum. Skeletal Radiol 2005;34(5):266–71.

81. Takahara M, Shundo M, Kondo M, et al. Early detection of osteochondritis dissecans of the capitellum in young baseball players: report of three cases. J Bone Joint Surg Am 1998;80(6):892–7.

82. Bowen RE, Otsuka NY, Yoon ST, et al. Osteochondral lesions of the capitellum in pediatric patients: role of magnetic resonance imaging. J Pediatr Orthop 2001;21(3):298–301.

83. Kijowski R, De Smet AA. MRI findings of osteochondritis dissecans of the capitellum with surgical correlation. AJR Am J Roentgenol 2005;185(6):1453–9.

84. Takahara M, Mura N, Sasaki J, et al. Classification, treatment, and outcome of osteochondritis dissecans of the humeral capitellum. J Bone Joint Surg Am 2007;89(6):1205–14.

85. Takahara M, Ogino T, Sasaki I, et al. Long term outcome of osteochondritis dissecans of the humeral capitellum. Clin Orthop Relat Res 1999;(363):108–15.

86. Loredo R, Sanders TG. Imaging of osteochondral injuries. Clin Sports Med 2001;20(2):249–78.

87. Peiss J, Adam G, Casser R, et al. Gadopentetate-dimeglumine-enhanced MR imaging of osteonecrosis and osteochondritis dissecans of the elbow: initial experience. Skeletal Radiol 1995;24(1):17–20.

88. Emery Kh VD, Laor T, Mussman A, et al. Gadolinium enhanced MRI in juvenile osteochondritis dissecans (OCD) of the knee: is it helpful for predicting the need for surgical therapy? Presented at the 46th Annual Meeting of the Society for Pediatric Radiology. San Francisco, May 10, 2003.

89. Dubberley JH, Faber KJ, Patterson SD, et al. The detection of loose bodies in the elbow: the value of MRI and CT arthrography. J Bone Joint Surg Br 2005;87(5):684–6.

90. Waldt S, Bruegel M, Ganter K, et al. Comparison of multislice CT arthrography and MR arthrography for the detection of articular cartilage lesions of the elbow. Eur Radiol 2005;15(4):784–91.

91. Schmidt-Rohlfing B, Schwobel B, Pauschert R, et al. Madelung deformity: clinical features, therapy and results. J Pediatr Orthop B 2001;10(4):344–8.

92. Cook PA, Yu JS, Wiand W, et al. Madelung deformity in skeletally immature patients: morphologic assessment using radiography, CT, and MRI. J Comput Assist Tomogr 1996;20(4):505–11.

93. Blanco ME, Perez-Cabrera A, Kofman-Alfaro S, et al. Clinical and cytogenetic findings in 14 patients with Madelung anomaly. Orthopedics 2005;28(3):315–9.

94. Vickers D, Nielsen G. Madelung deformity: surgical prophylaxis (physiolysis) during the late growth period by resection of the dyschondrosteosis lesion. J Hand Surg Br 1992;17(4):401–7.

95. Felman AH, Kirkpatrick JA Jr. Madelung's deformity: observations in 17 patients. Radiology 1969;93(5):1037–42.

96. Tuder D, Frome B, Green DP. Radiographic spectrum of severity in Madelung's deformity. J Hand Surg Am 2008;33(6):900–4.

97. Lovallo J, Simmons BP. Hand and wrist injuries. In: Stanitski C, DeLee JC, Drez D Jr, editors. Pediatric and adolescent sports medicine. Philadelphia: WB Saunders Co.; 1994. p. 262–78.

98. Alt V, Gasnier J, Sicre G. Injuries of the scapholunate ligament in children. J Pediatr Orthop B 2004;13(5):326–9.

99. Terry CL, Waters PM. Triangular fibrocartilage injuries in pediatric and adolescent patients. J Hand Surg Am 1998;23(4):626–34.

100. Bae DS, Waters PM. Pediatric distal radius fractures and triangular fibrocartilage complex injuries. Hand Clin 2006;22(1):43–53.

101. Abid A, Accadbled F, Kany J, et al. Ulnar styloid fracture in children: a retrospective study of 46 cases. J Pediatr Orthop B 2008;17(1):15–9.

102. Earp BE, Waters PM, Wyzykowski RJ. Arthroscopic treatment of partial scapholunate ligament tears in children with chronic wrist pain. J Bone Joint Surg Am 2006;88(11):2448–55.

103. Palmer AK. Triangular fibrocartilage complex lesions: a classification. J Hand Surg Am 1989;14(4):594–606.

104. Haims AH, Schweitzer ME, Morrison WB, et al. Limitations of MR imaging in the diagnosis of peripheral tears of the triangular fibrocartilage of the wrist. AJR Am J Roentgenol 2002;178(2):419–22.

105. Haims AH, Schweitzer ME, Morrison WB, et al. Internal derangement of the wrist: indirect MR arthrography versus unenhanced MR imaging. Radiology 2003;227(3):701–7.

106. Zanetti M, Bram J, Hodler J. Triangular fibrocartilage and intercarpal ligaments of the wrist: does MR arthrography improve standard MRI? J Magn Reson Imaging 1997;7(3):590–4.

107. Greene MH, Hadied AM, LaMont RL. Scaphoid fractures in children. J Hand Surg Am 1984;9(4):536–41.

108. Terry DW Jr, Ramin JE. The navicular fat stripe: a useful roentgen feature for evaluating wrist trauma. Am J Roentgenol Radium Ther Nucl Med 1975;124(1):25–8.

109. Cook PA, Yu JS, Wiand W, et al. Suspected scaphoid fractures in skeletally immature patients: application of MRI. J Comput Assist Tomogr 1997;21(4):511–5.

110. Waters PM. Operative carpal and hand injuries in children. J Bone Joint Surg Am 2007;89(9):2064–74.

111. Huckstadt T, Klitscher D, Weltzien A, et al. Pediatric fractures of the carpal scaphoid: a retrospective clinical and radiological study. J Pediatr Orthop 2007;27(4):447–50.

112. Cerezal L, Abascal F, Canga A, et al. Usefulness of gadolinium-enhanced MR imaging in the evaluation of the vascularity of scaphoid nonunions. AJR Am J Roentgenol 2000;174(1):141–9.

113. Chang CY, Shih C, Penn IW, et al. Wrist injuries in adolescent gymnasts of a Chinese opera school: radiographic survey. Radiology 1995;195(3):861–4.

114. DiFiori JP, Puffer JC, Mandelbaum BR, et al. Distal radial growth plate injury and positive ulnar variance in nonelite gymnasts. Am J Sports Med 1997;25(6):763–8.

115. Mandelbaum BR, Bartolozzi AR, Davis CA, et al. Wrist pain syndrome in the gymnast: pathogenetic, diagnostic, and therapeutic considerations. Am J Sports Med 1989;17(3):305–17.

116. Roy S, Caine D, Singer KM. Stress changes of the distal radial epiphysis in young gymnasts: a report of twenty-one cases and a review of the literature. Am J Sports Med 1985;13(5):301–8.

117. Liebling MS, Berdon WE, Ruzal-Shapiro C, et al. Gymnast's wrist (pseudorickets growth plate abnormality) in adolescent athletes: findings on plain films and MR imaging. AJR Am J Roentgenol 1995;164(1):157–9.

118. Tolat AR, Sanderson PL, De Smet L, et al. The gymnast's wrist: acquired positive ulnar variance following chronic epiphyseal injury. J Hand Surg Br 1992;17(6):678–81.

119. Shih C, Chang CY, Penn IW, et al. Chronically stressed wrists in adolescent gymnasts: MR imaging appearance. Radiology 1995;195(3):855–9.

120. Laor T, Wall EJ, Vu LP. Physeal widening in the knee due to stress injury in child athletes. AJR Am J Roentgenol 2006;186(5):1260–4.

121. Laor T, Hartman AL, Jaramillo D. Local physeal widening on MR imaging: an incidental finding suggesting prior metaphyseal insult. Pediatr Radiol 1997;27(8):654–62.

Index

Note: Page numbers of article titles are in **boldface** type.

mri.theclinics.com

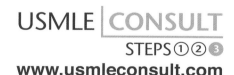

Our issues help you manage *yours.*

Every year brings you new clinical challenges.

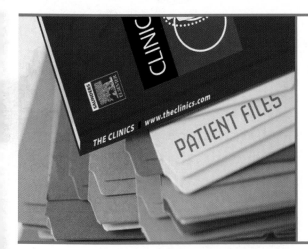

Every **Clinics** issue brings you **today's best thinking** on the challenges you face.

Whether you purchase these issues individually, or order an annual subscription (which includes searchable access to past issues online), the **Clinics** offer you an efficient way to update your know how…one issue at a time.

DISCOVER THE CLINICS IN YOUR SPECIALTY!

Magnetic Resonance Imaging Clinics of North America.
Published quarterly. ISSN 1064-9689.

PET Clinics.
Published quarterly. ISSN 1556-8598.

Radiologic Clinics of North America.
Published bimonthly. ISSN 0033-8389.

Ultrasound Clinics.
Published quarterly. ISSN 1556-858X.

Neuroimaging Clinics of North America.
Published quarterly. ISSN 1052-5149

eClips | CONSULT
Where the Best Articles become the Best Medicine

Visit **www.eClips.Consult.com** to see what 180 leading physicians have to say about the best articles from over 350 leading medical journals.

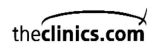
the**clinics**.com

Moving?

Make sure your subscription moves with you!

To notify us of your new address, find your **Clinics Account Number** (located on your mailing label above your name), and contact customer service at:

E-mail: elspcs@elsevier.com

800-654-2452 (subscribers in the U.S. & Canada)
314-453-7041 (subscribers outside of the U.S. & Canada)

Fax number: 314-523-5170

Elsevier Periodicals Customer Service
11830 Westline Industrial Drive
St. Louis, MO 63146

*To ensure uninterrupted delivery of your subscription, please notify us at least 4 weeks in advance of move.